PLAIN DOCTORING

Richard Moskowitz, M. D.

Selected Writings.
1983 – 2013

ISBN-10: 1482338017
EAN-13: 9781482338010

Library of Congress Control Number: 2013902237
CreateSpace Independent Publishing Platform
North Charleston, South Carolina

o

Table of Contents

Preface.

The following pieces span a period of 30 years, beginning with my first articles on homeopathy, and include excerpts from my two books and several essays on the philosophy of medicine in general. I've chosen them in part because they represent my main thematic interests over the years, and also because they address major issues of general import, in contrast with the more occasional pieces: shorter articles, political statements, book reviews, obituaries, letters, interviews, and the like.

But the main reason is that I still like them, both for what they say and how they say it, and have enjoyed re-reading them in the process of making and preparing this collection. Since looking back, reminiscing, and taking stock are among the special pleasures and privileges of growing old, making this collection has been a labor of love for me, a cherished memento of my home birth experience and my fortuitous stumbling into homeopathy, both of which profoundly changed both the shape of my career and the direction of my life, enabled me to practice medicine in a way that I could genuinely be proud of, and provided me with a radically different viewpoint that has helped me to clarify my thoughts about the medical profession and the healing endeavor generally. For all of these gifts I remain deeply grateful.

I have re read all of the articles in their entirety, edited them for typos, and taken the liberty of changing a word, sentence, or paragraph here and there; but in both form and content they are essentially the same as when I originally wrote them. As for the books, I likewise made a few minor changes in making my selection. With the pregnancy book, I chose the more down to earth clinical chapters, and limited myself mainly to the remedies and conditions for which I had actual case material, whereas with *Resonance,* I settled on the early chapters dealing with basic principles, to appeal to the general reader who, like me and everyone else, must surely remain mystified by the homeopathic phenomenon and all that has followed from it.

I. Memoir:
"Why I Became a Homeopath"

Why I Became a Homeopath*

My fundamental beliefs and attitudes about doctoring grew out of my experiences as a student in the 1960's, long before there was such a thing as "holistic medicine." Practical dilemmas first encountered on the wards of a large city hospital led me to study philosophy before going into practice, and have continued to shape my career ever since, throughout ***internship and more than forty years of clinical work.

In my school days I felt no particular calling to heal the sick, and there has never been another physician in my family as far as I know. Studious and scholarly by nature, I would undoubtedly have felt more at home in an academic discipline like history or philosophy than a worldly career such as medicine. Nor have I ever wholly overcome an instinctive distaste for the actual stigmata of illness, both the physical and emotional suffering and the tyranny they impose on loved ones and caregivers alike.

Why I chose a profession for which I had so little natural inclination, ambition, or special aptitude, and why I persevered in it in spite of repeated failures and disappointments, thus define a mystery, and suggest powerful unconscious forces at work. Framing the question in this way takes me back to my grandfather's death from renal failure around my sixth birthday, when intimations of mortality turned my life upside down. One night as I lay in bed, unable to sleep, my thoughts and fantasies coalesced into a vision of absolute clarity that I too was going to die, a fate from which no earthly power could save me. At my wits' end and desperate for solace, I burst into my parents' room, quite sure that I wasn't dreaming, and indeed awake as never before from the knowledge that death was *certain,* a standard of truth utterly new to my experience. From their bland dismissals and obvious reluctance to discuss it, I gathered that death was a mystery I would have to fathom by myself.

---

* "Why I Became a Homeopath," *Journal of the American Institute of Homeopathy* 89:74, Winter 1996.

Born with a crossed eye that resisted correction with glasses and orthoptic exercises, at thirteen I underwent cosmetic surgery that left me with a divergent squint both obvious and permanent. Equally powerless to achieve binocular vision or to stop trying to achieve it, I have never wholly adjusted to the resulting headaches, eyestrain, and automatic distrust of "experts," specialists, and high-tech solutions that have become almost second nature to me.

During the summer after my junior year at Harvard, while employed as a research trainee in biochemistry, I received a wake-up call that could and perhaps should have ended my medical career before it started. Justly famed for its pioneering work in animal genetics, the laboratory where I worked derived the bulk of its income from breeding and exporting pure strains of mice, rats, dogs, cats, monkeys, rabbits, and other species for biomedical experimentation all over the world. Extrapolating from the modest number of animals sacrificed in my own work, as well as that of my mentors and colleagues, I conjured up a rough estimate of the vastly larger total that we supplied to others for similar purposes, and thus came to appreciate the enormity of this terrible enterprise and my own undeniable complicity in it. Since then, no argument however subtle or forceful has ever persuaded me that human progress requires the systematic torture and killing of helpless creatures on such a scale and for such a purpose, or that valid standards of science or ethics could ever be built on such foundations.

In spite of these misgivings, I entered New York University Medical School in the fall of 1959, right on schedule. Most of our clinical work was performed at Bellevue Hospital, a venerable but antiquated institution that provided the most advanced diagnostic and treatment facilities *gratis* to anyone who needed them, along with substantial quotas of neglect and abuse from overworked interns and residents, and attentions both welcome and unwelcome from the students as we rotated through each service.

In those days, medical students were initiated into the mysteries of patient care by "drawing the bloods" for the day, a ritual happily long since dispensed with in most places. In charity hospitals maintained at public expense, indigent patients were routinely taken advantage of by us and the house staff in exchange for their care, and were expected to surrender unlimited quantities of blood for any tests that any of us were even remotely curious about. Even today, more than thirty years later, I can still almost hear the low, mournful wail that greeted us every morning, as the patients saw us coming with our implements down the hall. After days or weeks of experimentation on veins often weak and traumatized to begin with, our last resort was the dreaded femoral puncture, which took only a few seconds to execute, but left both victim and perpetrator holding our breaths until the huge syringes were filled at last.

Accustomed to thinking of illness as a particular episode or life experience that we come down with, work through, and eventually recover or possibly die from, I was wholly unprepared for a reality in which disease was the default condition, and a vast nexus of goods and services had been created to manipulate and exploit it. On those rare occasions when the beds were empty and the wards deserted, I imagined I could still smell the ineradicable miasma that lingered in the air, like the accumulated *residuum* of all diseases past and present. One of my favorite assignments was night call on the maternity service, where the miracle of birth occasionally squirted out before anybody had the chance to interfere with it. Listening to the chorus of women in labor from my cot in the next room, I often reflected on the word "obstetrics," derived from the Latin preposition *ob-,* meaning "against" or "in the way of," and the root *stet-,* meaning "stand" or "standing:" an obstetrician, etymologically speaking, was evidently a physician named and indeed celebrated for standing in the way of the birth process, for manipulating and controlling it for doubtless worthy purposes of our own.

On the medical wards, we were responsible for admitting all lobar pneumonia patients, usually alcoholics from the Bowery, for whom a high fever, productive cough, pleuritic pain, or some equally serious ailment was their only ticket to a warm bed and regular food on cold winter nights. In most cases, the sputum was loaded with *Streptococcus pneumoniæ,* an organism easily detected by microscopic examination and in those days wholly curable with minute doses of penicillin. Before initiating treatment, however, we were required to inoculate the specimen into the peritoneal cavities of two mice, which yielded an almost pure culture of the pneumococci when we sacrificed them two days later. Since the test

4

was largely academic, I only pretended to do it, not daring to raise the issue of animal testing, but unwilling to witness the atrocity myself.

Routinely enlisting us to perform their dirty work, the house staff merely pointed out that we could similarly lord it over our own crop of students when their turn came. In this fraternal spirit an intern once hit on me to pass a Rehfuss tube into the duodenum of a petite Puerto Rican woman whom he was working up for possible pancreatic disease. Basically a stomach tube tipped with a weighted metal ball to carry it through the pylorus into the small intestine, this little devil was practically impossible for an unanesthetized person to swallow without gagging. After three failed attempts, I found myself wishing that doctors be given a taste of their own medicine before being allowed to administer it to others. When the intern finally took over, he fared no better, and so proceeded to blame the victim, unleashing a torrent of abuse that included racist slurs like "stupid" and "animal" that required no translation. Pulling herself up in bed to her full height, this little lady suddenly and majestically grew in bearing and stature before my eyes, proudly rebuking his insolence, and vowing retribution if he ever molested her again. Not long after that, I spotted two burly, mustachioed young Latinos lurking about the ward and made myself scarce, but inwardly wished them well.

In like manner, the hospital dramatized the need for patient empowerment in the gnarled and twisted shapes it often assumed there, like the middle-aged black man with a chip on his shoulder who lived on the street, but knew more about emphysema and chronic lung disease than most of the doctors treating him for it, and could usually be found in the library boning up for our discussion of him on rounds the next morning. It took me a bit longer to understand that the inequality in rank and power that allowed us to do whatever we wanted and compelled our patients to obey and even thank us for it culminated in the actual propagation of disease, both indirectly, by spreading fear and doubt, and directly, through excessive use of diagnostic and treatment procedures with obvious power to harm.

One such example followed from the pet belief of a senior Professor of Surgery that the cause of chronic pancreatitis was spasm of the sphincter of Oddi, by producing reflux of bile into the pancreas, and hence chemical inflammation of the gland. After successfully creating a facsimile of the disease in experimental animals by applying electrical stimulation to the sphincter and clamping off the common bile duct behind it, he developed a protocol for human subjects that blithely crossed the frontier of ethical restraint into a gray zone where the only law was whatever the traffic would bear and whatever a tenured Professor could get away with.

Under his tutelage, Residents at the Surgical Clinic would select a quota of indigent patients with various digestive symptoms for "pancreatic studies," provided they were not yet diagnosed or claimed for other projects, like the Puerto Rican lady described above. Those who survived the ordeal of the Rehfuss tube might then become eligible for surgical insertion of a T-shaped catheter into the common bile duct, through which samples of bile and pancreatic juice could be taken for analysis, and radio-opaque dyes introduced for X-ray close-ups of the biliary and pancreatic duct systems, leading in some cases to cutting open the sphincter if it actually proved to be spastic.

While I like many others was slow to put it all together, it should not have been a surprise to anyone that traumatizing these highly delicate structures would often irritate and inflame them, thus provoking spasm of the sphincter, and eventually chronic pancreatitis as well. In this stepwise and almost imperceptible fashion, his careful methodology not only confirmed the theory that had inspired it, but also provided a continuous supply of experimental material, since once scarring had occurred, it usually proved irreversible.

Another memorable example of those years was the work of a well-known pediatrician, celebrated for his work with the virus of infectious hepatitis, now known as Hepatitis A, who conclusively proved for the first time what many had long suspected, that the disease is transmitted by mouth, through ingestion of contaminated feces, just like polio and other intestinal viruses. He too succeeded by his willingness to conduct dangerous experiments on individuals without their consent, in this case retarded children at Willowbrook State School, who could not speak for themselves and often lacked parents or guardians who were willing or able to speak for them.

Feeding stool samples from those with known infection to other inmates not yet sick, this doubtless sincere and even dedicated physician soon had irrefutable data regarding the portal of entry, incubation period, clinical course, liver enzymes, and every other known parameter of this major infectious disease. Some years later, when a citizens' group tried to blow the whistle on his research, which was conducted largely at public expense, he correctly pointed out that, because of overcrowding and poor sanitation, the disease was rampant at the school in any case, and was allowed to continue his work without interruption or even a reprimand.

Neither man was intentionally cruel or malicious, in the manner of serial killers who defy social norms, or torturers and war criminals who carry out atrocities or give in to coercion or social pressure under extreme circumstances. What they did was evil and indeed monstrous for precisely the opposite reason, that they were successful and even illustrious in a system which prizes their work so highly and rewards its achievements so richly that the distinction between valid science and criminal or immoral behavior is far less clear and the legal and moral standards regulating it are correspondingly ambiguous.

By my fourth year, as "matching day" for internships drew near, I realized that I could not bring myself to practice medicine in the way I'd been trained, and accepted a graduate fellowship in philosophy at the University of Colorado, in large part to try to find clarity and meaning in what I had just lived through. Long before I found words to articulate or concepts to explain it, I grasped on some deeper level that the mental sleight-of-hand involved in reducing illnesses to diseases and abnormalities, and using drugs and surgery to separate or remove them from the patient's body, is inherently fraught with ethical and practical risks that I could not accept on a routine basis, for no better reason than that that's how things were done.

Three years later, in 1966, I finally completed a one-year internship at St. Anthony's Hospital in Denver, including rotations of three months each in Medicine and Surgery, and two months in Pediatrics, Women's Health, and Emergency Medicine. With well over 500 beds and no Residents or permanent clinical Faculty, it was not designed or run as a teaching institution. Our instructors were simply the Attending Physicians using the hospital to admit and care for their private patients, on whose behalf we might be asked to complete an admission workup, insert an IV or venous cutdown, assist in surgery, or carry out any other menial tasks the Attending or Nursing Staff might require. In addition, indigent patients referred in from the ER or Outpatient Clinics, which we also staffed and ran, were assigned to our personal care under the nominal supervision of our Preceptor for each service.

In short, we operated for the most part under the old apprenticeship system, which grounded me thoroughly in how medicine was actually practiced, allowed me to learn at my own pace, and left ample room for close personal relationships with supervisors, attendings, nurses, and patients alike. But while generally knowledgeable and helpful if we could find them, our preceptors were often too busy with their own patients to be available when we most needed them. With only eight of us to cover the whole place, we were usually on our own, often in the dark, and wont to proclaim as a virtue the "see-one, do-one, teach-one" philosophy we were obliged to live by. While our patients undoubtedly appreciated and often benefited from our personal attention, they paid for it many times over by having to run the gauntlet of inferior care that followed from our having to learn everything pretty much by the seat of our pants.

In a typical vignette, my first D & C was ordered by my OB/GYN Supervisor for "diagnostic purposes" in a Welfare patient with a history of vaginal bleeding. Since the Hospital was owned by the Catholic Archdiocese and closely supervised by nuns, I was surprised when he told me not to bother with a pregnancy test, but I didn't argue. In the Operating Room, he took all the time in the world to show me how to administer paracervical anesthesia, dilate the cervix, and curette out the endometrial lining, but then grew oddly impatient during the procedure itself. "Moskowitz, get finished, already!" he kept barking at me, seemingly heedless of the fact that I was still removing handfuls of tissue, with no trace of the harsh, grating sound he had just taught me to wait for as the endpoint of the procedure. Once again I obeyed, but the Pathology report confirmed a pregnancy, and the next day we had to take her back and finish the job. Although he continued ever after to deny any prior knowledge or suspicion of it, both the illegality of abortion in those days and the woman's profound gratitude for what had happened pointed to our flawed collaboration as just about the only way for her to get the help she needed. Far more than any technical information, these were the lessons that stuck.

Another memorable experience grew out of my friendship with a patient, a Mexican guy in his mid-forties who had developed chronic thrombophlebitis of the deep veins of the calf as a result of the surgical ligation and stripping of his unsightly varicosities that he had been so eager for a year or two previously. I have yet to hear a convincing rationale for this purely cosmetic procedure, which by removing the superficial veins effectively doubles the load on the deep system, itself already compromised in many cases, and thus often brings about the same kind of chronic venous insufficiency that had more or less crippled this man with little hope of relief.

In time we became friends, and one day he invited me to his home in the projects to meet his wife, sample her famous *enchiladas,* and stay the night. In the wee hours of the morning, he woke me with an urgent plea to examine his aged father, who lived across the courtyard and was complaining of severe chest pain. As I entered his room, the old man was sitting up in bed, leaning forward with his hands clasped over his heart and a look of mortal terror in his eyes, a textbook picture of acute myocardial infarction.

Though equipped with nothing but my little black bag, and understandably reluctant to treat him at home, I dreaded even more subjecting him to the quasi-military atmosphere of the ambulance and Emergency Room, where his inability to speak or understand English made the risk of a serious or fatal complication loom even greater. So I gave him a shot of morphine, and within minutes he fell into a deep and peaceful sleep. By the time I left for work several hours later, he was resting comfortably in bed, obviously feeling much better, at which point his wife told me that he had recovered from at least three such episodes in the past, without any drugs or medical attention whatsoever. That made me wonder whether a lot of patients might not heal better at home, not only from heart attacks, but many other serious ailments as well.

As in most hospitals, the bulk of our instruction actually came from the nurses, who basically ran the place, but knew how to make it look as if they were following *our* orders rather than the other way around. Thus on a typical night in the ER, if a patient came in, say, wheezing from an allergic reaction, some version of the following dialogue would most likely ensue:

Nurse: *Shall I get the Benadryl, Doctor?*
Doctor: *Yes, thank you . . .*
Nurse: *How much, Doctor, maybe 50 mg. IM?*
Doctor: *Yes, that sounds about right . . .*

Along with much practical information of this type, we also learned from the nurses how to "play doctor," to enact the part of a physician in society, including roughly equal parts of bedside manner, educating the patient, and simply "breaking the news." Once I tried in vain to revive a 49-year-old man who had suffered a massive coronary in a Hospital corridor while awaiting elective surgery for a minor problem. With no idea of what had happened, his wife walked in just as he was being carted off to the morgue. Asking what the ice was for, she was told matter-of-factly, "We always pack 'em like that when they expire," her hysterical shrieks and sobs leaving me to grope for what few words of comfort I could come up with. From then on, the nurses often called me at such times, simply because I would take the time to speak with the relatives and make sure that they too were cared for.

Much as I enjoyed the thrill of performing surgery, and admired the technical skill and ingenuity that made it possible, at 6 in the morning it was always a challenge to get down enough breakfast to avoid feeling faint or nauseous at some point during the gastric resection or hysterectomy I was about to scrub in for. Although certainly in favor of chemical intervention and reconstructive or emergency surgery in acute or life-threatening situations, I already distrusted long-term drug treatment in most instances, and avoided elective surgery wherever possible, regarding them as a last resort rather than the model for what we were supposed to be doing. But they were still all I knew. Had anyone suggested acupuncture, homeopathy, or anything equally outlandish at the time, I'm sure I wouldn't have been in the least interested in or hospitable to it.

After completing my internship and licensure, I took my first job, a *locum tenens* covering for a busy GP who was taking a long-overdue vacation and had left strict instructions to his patients not to come in unless their problems wouldn't wait until he returned. Even so, I worked harder during those four weeks than at any comparable period before or since, beginning with Hospital rounds at 7 a.m., then office visits virtually non-stop until 9 or 10 at night, averaging at least 50 patients a day, 6 days a week, a schedule by no means unusual for a busy GP then or now. On top of that, I officiated at eight births, and covered the Emergency Room one night a week, when I could expect to be up into the wee hours admitting, working up, and following new patients without established physicians of their own.

On one such night, the ambulance brought in a heavy-set, 45-year-old Polish lady who spoke not a word of English and limped in bent over, holding her back, and groaning in pain. Suspecting a kidney stone, I palpated her abdomen and was surprised to find her far along in a pregnancy of which she herself was unaware. From her husband's crude translations, I learned that she had never been pregnant before, had had no period for 9 or 10 months, and simply let it go at that, not feeling or suspecting anything out of the ordinary, refusing to believe her husband when he told her the news, and indeed flying off the handle at both of us for making a joke at her expense.

When a vaginal exam revealed that she was also in advanced labor, I rushed her to the delivery room just in time to hand her a nine-pound baby girl who seemed perfectly normal in every way. Back in the nursery, however, she regurgitated whatever she drank, and a Barium Swallow and Upper GI revealed a tracheo-esophageal fistula, a life-threatening congenital anomaly that had to be repaired without delay. Both mother and child went home in fine shape in less than a week, but the greater part of this saga occupied just a few hours in the eventful life of my absent employer, whose seven-league boots I was struggling mightily to fill.

When he returned, I became House Physician at the Beth Israel, a smaller hospital nearby, where my duties were much the same as during my internship, doing chores and little favors for the nurses, the Attending Staff, and their patients, as well as assisting in surgery, being on call for any emergencies or special needs, and supervising the Old Folks' Home out back. Always a favorite part of my practice, working with the elderly demands mainly personal care and attention, with little expectation of radical cure, yet earns profound gratitude for any relief of pain, suffering, or the accumulated burdens of survivorship.

At the same time, I moved back to Boulder and began seeing patients in my little ground-floor apartment, mostly students, friends, and street people, as an experiment to make my practice more open, informal, and as consensual as possible. My procedure was to examine them as noninvasively as the situation allowed, using only the simplest tools, with as much give-and-take and direct participation as they seemed to want or could handle, making the diagnosis, to be sure, but then putting it aside, and waiting for their own individual need or history to suggest a regimen and plan of treatment most uniquely suited to them. While often difficult, and by no means uniformly effective, this approach was at least clean, honest, unlikely to cause harm, and kept me closely attentive to the doctor-patient relationship at every moment. Ever since then, these same priorities have continued to guide me in my search for a method and style of practice that could pass the test of time.

Meanwhile, as the War in Southeast Asia continued to escalate, I began to realize how thoroughly both my medical training and the culture of illness and disease that we all grow up with are steeped in the imagery of warfare and combat. With drug ads and hospital and charity fund drives all promoting the conventional wisdom that viruses and bacteria are simply invaders to be expelled and diseases enemies to be fought, most people were and indeed still remain ready, willing, and eager to use chemical weapons such as antibiotics, antihypertensives, antimetabolites, and other "magic bullets" against any complaint or abnormality that threatens or merely bothers them.

But when an American General openly boasted of destroying a village in order to save it, his words borrowed almost *verbatim* from the cancer specialist, the gruesome footage of such exploits transformed what had formerly seemed like a mere figure of speech into a systematic philosophy of militarism for its own sake, with a gratuitous ferocity that began to shock even its own proponents. In that way it dawned on me that I'd been trained as a soldier to fight in the front lines of an endless war against disease, armed with the latest weapons to shoot down and kill all symptoms and abnormalities whenever and wherever they showed themselves. Once again, as in medical school, I prayed for the courage and the opportunity to desert my post and fight no more.

By then I was practicing what I would call "minimalist" medicine, that is, giving out liberal helpings of education and advice, while doing as little as possible of a drastic nature, seeing my rôle as mainly guiding people through the medical system and protecting them from being hurt too badly. These are still important priorities for me; but back then, with fewer and fewer procedures available that did no harm and made sense to me in other than acute or extreme circumstances, I had little to offer my patients when their illnesses got worse, while my growing estrangement from the profession as a whole made it increasingly difficult and unpleasant for me to practice at all.

Applying to a Boulder hospital for admitting privileges, I quickly discovered that my antiwar views and unorthodox style of practice had alienated many of the doctors in town. On the advice of a friendly internist, I introduced myself to as many of them as were willing to meet me, and was narrowly approved by just one vote; but the Board of Trustees simply overruled them the next day, evidently alarmed by the fact that what they feared or imagined I stood for had split the Medical Staff right down the middle.

Then in April of 1969, with my confidence and self-esteem at their lowest ebb, a simple request from out of the blue helped me see things more clearly, and showed me a path I could follow. Due to give birth in a month, a woman I knew very slightly telephoned to ask if I would come to her house to help with the labor, which none of the OB's in town would even consider. Although I'd never heard of anyone doing such a thing, or imagined that anyone would even want to, and was keenly aware of my own feelings of insecurity, with no nurses to hand me instruments and no hospital to back me up, I sensed in my desperation that here at last was something I could do as a physician without doing harm to people or telling them how to live.

When her time came, I'd intended to perform a vaginal examination as soon as I arrived, to assess how the labor was progressing, and I'm still not sure if it was the candlelight, or the Bach playing softly, or the rapt expression on all their faces; but somehow I got it that the exam was a routine procedure I'd been trained to do, rather than anything that Dorothy herself really needed or was asking for. After a lot of soul-searching, I decided that if anything went wrong, I had to be able to trust myself to figure out what needed to be done at the time, and that the best thing to do at the moment was to sit down, be quiet, and pay attention like everyone else. Mostly without words, Dorothy taught me

13

pretty much the whole course that day, although I'd still like to know how, where, and from whom *she* learned it, since her first child had been born under general anesthesia nine years before.

Her son Adam was born at dawn, with mother and child bathed in a soft halo of light all around them, like a Madonna of Raphael or Filippo Lippi; and we all saw it and gazed at it and her, the baby, and each other, as I imagine human beings have always done since the beginning of time. In no way uncanny, strange, or outside the realm of natural law, Adam's birth was a miracle in precisely the opposite sense, of something happening in full awareness, which only our customary inattention would need to single out, and only our remembering what all other animals have never forgotten bespoke a real deliverance.

Her daughter Erica announced her intention to take the placenta to school; but when her friends came by and pooh-poohed the idea, she wrapped it in a plastic bag and stuffed it under her coat, like a reluctant conspirator carrying an oversized bomb. A short time later, the school nurse telephoned in a panic, so I stopped by to fetch it on my way home. Assuring me that she wasn't really *against* "this sort of thing," she explained with some embarrassment that they didn't have refrigeration for it, that she'd have had to ask the principal, who happened to be out of town, and that she could lose her job if she acted on her own. I wish I'd had the presence of mind to ask her what she thought of a state of affairs in which she could lose her job for talking to a bunch of schoolchildren about giving birth to a baby, or indeed what her job *was* if not that. But I didn't. The holy relic lay in state on my coffee table for a week without the slightest odor or trace of putrefaction, like the dead bodies of certain gurus and saints of popular legend.

Adam's birth first gave me a glimpse of how I could function as a physician, a way that still works and makes sense to me. Even the most enlightened hospital has to make rules for people, to act as if it knew what's best for them, better than they do themselves, while as a guest in Phil and Dorothy's home it was no longer appropriate for me to tell them what to do or how to live their lives. Indeed my rôle was no longer to *do* anything in particular, but simply to *be there* for them in whatever way seemed useful at the time, to help them make whatever decisions they needed to make, and to complete the natural process that was already under way.

14

For a long time I guarded the memory of that experience like a precious jewel; it never occurred to me that anybody else would try to do such a crazy thing. Moving back to New York in search of new directions, I took a full-time position on the Medical Staff of a Neighborhood Health Clinic in Brooklyn that was created as an outpost of President Johnson's "War on Poverty." With a clientele that was mainly poor and black, and lived in the slums of Red Hook, our spanking-new facility was incongruously located in upscale Brooklyn Heights and included a fleet of reconditioned taxis to ferry our patients from the bottom of the socio-economic ladder to the top and back again.

Gratified that our budget at least provided for home visits, one day I was sent to the projects to see an old man in his nineties who was too ill to travel. As I entered the bedroom, he spotted my silvery moustache and rose smartly to attention, saluting me as if I were General Pershing, his Commanding officer, and he still a doughboy in the First World War. But before I could play along, he doubled over in pain, and while easing him back into bed I could feel the vast bulk of his liver, studded with hard, metastatic nodules in an obviously terminal state. Confiding to his wife that he had cancer and would undoubtedly die soon, I offered to find her a housekeeper to make them both more comfortable in the brief time remaining; but she was over eighty herself, with major health problems of her own, and wouldn't hear of him dying in that wretched little apartment, insisting that we admit him to the hospital and care for him there as best we could.

As a satellite of the vast Kings County Medical Center, our Clinic was required to admit all inpatients to Long Island College Hospital, its local affiliate, and to surrender all authority over their care to the interns and residents in training there. Determined at least to meet and talk with them first, I argued that since both the diagnosis and the outcome were already certain, the most humane and sensible option was to give him plenty of morphine, make him as comfortable as possible, and let him die in peace. But the House Staff greeted my suggestion with disbelief, as if it were a relic from the Stone Age. Just as I feared, they were determined to perform a liver biopsy and begin chemotherapy, purely as a training exercise, knowing that the drugs were toxic, debilitating, and of no lasting benefit, and that the procedure itself would very likely result in pneumonia and a miserable death, as in fact it did.

By the summer of 1970, I'd had enough, and once again sought refuge out West, renting a cabin high in the mountains above Boulder. No sooner had I arrived than women began calling me to help with their home births, and before long I was as busy as I could be, attending maybe 40 births by spring, and about 150 in the three years I lived there, time enough to watch Dorothy's romantic idea catch on and spread like a prairie fire through the subculture. Without an office, nurse, appointments, or even a telephone at first, I was totally available to my patients if they could find me, an arrangement that, while clearly unsuitable for some, fit in quite well with the frontier ethos and flourishing grapevine of that time and place.

The way it worked was that patients made it their business to know or find out where I was at all times, while I taught them the basics of emergency childbirth in case I didn't make it, and dropped in on anyone close to term whenever I came to town, a journey of twenty miles over rough mountain roads that in winter became an arduous and sometimes thrilling adventure. The best part was what happened when I got there, whether finding the labor already in progress, or being treated like an honorary member of the family for a while, or at least being rewarded with a hot meal, good company, and a warm bed for the night.

In any case, I never missed a birth, lost a baby, or needed to take anyone to the hospital in those days, a record that I can't explain and certainly never equaled or even came close to in later years, when I opened an office, hired nurses and receptionists, hospitalized people when I had to, and witnessed my full share of complications like everybody else. Only in retrospect can I fully appreciate how fortunate and indeed in a state of grace I must have been, as if blessed by the vision that Dorothy had bestowed on me, and determined to do everything in my power to be worthy of it. Whatever the reason, it cannot have been any particular skill or affinity on my part, since I had only a rudimentary knowledge of pregnancy and childbirth, felt even more keenly than my patients my unworthiness to supervise this most womanly activity, and could only justify it as an anomaly of medical history, which the home birth movement itself would and did eventually rectify.

Many of those births still remind me of the wide-open, experimental atmosphere and flair for self-discovery that seemed so characteristic of those years. Bored with successful careers in the New York theater and art scene, one newly-married couple set out on their honeymoon in an old school bus that they had transformed into a romantic bower of velvet hangings, silk brocades, and other offerings of beauty and magic to the new life they dreamed of. Aiming for California like so many others, they never made it past the mountains, where they ran out of cash, discovered they were pregnant, and fell under the sway of Chögyam Trungpa Rimpoche, the charismatic Tibetan master who lived and taught nearby.

Taking advantage of electric and water hookups at a friend's house in town, they continued to live and hold court in the bus, where we met to prepare for the birth. As the labor began one raw November morning, dozens of friends and well-wishers gathered in the house and began carousing and drinking heavily to celebrate the event as if it had already taken place. By nightfall, Maggie was tired and panting rapidly, but her cervix was still only minimally dilated, and all the patience and encouragement I could muster failed to help her over this seemingly huge and insurmountable obstacle. With her labor at a standstill, I went back into the house, and solemnly announced that she needed the collective energy and moral support of everyone there, without any clear idea of what I actually had in mind. As if on cue, they filed out into what had become an icy drizzle, lined up alongside the bus, and began chanting the sacred syllable in a loud, insistent drone that sounded as if it would continue until something pretty impressive happened.

Thus summoned to what would become perhaps the greatest performance of her career, the former actress quickly revived in the presence of her audience, inviting everyone inside the bus, passing out candles, and no longer in any doubt about what to do next. Opening the *I Ching* at random, I read aloud from the first hexagram I turned to; and although I have no memory of the actual passage, it elicited a chorus of nods and murmurs as if cosmically appropriate to the occasion. Taking hold of two ropes that her husband Don had hung from the ceiling for just this purpose, Maggie pulled herself up to a squatting position on the bed and began bellowing like a heifer with each contraction, although she was still by no means fully dilated, felt no definite urge to push, and

17

taught herself as if by sheer force of will how to recognize and direct an instinct that still lay hidden deep inside her. When her daughter finally emerged, weighing almost eleven pounds, her prodigious size made the physical and moral difficulties of her birth seem almost legendary in Maggie's heroic mastery of them.

These early experiences also taught me to respect my patients' life choices even when I disagreed with them, questioning and at times arguing when I felt strongly, but in the end giving them the say about the kind of health care they wanted. With no past experience to guide me, I fretted a lot about the nutritional state of a macrobiotic couple who held forth as if they exemplified the highest moral virtue through their spiritual understanding of food; but I did enjoy the dinner they set before me well enough to persuade me to work with them. As it happened, the labor and the birth went off perfectly; and although the baby was smaller than average, as I've since come to expect, she grew to be as strong and healthy as anyone could wish.

Over the next twelve years, I attended somewhat more than six hundred home births; and the model of doctor-patient relationships that emerged from them is as relevant today in my office practice as it was then in the field. I feel as proud as of anything else I have ever done to have helped these families come together and bear their children in a manner and setting of their own choosing, and in spite of the generally lackluster support and at times active opposition of the medical community.

Through its gentle, family-centered atmosphere, home birth also promoted and left ample room for self-healing in other ways, and encouraged me to explore subtler and less aggressive modes of treatment in my medical practice as well. With my background and interest in biochemistry, I naturally gravitated to the study of plant and folk remedies, and soon began combing through old herbals, learned to identify various local species, made infusions, poultices, ointments, and suppositories, and tried them on myself and my patients. In these investigations my chief mentor was Hanna Kroger, an old German woman who had emigrated to the States after the War, owned a health food store in town, and had a large, devoted following that included young and old alike. Bothered by a broad range of ailments, customers she knew and trusted would follow her into a small back room, where she dowsed with a pendulum for a variety of energy disturbances, and the naturopathic treatments that she felt were best suited to them, consisting of vitamins, herbs, supplements, and even homeopathic remedies, which I first heard of in her shop. At times she would also send saliva and hair samples to an even more aged colleague in Albuquerque, who claimed that she could detect trace amounts of toxic wastes, parasites, and other pathological residues by using some kind of radionic device that she talked about in hushed tones.

Although most of what Hanna did seemed like hocus-pocus to me, she also introduced me to the realm of esoteric phenomena that intuitively I knew existed but had never directly witnessed or experienced myself. Whenever I tagged along with her, she would show me things that I couldn't believe or understand, yet stimulated me to imagine what the world would have to be like if they were true. About two months after giving birth, one of my patients called late at night because of severe abdominal pain that had developed that afternoon, after returning from a long trip to her in-laws to show off the baby. On pelvic examination, I felt a taut, bulging mass the size of a tennis ball in the area of her right ovary, which clearly needed to be removed surgically without delay; but she refused to go to the hospital unless I first called Hanna, who was herself reluctant to come and needed some coaxing on my part.

Upon entering the room, she went straight to the bedside, knelt by the left side of my patient, and began to pray, placing the palm of her left hand gently on the abdomen over the cyst, and allowing her right arm to dangle by her side. After a few minutes, Hanna's body began to shake convulsively, so much so that I fancied I could sense a current of energy passing up her left arm, across her chest, down her right arm, and out her free hand. Proceeding methodically to the other side of the bed, she then placed her right index and middle fingers on the right pubic ramus, which she identified as a pressure point for the right ovary, and pressed down firmly on it, eliciting a mighty jolt and shriek of pain from my patient, who all but levitated out of bed, but then settled back down into quiet moaning and whimpering for about fifteen seconds, after which she fell silent. Similar pressure on various other points elicited no more than a brief wince or two, after which Hanna rose and left, prescribing nothing more esoteric than a molasses douche and a day in bed.

19

Re-examining her immediately afterward, I was amazed to discover that both the pain and the cyst had completely disappeared, and I can vouch for the fact that they never came back in the two years I kept track of this woman before leaving the area. Since then, I've seen my share of ovarian cysts dissolve in a few hours or days with remedies, but never an instantaneous cure of a surgical emergency to rival this one, which taught me that healing is possible even when we least expect it, have no idea what form it will take, and can never adequately explain it by any doctrine, concept, or method, however scientific it may be.

In 1973, I moved to New Mexico to study acupuncture with Sensei Masahilo Nakazono, a Japanese master who also taught aikido and practiced Shinto, the ancient religion of his country, by chanting "the sacred sounds" whereby his earliest proto-human ancestors were said to have expressed and communicated their feelings directly, without the mediation of spoken or written language. While beginning to train a few Western students, he had been chosen to preside over the newly-created State Board of Acupuncture after curing a number of legislators of serious ailments. Although his religious practice and authoritarian style always remained foreign to me, and I never got used to seeing patients two or even three times a week for months at a time, I revered him as a teacher and healer, and was often in awe of his skill and charismatic power to heal patients who were seriously or even gravely ill.

I deeply respect and admire Oriental medicine for its systematic philosophy of the organism as a unitary life-energy principle, operating prior to any subdivision of it into thoughts and emotions, on the one hand, and organs, cells, and molecules on the other. By learning to palpate subtle variations in the radial pulses, using nine positions on each side, a skilled practitioner can assess the energy state of the internal organs based on the condition of the "meridians" or longitudinal energy currents on the body surface that are thought to correspond to them. Thereby avoiding the Western "mind-body problem" entirely, traditional acupuncture diagnoses and treats illness uniquely and globally in each patient as an integraed energy system, and can relieve pain and suffering, cure illness, and restore and promote health on a deeper level and with subtler methods than Western medicine, with all of its heavy artillery, seems capable of or even much interested in. As my introduction to

20

energy medicine, acupuncture continues to open up new paths in my thought and practice, and I will always be grateful to the Sensei and honor his memory for sharing his truths so generously with me.

A few motnhs later, I stumbled into homeopathy. After poring over an old text I found in a used bookstore, I got no further than wanting to try *Apis mellifica,* the honeybee, for a patient who was highly sensitive to bee stings, and telephoned an aged homeopath I'd heard of back East to ask if that would be an appropriate prescription. "Well, sonny boy," he replied in his economical Vermontese, "I think you'd better come to our summer school!" I decided to give it a try, but neither the backwoods state college where the course was held nor the advanced age and semi-retired status of the doctors who taught it augured well for the future of the method. Few of them were still earning a living from practicing it, as if the whole generation of active, full-time practitioners that should have preceded us had never materialized. The course itself lasted only two weeks, after which they turned us loose to practice what we had learned. With no full-time schools, clinics, or teaching hospitals to its name, and very few retail pharmacies to send patients to, it was a stretch to imagine that American homeopathy could survive much longer.

Yet from the moment I entered that class, I knew that it was exactly the kind of thing I'd been hoping and looking for, and that I could happily devote the rest of my professional life to studying and practicing it. Long before I'd taken remedies myself or seen them work in a patient, it made sense to me as both a philosophy, a coherent body of thought with basic assumptions that rang true, and a detailed, systematic methodology that followed from them. It even showed me a better way of doing what I was already trying to do: making the diagnosis, and then putting it aside, allowing the distinctive patterns of my patients' illnesses to suggest proper treatments for them. Reframing illness as the attempt of the organism to overcome whatever is keeping it off balance, homeopaths identify the individualizing features of each patient's symptom-picture, and administer ultradilute doses of the medicine that most closely matches it to strengthen and resonate with the process of self-healing that is already under way.

Far from repudiating allopathic medicine because of it, I chose homeopathy because it charted a clear path through the hidden risks and self-imposed obstacles that had kept me from practicing medicine at all for such a long time. As to whether it really *works,* I offer the whole of my career since then as evidence that it does, having used it more or less exclusively for the past twenty-three years with never a cause to regret it. My first patient was myself, waking from a concussion after a head-on collision with a drunk driver, bleeding from a scalp laceration, and in considerable pain from several rib fractures. Sitting erect in the ambulance, I felt dazed but otherwise tolerably OK until the EMT deposited me onto a Gurney at the ER, flat on my back, helpless, and immobile, the slightest change in position sending stabs of pain through my chest that sapped my strength and will to recover. When my nurse arrived to take me home, I took from my bag a powder of *Arnica* 200, put a few granules on my tongue, and within a few seconds was able to lift my bloody shirt over my head and take it off without her help, an incredible feat under the circumstances. Feeling no more pain for several days, I recovered without further incident.

That first winter, I saw mostly acute illnesses, i.e., colds, flu, Strep throats, bronchitis, and other incidental complaints of pregnant women and their families, who formed the backbone of my practice at that time. Whenever a patient needed medicine, I rummaged around in my books until I found one that seemed suitable, and both of us were often quite pleasantly surprised at how quickly and effectively it worked to relieve pain and suffering, to impart a feeling of strength and well-being, and to cut short the natural course of the illness. Soon I began trying remedies at births, too, with similar results: at times none, often good, and sometimes miraculous.

One such was the experience of a twenty-year-old woman, pregnant for the first time, who gave birth to a girl after a prolonged second stage. Although well-formed and weighing over eight pounds, the baby was covered with thick, greenish-black meconium, took one gasp, and then breathed no more. When brisk suctioning of the nose and mouth produced only more of the same sticky stuff, I tried and failed to intubate or even visualize the trachea, while the child lay pale, limp, and motionless, with a heartbeat of only 40 per minute, responding feebly to mouth-to-mouth resuscitation, but unable to breathe on her own. I put a tiny powder of *Arsenicum album* 200 on her tongue, and almost instantaneously she awoke with a jolt, crying and flailing, her heart beating vigorously at 140 per minute, and her skin glowing pink with the flame of new life, the whole evolution requiring no more than a few seconds. Experiences like these are inscribed for life in every practitioner's mind.

Since 1974, I have practiced homeopathy more or less exclusively and according to the classical method, prescribeing only one medicine at a time for the whole patient. Those I fail to help I refer to another homeopath if possible, and for more drastic treatment when necessary. If practiced conscientiously, the method poses minimal risk of harm, and allows me to develop my skills through experience and to learn and grow at my own pace. Since I can see only as many people as I can see, and learn only as fast as I can learn, most of my patients understand and readily forgive the fact that expertise is acquired little by little, and at the cost of numerous mistakes and failures. On the other hand, I have also been able to help people in ways and situations that would have been inconceivable to me before.

I'm thinking of a 34-year-old woman who came to see me shortly after we moved to Boston, with a history of severe and painful endometriosis since her teens. Already a veteran of four surgeries to remove large, blood-filled cysts from her bladder and ovaries, and several courses of male hormones to correct the hormone imbalance, she came solely to restore her menstrual cycle, having long since abandoned any hope of childbearing. Intensely painful throughout her teens and twenties, her periods had become scanty, "dead," and dark-brown as a result of so many operations and years of hormones and oral contraceptives in the past; but with treatment they became fuller and richer, and within six months she was pregnant. When I next saw her for a different ailment eight years later, she had produced two healthy children after uncomplicated pregnancies and normal, vaginal births and had remained in good health ever since. While no one can ascribe such an outcome to a remedy or any other agency in precise, linear fashion, my patient has never stopped thanking me for it, reason enough to be grateful for a process by its very nature persuasive and catalytic rather than forcible or compulsory.

I can readily understand the skepticism and incredulity in the eyes of my patients after the long interview, when I put a little bit of "fairy dust" on their tongue and ask them to come back six weeks later. What we call the "Law of Similars" has never attained general acceptance in medicine, and even those of us who use it every day regard it as a mystery. Still less satisfactorily has anybody ever explained how a medicinal substance diluted beyond the molecular limit of Avogadro's number could possibly have *any* effect on a patient, let alone a curative one. But the standard argument that homeopathic remedies are merely placebos cuts both ways. For quite apart from *how* they do it, the extent to which people are able to heal themselves without drugs or surgery, whether through acupuncture, homeopathy, placebos, faith healing, or the laying-on of hands, proportionately reduces the need for costlier and more drastic methods and deflates the extravagant promotional claims made for them.

I do not believe and have never taught that homeopathy is the only way to heal people or the best way for everyone. By no means a panacea for all ills, it has substantial limitations of its own, some of them inherent and others that will need to be reassessed in the light of a new science of energy medicine that is still in its infancy. I practice it mainly because it is the philosophy and method best suited to my own history and personal style. Even when it is better understood, I doubt that it will ever become the dominant mode of treatment for this or any other society; and indeed if it did, I might begin to lose interest in it. Since nobody has all the answers, and everybody has some of them, it makes the most sense for all of us to work together, discovering our several truths wherever we find them, and celebrating beauty for its own sake.

II. Writings on Midwifery:

Homeopathic Medicines for Pregnancy and Childbirth (Excerpts)

"Some Thoughts on the Beginnings of Life"

Homeopathic Medicines for Pregnancy and Childbirth*

From Introduction.

This book grew out of two improbable revivals of the past twenty years. One is the home birth movement, which despite powerful medical opposition has already effected important changes in the sociology and politics of women's health in the United States. The other is classical homeopathy, likewise against all odds, which has proved surprisingly versatile and popular as a primary-care vehicle for health professionals and lay people alike. What both movements have in common is a commitment to gentler, more natural models for health care and the healing relationship.

I have used homeopathic remedies since 1974 in more than 800 pregnancies. I have found them to be wonderfully safe and effective in many situations where more drastic methods are not required. Yet there exists no basic work in English on homeopathy in pregnancy and childbirth that would be helpful in contemporary home, hospital, or birthing center settings. That is the need I have tried to satisfy.

I have decided to give primary emphasis to homeopathic self-care of common functional problems that tend to correct themselves spontaneously. In part that is because they are most amenable to the action of natural remedies and therefore least likely to require drugs or surgery. They are also the complaints that I have encountered most often in my own experience, which has been limited mostly to home and office settings.

But the most important reason is my conviction that self-healing is the very heart of what health care is all about, and that self-care provides the proper model for client-professional relationships as well. Though at present the book will likely appeal primarily to a lay audience, I hope and

---

* *Homeopathic Medicines for Pregnancy and Childbirth,* 288 pp., with Index, North Atlantic Books, Berkeley, CA, 1992.

expect that eventually it will prove useful in hospitals, birth centers, and academic training programs for childbirth professionals of every type.

I should add that I hold no brief for homeopathy as a panacea for all ills, or to the exclusion of other methods. I offer it exactly as I found it -- as an elegant and useful technique that deserves to be better known, understood, and used by all. But it should not be considered an alternative to or substitute for trained, experienced professional help. Nevertheless, there are many common situations where its tiny and infrequent doses make it more attractive than powerful and potentially toxic pharmaceutical drugs, whose safety in pregnancy and childbirth is always an issue and must often be extrapolated from animal models.[1]

The actual technique of homeopathy involves the use of highly diluted remedies in a manner still not wholly understood. The skepticism and doubt that the method very properly arouses are best answered by the same test that all patients have always used, namely, does it *work*, does it really help people to heal themselves? I offer this body of experience as evidence that it does. Recent double-blind studies have also confirmed that homeopathic remedies given late in pregnancy tend to shorten labor and prevent dysfunctional patterns and other complications more effectively than placebo alone.[2]

The effectiveness of homeopathy in treatment also helps encourage more humanistic and patient-centered models for thinking about the healing process in general. Simply including patients' subjective experience in the definition of health and illness endows their admittedly anecdotal stories with explanatory and indeed mythic power that no mere statistical analysis or "placebo effect" can match. For all of these reasons, I will feel amply rewarded if pregnant women will simply try homeopathy and see for themselves.

What follows is in no sense a comprehensive textbook of homeopathy in pregnancy and childbirth. The homeopathic *Materia medica* already comprises over two thousand remedies, every one a possible candidate for inclusion here. My intention is simply to develop a kit of basic remedies and enough methodology to help people get started in using them. I have therefore limited myself to those common remedies and conditions with which I've had the broadest personal experience as a solid foundation to build on.

The book is a "primer" in that sense, intended for beginners in homeopathy, both lay and professional, as a basis for further study. It consists of three sections: 1) a brief introduction to the homeopathic philosophy and method; 2) a condensed *Materia medica* of 25 important remedies; and 3) an outline of common problems of pregnancy and childbirth, with cases and remedies, including some not previously discussed.

Wherever possible, I have tried to illustrate the text with actual vignettes from my own experience, because knowledge of the remedies is built to a great extent on the distinctive features of real people. Looking back on this unforgettable chapter of my life has also been a great pleasure to me, and will hopefully serve to make it more vivid for others as well.

NOTES.

1.Cf. Brackbill, Y., et al., *Medication in Maternity,* International Academy for Research in Learning Disabilities, Ann Arbor, 1989, pp. 43-129.

2.Dorfman, P., et al., "Preparation for Childbirth by Homeopathy," *Cahiers deBiothérapie* 94:77, 1987.

From Chapter 9, "Late Pregnancy."

Genital Herpes.

The herpes viruses present a special problem because of the potential risk that the mother may pass it to the fetus *in utero* or to the baby as it exits from the vagina. Although herpes infections are quite common during pregnancy and quite rare in the newborn, it is often very serious and sometimes fatal when intrauterine or vaginal transmission occurs. While the mother's first lesion is by far the most dangerous, and previously infected women usually show antibodies in the amniotic fluid, even recurrent lesions have been implicated in some instances. In any case, to be on the safe side, most obstetricians still advocate elective Caesarean section for women with active lesions discovered within 4-6 weeks of the due date.

Although women with genital herpes in pregnancy will often benefit from homeopathic care, consultation with a physician or nurse-midwife is strongly recommended, and self-care for lesions appearing late in pregnancy should be combined with regular prenatal care and laboratory examination, given that many suspected lesions are unconfirmed by culture. Naturally, if there are no active lesions, and the parents are prepared to accept responsibility for the outcome, the final decision about a home birth rightfully belongs with them.

Sepia, trituration of the ink, *Sepia officinalis,* the cuttlefish.

The leading remedy for herpes of the vulva, labia, and vagina, *Sepia* will ordinarily be indicated by its typical general features, but may also be tried when more precise indications for it or any other remedies are lacking. (See Chapter 4.)

Phosphorus, saturated solution of elemental phosphorus in alcohol, P.

Here too, the general features of the remedy -- burning pains, thirst, fears, hypochondriasis, etc. -- will usually be prominent, and a lot of reassurance will be required. (See Chapter 7.)

> *Case 9.4.* Ten weeks into her first pregnancy, a 29-year-old woman was very excited and in resplendent health, but spooked about genital herpes. Already a veteran of six lesions in her pubic hair, the most recent had been just two weeks earlier; and as her imagination raced ahead to every possible future scenario, her big, lustrous, black eyes stayed riveted on me for protection. She was happily married and had no other medical problems. After a round of *Phosphorus* 200, everything went smoothly until about 35 weeks, when she reported two new lesions less than a week apart, both less prominent and intense than usual, but still worrisome. After a Pap smear and several cultures were negative, I gave a dose of *Phosphorus* 1M, and we decided to proceed with the home birth, which went off beautifully, without a hitch. . .

Mercurius, triturate of pure metallic mercury, quicksilver, Hg.

The great anti-syphilitic drug of Hahnemann's time, *Mercurius vivus,* his own preparation of metallic Hg, remains widely used in homeopathy for the treatment of destructive or ulcerating lesions anywhere in the body, with foul, slimy, debilitating excretions or discharges from any orifice. In the mouth, where Hg amalgam fillings may actually contribute to the problem, indications for the remedy include excessive salivation, foul breath, painful or abscessed teeth, , and herpetic or aphthous ulcers. In the vulva or vagina, it may be useful for herpes or other infections with ulceration or offensive discharge. Also a leading remedy for dysentery, *Mercurius* should be considered for patients with bone pains, night sweats, and unwholesome discharges anywhere, especially when intensified during the nighttime hours.

Thuja, tincture of fresh, green twigs of *Thuja occidentalis,* arbor vitæ.

Identified by Hahnemann with another of the great chronic disease styles, this shrub is indicated for patients whose symptom-picture is dominated by excessive growth or proliferation of tissue, e. g., warts, moles, cysts, tumors, and hyperplasia, and by a history of gonorrhea or other genital infections suppressed but not cured by allopathic treatment.

> *Case 9.5.* Early in her first pregnancy, a woman of 32 came in for her initial visit worried mainly about genital herpes. Most of her 10 previous lesions had been on the vulva, the most recent only 2 weeks ago. As a child, she had had numerous warts on her hands and knees, all of them frozen off with liquid nitrogen, as well as a Bartholin cyst that was drained surgically a few years back, and several positive Pap smears for cervical dysplasia. Although in excellent general health, she had suffered from insomnia for many years, and was otherwise almost painfully reserved about her personal life.
>
> With a dose of *Thuja* 200, she had no lesions for many months, even after typical premonitory symptoms on two occasions, which had never happened before. At 32 weeks she developed an atypical lesion that tested negative twice; so we repeated the remedy and opted for the home birth, which went off beautifully. . . .

Two Important Remedies for Late Pregnancy.

Two medicines are indicated for so many second- and third-trimester ailments that they could almost be thought of as "constitutional" remedies for late pregnancy itself. Although often prescribed in the early months as well, they are particularly significant for maternal physiology once placental development is well-established, and both should be thought of on the basis of their overall symptom-picture as much as for any specific complaints.

Sulphur, triturate of elemental sulfur, brimstone or flowers of sulfur, S.

A constitutional remedy *par excellence* for many types of acute and chronic illness, *Sulphur* corresponds beautifully to the additional metabolic demands of pregnancy, when increased cardiac output is required, pre-existing tendencies are often heightened, and even well-established patterns may need to be modified or changed. Often traceable to excessive and unregulated heat production, *Sulphur* complaints tend to be characterized by excessive intolerance of warm rooms, warm clothing, or becoming warm in bed, and to manifest in a rough, crude, or uneven way, involving some areas much more strongly than others. No matter what the presenting complaint, most *Sulphur* patients will also exhibit other typical features, like burning pains, itching, and redness, all aggravated by heat and relieved by cold, with extreme thirst for cold drinks, ravenous hunger or faintness, especially around 11 a.m., and intense cravings for sweets and alcohol. (See Chapter 7.)

> *Case 9.14.* At 16 weeks in her first pregnancy, a 31-year-old woman came in feeling "run-down" and faint, particularly in the heat. Given her history of major depression following her mother's death, she seemed remarkably good-natured and even ebullient in the office, engaging in rough banter with her husband and laughing uproariously at her own infirmities. Heavily built and rather slovenly in appearance, she ate enormous meals with gusto, washed them down with large quantities of water and soda, and felt faint if she waited too long in between. Already a little edematous and water-logged, she was also often awakened in the night by dryness and itching in her nose. After *Sulphur* 1M, her energy seemed more balanced, her appetite less extreme, and she finished out her pregnancy in good shape, giving birth at home without difficulty. . .

Kali carbonicum, triturate of the salt, potassium carbonate, K_2CO_3.

Easy to overlook but not difficult to recognize, the picture of *Kali carb.* tends to fit patients who seem crabby, vague, and evasive in telling their symptoms. Yet despite their sometimes humdrum character and unappealing presentation, the complaints are usually sufficient to point to the remedy once it is thought of.

First, the remedy is full of nagging, stitching pains, "side aches," and lumbago, in which the painful areas need to be rubbed or pressed hard for relief. Second, both the patient herself and most of her particular

31

symptoms tend to be aggravated in the wee hours of the morning, especially from 2 to 4 a.m., making *Kali carb.* an important remedy for insomnia late in pregnancy. Whether awakening to urinate, from pain or anxiety, or with no other symptoms at all, the patient may be unable to get back to sleep, perhaps troubled by family matters or vague doubts and fears that remain ill-defined. Many patients needing *Kali carb.* are tormented by diffuse or free=floating anxiety, especially when alone and unoccupied by the chores of everyday life. Also chilly and sensitive to cold, it is an excellent remedy for almost any ailment in late pregnancy with the above features. It has seen good service in the treatment of cough and catarrh, pneumonia, bronchitis, and in delayed or prolonged convalescence following any severe or debilitating illness, with chronic fatigue, anemia, and weight loss.

> *Case 9.16.* Six months into her second pregnancy, a woman of 30 came for her regular prenatal visit complaining of heartburn, insomnia, and sporadic, flu- like episodes of weakness that would overtake her suddenly and force her to lie down for perhaps 30 minutes at a time. Most noticeable after eating or even drinking tea with honey too late in the evening, the heartburn often woke her at 3 a.m. Yet most of the time she enjoyed her favorite meat and sausage dishes with impunity, and she also regularly awoke at that hour without any heartburn, feeling chilled even under the covers, and worrying about their shaky finances and how she would manage to care for the baby. All of these symptoms were narrated in a whining, monotonous style, as if calculated to bore the listener. After a round of *Kali carb.* 200, her sleep and energy improved, the other symptoms receded into the background, and she had a quick and easy home birth with no complications. . .

From Chapter 10, "Labor and Childbirth."

The intensive work of childbirth is ordinarily completed within a few hours and easily forgotten after months of gestation and the years of parenting to follow. Yet it remains the ultimate emotional and physical challenge that most pregnant women anticipate and prepare for, the biological "moment of truth" wherein all their hopes and fears for themselves and their children are concentrated and put to the test.

In a fast or easy labor, the successive stages often overlap or merge smoothly into one another, such that changes in breathing, vocalization, feeling-tone, and body language are adequate to monitor its progress without repeated vaginal exams or other intrusive medical procedures. When the process becomes "stuck" or simply requires a longer time, definite stages are accurately identified and clinically useful as well. I have therefore retained the concept of stages in the loose sense of milestones to be passed by each woman in her own time and her own way, rather than as standards or expectations of performance or behavior. . .

"False" Labor.

Meaningful only after labor has actually stopped, the term suggests a credible imitation of the real thing, with more or less strong and regular contractions that may continue for several hours but fail to progress beyond a certain point. Unlike premature labor, it typically occurs more or less at term, with a viable baby inside. Most cases I can recall were in second or later pregnancies, when I'd spend the night at the house to be on the safe side, but the morning would bring no more than the same sporadic contractions that had been happening for days or weeks already.

Although a genuine nuisance for all concerned, false labor seems to be a normal variant, even a kind of rehearsal that can actually shorten the rest of the labor when it finally kicks into gear, almost always within a few days to a week at most. . .

Case 10.7. After an uneventful second pregnancy and a long night of false labor the week before, a woman of 25 called me again in the wee hours of the morning, this time greeting me with twin daughters in her arms when I arrived. "You're a little late, Doc!" she teased, her high spirits charming away my embarrassment at not having spotted the twins beforehand. Her uterus remained hypotonic after the birth, however, and she continued to bleed rather heavily, feeling faint and chilly, yet wanting the windows wide open for relief. *Pulsatilla* 30 was speedily effective in this typical situation: shreds of membrane and placental fragments were expelled, the bleeding slowed to a trickle, and her pulse and blood pressure reverted to normal levels. After that little scare, the rest of her postpartum course proceeded without difficulty.

Late Onset and Postmaturity.

Although such calculations are again unavoidably imprecise, pregnancies continuing well past term call for more careful attention. Postmaturity includes many of the same issues as prematurity and dysfunctional labor, and is covered by many of the same remedies. As always, their effectiveness in initiating labor depends on both their overall "fit" and detailed similarity with the total symptom-picture of the patient.

Whether handed down by friends or relatives, or previously experienced or imagined by the patient herself, obsessive fears or "horror stories' about labor, birth, or parenting may prevent labor from starting or interfere with its progress.

> *Case 10.1.* In labor for the first time, a woman of 28 was already fully dilated when I got there, with the baby's head halfway down the vagina. Thinking only to applaud her achievement, I exclaimed, "That's wonderful, Angela; it looks like the baby will be born within the hour!" No sooner had I spoken than my words seemed to have precisely the opposite effect, of stopping her labor in its tracks; and when I examined her, by some feat of sorcery that seemed physically impossible, the cervix had reappeared and pulled the head back up into the uterus, and no remedy I gave her would persuade it to relax its hold. As we talked, it became clear that she simply needed more time to process her so far subservient role in her husband's tight-knit, clannish family; and she gave birth easily a few hours later, once this important inner work was well under way. . .

Failure to Dilate: Prolonged, Difficult, and Dysfunctional Labor.

Although likewise vague and imprecise, these terms refer to common problems that most people can learn to recognize. Any remedy may be useful at any stage of labor, but the overall symptom-picture consistently yields better results than a prepared recipe. Finally, even well-selected remedies don't always work. The reader should beware of wishfully thinking that remedies alone can eliminate suffering, and of overlooking the obvious possibility that we can get stuck at any point, and healing may simply fail to occur.

Caulophyllum, tincture of the root, *Caulophyllum thalictroides,* blue cohosh.

This remedy tends to work best early on, where the uterus and indeed the patient herself are exhausted out of proportion to any obvious work done, and lacking more distinctive features of other remedies. The uterus feels soft, even at the height of the contraction, the labor fails to progress, the woman is oddly and profoundly exhausted. Typically short and unstable, the contractions may be feeble and infrequent, or sharp and spasmodic, and are felt low in the pelvis, rather than at the top or fundus of the uterus, often accompanied by trembling, shaking, and nervous excitement as well. With these warning signs, the remedy may be given right at the beginning, without requiring a vaginal exam to confirm them. (See Chapter 3.)

> *Case 10.3.* After a hospital birth under general anesthesia, and a second born prematurely at 30 weeks, a woman of 28 had a healthy and uneventful third pregnancy, except for some bleeding and cramping in the last trimester. She went into labor right on schedule, but very desultorily at first, with very weak contractions felt low in the pelvis. With the aid of *Caulophyllum* 30, she soon went into active labor, and gave birth within the hour, although needing the remedy again for flabby contractions and bleeding afterwards. The rest of her postpartum course was entirely normal. . .

Cimicifuga, tincture of the root, *Cimicifuga racemosa,* black cohosh.

While similar in type to those of *Caulophyllum,* the contractions of *Cimicifuga* tend to be more violent and are often accompanied by other even more disturbing symptoms. The patient may appear gloomy, dejected, or morose, with persistently negative thoughts, doubts, and fears about her ability to continue. In more advanced cases, fears of insanity or psychotic ideation and behavior may present a truly alarming picture. In addition, there is usually evidence of fragmenting on the physical level, in the form of alternating symptoms, grimaces or coarse involuntary movements, or severe headaches or neuralgias that interrupt the continuity of the labor. (See Chapter 3.)

> *Case 10.4.* After two abortions, a woman of 29 married and became pregnant again easily, opting for a home birth in part because of irrational fears of the hospital, stimulated by films like "One Flew Over the Cuckoo's Nest." The pregnancy was healthy and uneventful, as was most of the labor; but she

"lost it" during transition, when the unrelenting pain revived her old fears of hospitalization. *Cimicifuga* 200 calmed her almost instantly, and she gave birth soon after without further difficulty. . .

Pulsatilla, tincture of the fresh flowering plant, *Pulsatilla nigricans,* the windflower.

Useful at every stage of pregnancy and labor, *Pulsatilla* will usually be thought of because of the general symptoms, such as emotional and/ or vasomotor instability, and marked improvement from drinking fluids, exposure to cool, fresh air, and simple affection and caring. Although commonly indicated during labor, it should not be overlooked for problems with bleeding, retained placenta, or other postpartum complaints. (See Chapter 4.)

> *Case 10.6.* After a healthy first pregnancy greatly benefited by *Sulphur* 1M in its final months, a 30-year-old woman had a short, easy labor until the second stage, when the baby got "stuck" at a +1 station, her contractions stalled, and she became cross and weepy. When *Chamomilla* 30 produced no benefit, she asked for fresh air and some quiet time with her husband, which together with *Pulsatilla* 30 helped her push the baby out with no further delay. . .

Chamomilla, tincture of the whole fresh plant, *Matricaria chamomilla,* chamomile.

Extreme sensitivity to and intolerance of pain are the hallmarks of this remedy, whatever the condition. In labor, the patient is likely to be cross and irritable whenever the pain is intensely felt, demanding inordinate attention and support yet unable to accept, acknowledge, or make use of them when offered. The bowels may be disordered as well, with loose stools, flatulence, or simple hypermotility. (See Chapter 5.)

> *Case 10.9.* After an uneventful first pregnancy, a 29-year-old woman was already in active labor when I arrived, running short laps around her tiny living room and forbidding me to get close enough to examine her or listen to the baby. She did want something for the pain, however, so I gave her a few doses of *Chamomilla* 30 whenever she slowed down long enough to take them. Without delay or fanfare, or indeed any friends or relatives to help her, she soon gave birth in her bed with her pets in attendance, and only her thanks for it afterwards to suggest that the remedy had played any role. . .

Nux vomica, tincture of the seeds, *Strychnos nux vomica,* poison nut.

Often overlooked in favor of the usual "female" remedies, *Nux vomica* has come to the rescue in many instances of rectal or bladder dystocia, where the labor is obstructed by a full bladder or rectum, with painful and ineffectual urge to urinate or defecate, owing to spasm of either or both sphincter muscles.

At any stage of labor, the remedy should be thought of when the patient feels a strong but unproductive urge to go to the toilet with the contraction, especially if other typical elements are present, such as irritability, overstimulation, and craving for or intolerance of coffee, tobacco, alcohol, and other stimulants. . . (See Chapter 6.)

Resuscitation of the Newborn.

When the baby is born, the umbilical cord may be left ubdisturbed until it stops pulsating and the placenta separates from the endometrium, typically with a substantial gush of blood. Even then, there is no rush to cut it, since the umbilical vessels promptly close of their own accord. Obviously, if the cord is wound tightly around the baby's neck, it should be clamped and cut immediately, without waiting for the shoulders to be born.

The health status of the baby should be assessed immediately, utilizing the Apgar score of five vital functions at 1 minute and 5 minutes:

1) *heart rate* (score 2 for over 100/min., 1 for below 100, 0 for no heartbeat);

2) *respiratory effort* (2 for vigorous cry or regular breathing, 1 for slow or irregular, 0 for none);

3) *color* (2 for pink, 1 for pink body and blue extremities, 0 for all blue, gray, or white);

4) *muscle tone* (2 for active movement, 1 for flexion of extremities, 0 for lying limp and motionless); and

5) *reflex irritability* in response to nasal suctioning (2 for cough or sneeze, 1 for grimace, 0 for no response).

Newborns with scores of 7 to 10 are considered normal and require no resuscitation; those with scores of 4 to 6 are mildly to moderately depressed, and will often recover with simple suctioning and brief resuscitative efforts; and those with scores of 0 to 3 are severely depressed, at high risk of death or irreversible brain damage, and require immediate transfer to a newborn ICU.

In conjunction with first-aid measures, homeopathic remedies can play a valuable role. For newborns, I prefer the tiny #10 granules delivered from the moistened fingertip, perhaps 10-20 per dose, directly on the tongue. In critical situations, the remedy may be repeated every 10 seconds and changed if there is no effect after 2 doses.

Arnica, tincture of the fresh plant, *Arnica montana,* leopard's bane.

The remedy par excellence for blunt trauma to the soft tissues, *Arnica* is also unsurpassed for reactivating stunned autonomic reflexes, and should be considered for the baby as well as the mother after a traumatic birth, especially with bruising or cephalhematoma. In such cases, *Arnica* given promptly after the birth can be lifesaving.

> *Case 10.12.* After prolonged back labor and hours of pushing in a persistent posterior presentation, a 23-year-old woman gave birth to her second child, a boy, who seemed a little dazed and unresponsive at first, with an Apgar of 7 and a large hematoma on the forehead. After a single dose of *Arnica* 200, he revived in a few seconds. By the time I left a few hours later, the bruising was no longer visible; and he had no further problems afterward.

Carbo vegetabilis, triturate of wood charcoal, carbon, C.

A leading remedy for inadequate oxygenation of the tissues, *Carbo veg.* is especially useful when the baby is mildly or moderately depressed, cyanotic, and slow to respond, but still capable of some unassisted respiratory effort. (See Chapter 6.)

> *Case 10.13.* After a hospital birth complicated by heavy bleeding, and an abortion at 16 weeks, a woman of 34 got pregnant again and was plagued by nausea that persisted into the later months, along with other digestive complaints of long standing, chiefly an intolerance of overeating and rich food. In labor, she dilated uneventfully, but had great difficulty pushing the baby out owing to edema of the vaginal wall, and finally succeeded only after a

midline episiotomy under local anesthesia. Her daughter weighed 8 pounds, but was moderately depressed, with an Apgar of 6, feeble respiration, and a heart rate of 60 per minute. Brisk suctioning and paraspinal stimulation helped a little, but one dose of *Carbo veg.* 200 quickly elicited the loud cry we were waiting for; she pinked up within seconds, and continued to thrive after that. . .

Arsenicum album, triturate of arsenious trioxide, As_2O_3.

In the absence of more distinctive indications for other remedies, *Arsenicum* is the best remedy in my experience for severely depressed babies who appear lifeless, with little or no color or respiratory effort and would otherwise be destined for intensive care. Although infrequently cited in the literature on newborns, it does correspond well to auto-intoxication and complaints incident to the dying process.

> *Case 10.16.* After a healthy first pregnancy disturbed only by a series of vaginal infections, a woman of 24 went into labor and achieved full dilatation with no difficulty; but the baby, who had remained in the vertex presentation all through the pregnancy, had evidently turned since the last prenatal visit and was now clearly breech. Descent and expulsion were easily achieved, with some rotation of the legs to deliver the shoulders; but the boy, though mature and well-formed, lay pale and motionless despite vigorous suctioning, and did not breathe at all. Fortunately, the heartbeat was still strong, and he pinked up immediately after a dose of *Arsenicum album* 200 and a few good cries. . .

Retained Placenta.

Many women cease having contractions for a short time after giving birth; with a normal amount of bleeding, it is unnecessary to try to extract the placenta before they resume. The simplest way to facilitate them is to give the baby to nurse as soon as possible, to signal the pituitary to release enough oxytocin for the final tasks of labor. If the baby is unable to nurse satisfactorily, a spouse, friend, or loved one may be called upon to substitute.

Placental separation often occurs within a few minutes after the birth, and is usually announced by a sudden gush of blood. In most cases, descent into the vagina and expulsion are readily accomplished with a few good contractions, again centered in the fundus or top of the uterus, which hardens perceptibly after each one, but now also remains fairly hard in between.

Homeopathic remedies can be as helpful in this third stage of labor as before, both to stimulate more efficient contractions and to promote hemostasis after the placenta is out. . .

Pulsatilla.

Prescribed on the basis of its general features, as always, *Pulsatilla* fits patients with the typical vasomotor instability and improvement from open air, drinking fluids, and simple affection and loving care. (See Chapter 4.)

> *Case 10.17.* After a successful home birth and a miscarriage, a 29-year-old woman completed her third pregnancy without any health difficulties to speak of. The labor was very short, and she gave birth to a son easily, with no tears; but the placenta stubbornly refused to come out. One dose of *Pulsatilla* 30 enabled me to lift it out with a little fundal pressure. Bleeding was insignificant, and she had no further problems.

Sepia.

While classically associated with bearing-down sensations and other general characteristics, *Sepia* is also the remedy I've used the most for retained placenta in the absence of other distinctive or guiding symptoms for other remedies. (See Chapter 4.)

> *Case 10.18.* After an ectopic pregnancy, a woman of 31 was in good health for her second one, except for some brown spotting in the early months that *Kali carb.* and *Sepia* took care of. At term, her membranes ruptured, and she soon went into labor and gave birth to a son; but after separating normally, the placenta wouldn't come out. *Pulsatilla* 10M elicited strong contractions, but still the placenta wouldn't budge, until I gave her *Sepia* 10M, when it slid out easily, with no resistance. . .

Postpartum Bleeding.

Excessive postpartum bleeding is usually passive and insidious, due to uterine hypotonicity, and may be difficult to recognize in the home setting until a great deal of blood has been lost, since even a normal amount (400-500 cc.) can elicit reflex faintness and low blood pressure at first indistinguishable from more serious forms of shock or circulatory collapse. A retained placenta or placental fragments may also interfere with hemostasis and thus promote bleeding.

In any case, the remedy indicated by the totality of symptoms will usually be effective, and may also suggest possible contributing factors, such as dysfunctional labor, uterine atony, traumatic birth, or a pre-existing bleeding tendency. Naturally, in serious or advanced cases, manual or surgical removal of the placenta, blood transfusion, and other emergency measures may also be required. . .

Cimicifuga.

The chief indications for this remedy include dystonic uterine contractions, accompanied by fears, negativism, or dejection; grimaces or choreiform movements; and headaches, neuralgias, and joint pains. It should be considered when a bizarre alternation or freaky, random jumble of symptoms evoke a sense of physical, mental, and emotional fragmentation that feels alarming, not least to the patient herself. (See Chapter 3.)

> *Case 10.22.* After a difficult first pregnancy hampered by endless doubts and complaints, a 28-year-old woman finally went into labor. At the peak of the first stage and again in the second, her old defeatism came back in a big way, but resolved each time with the help of *Cimicifuga* 200. The birth of her nine-pound son and massive placenta were followed by a substantial amount of thin, liquid blood, which slowed to a trickle after *China* 200. Once her pulse and blood pressure had stabilized, I suggested *Cimicifuga* 200, up to 4 times a day as needed, and she reported minimal bleeding and discomfort, with no further emotional difficulties. . .

Arnica.

Arnica will often be the remedy of choice for excessive bleeding following an precipitate or traumatic birth, prolonged or difficult pushing, an unusually large baby, shoulder dystocia, difficult forceps extraction, or simple bruising, soreness, and depression of normal hemostatic reflexes:

> *Case 10.23.* Following a successful hospital birth, a woman of 37 opted for a home birth the next time, and went into labor and delivered so fast that I barely made it in time. A tiny laceration was repaired, but she continued to

bleed rather heavily. I gave Arnica 30 q 2 hours for 4 doses, and q.i.d for 2 days after that, with excellent results: the bleeding quickly subsided, and she had no further problems.

Sabina, tincture of the fresh, young branch tops, *Juniperus sabina,* the savin tree.

One of the leading remedies for postpartum bleeding, *Sabina* is especially useful in heavily-built patients with a florid complexion, flushing of the face, and intolerance of heat. The bleeding is typically forceful and gushing, with bright-red blood and dark clots, and many patients complain of girdle-like pains from sacrum to pubis in the process of expelling them. Retained placenta or after-pains may also complicate the picture.

Sabina is also useful in late bleeding or hemorrhage a week or more after the birth, and for subinvolution or bleeding that continues until the time of the 6-week visit, in the absence of specific indications for other remedies. (See Chapter 8.)

> *Case 10.24.* A 22-year-old woman gave birth to a 6-pound baby girl, her first child, after a short, easy labor, with both her mother and husband in loving attendance. The placenta came out easily, even before the cord was cut, and appeared intact; but she bled quite heavily afterwards, and 2 doses of *Sabina* 30 were needed to stabilize her blood pressure and reduce the flow to more manageable levels. When the fundus remained soft despite my efforts to massage it, even after *China* 200, I emptied the uterus manually, removed several large clots and membranous fragments, and was finally able to leave her with *Sabina* 30 q 3 hours. From then on, she made a speedy recovery and had no further problems.

China, tincture of the dried bark, *Cinchona officinalis,* quinine bark.

The botanical source of quinine, and the object of Hahnemann's first proving, from which homeopathy was originally developed, *China* was then and remains even today a splendid remedy for the treatment of malaria and other intermittent fevers with chills, bone aches, dizziness, and sweating.

In homeopathy it is also invaluable for passive uterine bleeding secondary to muscular fatigue and general exhaustion , with persistent oozing of dark, thin, or even watery blood. In such cases, the leading indications are much the same shock-like symptoms as would be expected from excessive blood loss: faintness, thirst, and extreme chilliness, with nervous shivering and relief from warmth in any form. Other confirmatory symptoms may include gassy abdominal distention, headache, neuralgia, and after-pains, with heightened sensitivity to drafts, touch, noise, or other external stimulation.

China is also unequalled as a restorative later in the postpartum period for persistent weakness or exhaustion following excessive loss of blood, and more generally for any ailments traceable to loss of other body fluids as well, such as prolonged nursing or diarrhea and gastroenteritis with dehydration. (See Chapter 8.)

> *Case 10.25.* Despite a history of chronic fatigue and considerable anxiety about her health, a 25-year-old woman remained quite healthy throughout her first pregnancy, with help from *Pulsatilla* and a good deal of reassurance. After a labor that seemed in retrospect almost too easy, she gave birth to a seven-pound daughter, followed by a hugely oversized placenta and large volumes of dark, watery blood that poured out of her as if from a faucet. *China* 200 all but stopped the flow within a few seconds, but she needed several more doses before I could safely leave, with her blood pressure and pulse hovering around 90/60 and 120 per minute for several hours. On nothing but iron supplements for a month, she recovered quickly, with no problems or sequelæ; and her energy returned to normal levels well before the time of her 6-week visit. . .

From Chapter 11, "The Newborn Period."

After-Pains.

Under hormonal stimulation, and especially in response to nursing, the postpartum uterus continues to contract down on itself for many days, maintaining hemostasis and gradually reverting to its non-pregnant size. Usually painless, these contractions can be assessed using the same standards as for labor, the more painful and dysfunctional varieties being likewise felt primarily in the lower segment and often associated with excessive bleeding as well. The appropriate remedies and indications are also much the same as for dysfunctional labor and postpartum bleeding (See Chapter 10) . . .

Cimicifuga.

An important remedy for after-pains, *Cimicifuga* has violent spasms and neuralgias felt low in the pelvis and often unstable, darting about or alternating with other symptoms, such as insane fears, dejection, or coarse involuntary movements, in a manner evocative of physical and mental fragmentation. (See Chapter 3.)

> *Case 11.1.* A 23-year-old woman became pregnant two years after an abortion that was followed by excessive bleeding and a pelvic infection, an experience so unpleasant that the thought of repeating it made her violently dizzy and nauseated with guilt and self-reproach. In excellent health until the final weeks, as the birth drew near she began complaining of fatigue, restless sleep, and scary dreams in which she would be forced to endure various penitential ordeals for the baby to survive unharmed. *Pulsatilla* 1M was wonderfully soothing to her, and she gave birth to a fine son after a short, easy labor, with no bleeding or tears. Later that day she phoned because of severe after-pains that evoked many of the feelings she remembered from the abortion, and here *Cimicifuga* 200 was splendidly effective, although it had to be repeated several times in the next few days. An episode of painful uterine bleeding and clotting one month later stopped almost immediately after taking the same remedy, and she had no further difficulties. . .

Paralysis or Prolapse of the Rectum and Bladder.

Often foreshadowed by a family history or tendencies already evident in the past, excessive stretching or tearing of the suspensory ligaments of the pelvis during the birth can result in actual prolapse or retroversion of the uterus. Injury or surgical trauma to the supporting tissues of the bladder or rectum can similarly lead to prolapse of the rectum through the anal opening, paralysis of the bladder or rectum, or cystocele and/ or rectocele with sagging of the bladder or rectum and prolapse into the vaginal vault. Although surgical repair may be helpful when necessary, many will correct themselves spontaneously or can be greatly relieved with homeopathy if recognized and treated early enough.

Sepia.

The first remedy to be thought of for abnormal heaviness or dragging, pulling, or bearing-down sensations in the pelvic organs, *Sepia* is unequalled in the treatment of uterine prolapse or retroversion, and in many other postpartum complaints as well. Other typical features, like irritability with loved ones, wanting to be left alone, nausea better from eating something, and a strong need for physical exercise, will help to confirm the selection. (See Chapter 4.)

> *Case 11.2.* After a home birth with late postpartum bleeding that stopped promptly after *Caulophyllum* 200, a woman of 29 became pregnant again, and once more enjoyed excellent health from the beginning. Although greatly annoyed by periodontal disease, heartburn, and overheating in the final months, she responded beautifully to *Sulphur* 10M, and her labor was fast and easy, like the first. The next day she called back distraught because of "an enormous weight" that proved to be the uterus protruding out of the vagina and felt even worse when she urinated. After manual repositioning, I gave her *Sepia* 200, 3 doses in 24 hours, and by then the prolapse had corrected itself without mechanical support and did not recur. The rest of her postpartum course was uneventful. . .

Opium, tincture of the gum, *Papaver somniferum,* opium poppy.

One of the great medicines of human history, opium is a potent narcotic analgesic rivalled only by its own alkaloids, morphine and codeine; by semi-synthetic derivatives, like heroin and dilaudid; and by wholly synthetic analogues, mainly Demerol and methadone, all of which act on special receptors for opiate-like "endorphins" produced in the brain itself. Homeopathic *Opium* is useful for ailments associated with painlessness, stupor, and coma, and also for shock and paralysis of the urinary bladder and/or intestines following Caesarean section, hysterectomy, or other major surgery under general anesthesia. (See Chapter 10.)

> *Case 11.3.* Three weeks after a seemingly normal hospital birth in another town, a woman of 32 developed severe abdominal pain, and a friend of hers prevailed on me to see her at home because she was "too sick to move." On entering the house, I was greeted by the stench of a massive pelvic infection emanating from behind the closed door of her bedroom over 30 feet away. With a fever of 102° and a pulse of 120 per minute, the patient lay close to death, her abdomen rigid and immobile, and her sensorium clouded and dreamlike.
>
> Giving her a dose of *Pyrogenium* 200, I sent her to the hospital by ambulance, and she underwent an emergency hysterectomy that cost her both tubes and ovaries as well as her uterus; but she did amazingly well until the third day post-op, when Intensive Care reported a urinary output of only 200 cc. in

the past twelve hours. Even on massive doses of Demerol, she was alert and apprehensive when I saw her, perhaps realizing only then how close to death she had been. I gave her one dose of *Opium* 200, and 2 hours later she had diuresed over 600 cc. Her output remained normal thereafter, and she made an excellent recovery.

Ruta, tincture of whole fresh plant, *Ruta graveolens,* rue.

Most commonly used in first aid for sprains, bone bruises, and injuries to the periosteum and other connective tissues, *Ruta* is also excellent for prolapse of the rectum following childbirth, which often corrects itself even without remedies but will do so much more quickly with their help:

> *Case 11.4.* After some early nausea, a woman of 26 was disabled for much of her first pregnancy by her old back pain, a stretching or pulling sensation that was aggravated by sitting, relieved by hot baths, and as her labor approached was as bad as it had ever been. At home with only her husband and several close friends in attendance, she had a remarkably short and easy labor, and gave birth to a 7-pound son without any difficulty; but by the next day they called me for the first time because her rectum was protruding from the anal canal by an inch or two. *Ruta* 200 was superbly effective for this extremely distressing situation; the prolapse corrected itself completely within a day and a half, and her back improved considerably as well.

Phlebitis.

Inflammation of the deep veins of the thigh and calf is not uncommon in the hospital, especially after C-section, and also occurs sporadically at home, but is usually preventable by early ambulation as soon as possible after the birth. Beginning as soreness and purplish swelling along the track of the affected veins, phlebitis may progress to swelling and pain of the entire area, with palpable or visible clots, and often fever, chills, and malaise as well. Early treatment is imperative, because of the risk of acute pulmonary embolism and chronic venous insufficiency. . .

Hamamelis, tincture of the stems and twigs, *Hamamelis virginica,* witch hazel.

Unsurpassed for simple injury or traumatism to the veins from childbirth or any other cause, *Hamamelis* is the remedy of choice when phlebitis appears imminent or threatening, or there are no clear or distinctive indications for other remedies.

> *Case 11.5.* A 32-year-old woman finished her second pregnancy in good shape after a period of depression early on that was helped a lot by *Natrum mur.* and *Sepia.* The labor was more difficult than either of us expected, especially the last two hours of strenuous pushing, for which she was unprepared and out of condition. Within 48 hours she developed a fever of 101.6° with chills, sweats, and tenderness of the left femoral vein, by then clearly visible and palpable as a thick blue cord extending halfway down her thigh. This ominous situation was quickly defused with *Hamamelis* 200, the inflammation subsiding after the first dose; within 12 hours she was fully recovered, with no recurrences or sequelæ, and the remainder of her postpartum course was uneventful.

Postpartum Infection.

Originally a disease of poor sanitation and still an important cause of maternal deaths in the third world, postpartum infection in the US today is overwhelmingly a disease of hospitals, where the routine use of potent antibiotics selectively breeds highly-resistant organisms. In healthy and well-nourished home-birth populations, major infections are relatively rare, provided the midwife is careful not to introduce unfriendly foreign bacteria into the vagina. Other risk factors include retained placental fragments, difficult or traumatic birth, poor nutrition and personal hygiene, and pre-existing illness with a weakened immune system.

Bryonia, tincture of the root before flowering, *Bryonia alba,* wild hops.

A leading remedy for appendicitis, *Bryonia i*s invaluable in all forms of peritoneal infection, with pain aggravated by the least movement, mild delirium or stupor, thirst, and similar aches and pains elsewhere in the bones, muscles, and joints. (See Chapter 6.)

> *Case 11.6.* After a successful home birth, a woman of 28 became pregnant again with a Lippes loop still in place that I was unable to remove. Though bothered by diarrhea, leg cramps, and varicose veins for much of her pregnancy, she improved with *Calcarea carb.* and remained generally healthy otherwise. After a short, easy labor, she produced a strapping nine-pound daughter with no problems of any kind, but the IUD was still nowhere to be found.

47

Two weeks later, after a steak dinner, she developed a burning pain in the stomach, followed by weakness, muscle aches, and severe pain lower in the abdomen. When I saw her the next day, the pain was sharply localized to the right lower quadrant over McBurney's point, felt worse from a deep breath or the slightest movement, and was accompanied by a fever of 101.2°, chills, and a pulse of 120 per minute. The painful area was exquisitely tender, but there was no guarding or rigidity elsewhere. After a few doses of *Bryonia* 200, this whole appendicitis-like illness evaporated in less than 36 hours. Her IUD was later found embedded deep within the uterine wall and had to be removed surgically.

Pyrogenium, tincture of purulent material from an abscess or rotting meat, pus.

An epitome of homeopathic philosophy, *Pyrogenium* is a by-product of illness that has been tamed by dilution and succussion into a harmless and useful medicinal agent. Derived from ordinary pus, it is indispensable in the treatment of severe or fulminant infections like peritonitis, endocarditis, or septicemia, particularly in immunocompromised patients at the mercy of their own resident bacteria or fungi, when antibiotics alone may be insufficient.

Above all, it is unrivalled in its ability to prevent or reverse incipient or threatening postpartum infections associated with retained decidual or placental fragments. If the lochia turns foul or the woman develops fever and chills a few days after giving birth, *Pyrogenium* 200 will often abort the illness before more ominous symptoms appear, and most patients will recover completely without complications or sequelae requiring more drastic measures.

In more advanced cases, its specific indications include putrid or cadaverous odors, depressed sensorium, generalized aching and soreness, and paradoxical slow-ing of the pulse as the fever rises, and acceleration as the fever subsides.

Case 11.7. After an unhealthy first pregnancy complicated by malnutrition, a 24-year-old woman gave birth to an undersized baby that required *Carbo veg.* 200 and some resuscitation. She also bled a fair amount afterwards. Three nights later she telephoned to report fever, chills, and violent cramps in the lower abdomen extending into the thigh. On examination the temperature was 101.4°, the pulse 132 per minute, and there was marked tenderness over the left ovary and lower abdomen generally, with guarding and rebound. The lochia was unremarkable, but she was nauseated and unusually thirsty. My treatment consisted of *Pyrogenium* 200 four times daily and a solemn promise to drag her to the hospital if she got any worse. She slept peacefully for the rest of the night, and awoke the next morning drenched in sweat but with no fever, chills, or thirst to speak of, and very little pain. By that evening, the illness was over, and she nursed her baby for many months without further difficulties. . .

Depression and Emotional Difficulties.

In the newborn period, hormonal mechanisms related to nursing and involution can easily magnify the normal stress of adjusting to a new baby, a task for which the classic nuclear family may also lack adequate resources. In any case, many of the emotional issues that were manifest during the pregnancy may reappear with added poignancy after the birth, and many of the remedies and their indications are likewise similar to those already described (See Chapter 8). . .

Ignatia, tincture of the seeds, *Ignatia amara,* St. Ignatius' bean.

This remedy is often indicated in acute situations colored by grief, sorrow, or disappointment, resulting in emotionally or anatomically "impossible" or contradictory symptoms. Other signs of an overly sensitive or irritable nervous system should also be present, such as insomnia, craving for or intolerance of drugs and stimulants, or simple "nervousness:"

Case 11.9. A married woman of 19 conceived as soon as she stopped taking her birth-control pills, became severely nauseated, and was greatly relieved by stopping all coffee, alcohol, and tobacco, all of which she had used regularly for several years. Although still grieving over her parents' divorce four years earlier, she remained in good health throughout the pregnancy, worked right up to the end, and gave birth to an 8-pound daughter without any difficulty. At 10 days of age, however, the baby had already lost a pound and a half and appeared acutely dehydrated, nursing well at first, but screaming and pulling away after a few seconds, while the mother although clearly unnerved by what was happening, ate very little and seemed almost eerily calm and serene while she tried in vain to nurse. Fortunately, the baby began to thrive on bottle feedings, which the mother likewise accepted with the same apparent nonchalance as before. Because of all these discrepancies, I gave her a round of *Ignatia* 200, 3 doses in 24 hours, and to my great amazement she regained her appetite within a week, the baby began gaining weight on nothing but her breast milk, and in the months that followed they both did well without needing any remedies or further assistance of any kind. . .

Jaundice.

Owing to immaturity of the liver, many healthy infants become jaundiced for a few days, usually beginning around the third day of life. Although this so-called "physiologic" jaundice is self-limiting and in no way injurious, the serum bilirubin not infrequently reaches 15 mg. per 100 ml., a level also seen in cases of Rh or ABO incompatibility. Bruising from a difficult or traumatic birth may further intensify the jaundice and cause it to appear sooner.

In the case of blood-group incompatibility, which may require intensive light therapy and exchange transfusion for the worst cases, the jaundice usually appears earlier, often at birth, and reaches a higher peak level within 24 to 36 hours, while the baby may appear sickly and be unable to nurse, the sensitized peripheral blood contains antibodies to Rh, ABO, or other red-cell antigens, and evidence of increased red-cell destruction, chiefly a high reticulocyte count.

Physiologic jaundice, on the other hand, is not dangerous and requires no treatment unless it persists or is unusually intense. Even in such cases, frequent nursing and additional hydration will help flush out the bilirubin quite effectively. Weather permitting, covering the baby's eyes and exposing the skin to direct sunlight for four 20-minute periods daily is a simple and effective alternative to ultraviolet phototherapy in the hospital, while on overcast days a blue incandescent bulb or "grow light" serves almost as well. Homeopathic remedies are also very helpful.

Natrum sulphuricum, triturate of the salt, sodium sulfate, Na_2SO_4.

An important remedy for asthma, allergies, and other ailments that are intensified in hot, humid weather, *Natrum sulph.* is often used empirically in the absence of more specific indications for the treatment of physiologic or hemolytic jaundice in the newborn.

Case 11.18. In a difficult first labor that I was unable to help much with remedies, a woman of 24 made rapid progress in the hospital with Pitocin in IV drip, the birth following with considerable force. The baby was born in good condition, with no distress and perfect Apgar scores, but turned quite yellow after 12 hours, with a bilirubin of 5 mg. per 100 ml. Since he was already nursing and gaining weight, we were content to observe him. On the third day, the bilirubin reached 14 mg., so I gave him a round of *Natrum sulph.* 200, three doses in 24 hours, the jaundice faded rapidly, and he continued to thrive. . .

Colic and Milk Intolerance.

More prevalent in bottle-fed babies, colic or painful intestinal cramping typically occurs within an hour after feeding and tends to subside as the digestive tract matures, ordinarily around three months of age. Colic is also seen in babies who nurse, many of whom are cured or improve dramatically when the mother eliminates milk and other dairy products from her diet; others will not be benefited, or may tolerate cow's milk without difficulty. Rarely an infant may become sensitized to its own mother's milk and need to be fed with formula for a few days or nursed by someone else.

In addition to a trial of eliminating dairy from the mother's diet, homeopathic remedies are often wonderfully effective in the treatment of infantile colic, with none of the drowsiness, sedation, and other side effects of pharmaceutical drugs.

Chamomilla.

A leading remedy for colic or periodic irritable crying in the early months, *Chamomilla* comes closest to the routine experience of most colicky babies that their parents would dearly love to forget. At the center of it is simple intolerance of pain in the form of anger, outrage, or extreme irritability, which can themselves aggravate and prolong other associated complaints.

Typically red-faced and infuriated by pain, the child needing *Chamomilla* may kick and scream loudly, or in some cases wiggle, squirm, and pull away from the breast even while nursing; although comforted somewhat by being carried about or taken for a ride in the car, they are apt to resume just as forcefully when put down to sleep or rest. Often accompanied by flatulence or noisy commotion in the bowels, the stools range from loose and greenish to offensive diarrhea. Yet apart from and in between these episodes, many colicky babies are notoriously healthy and happy otherwise, nursing well and gaining weight normally. (See Chapter 5.)

> *Case 11.20.* A woman of 32 had her first baby in the hospital with no trouble, but the boy developed colic at about 4 weeks of age. With a history of lactose intolerance herself, the mother eliminated all dairy from her diet, and the baby did improve a lot; but a week later he had his worst attack so far and had since been prone to hours of frenzied crying every evening after nursing. Quite happy and prosperous at other times, he would suddenly yell and scream inconsolably unless carried about by his mother, while his intestines often contributed noisy protests of their own. For some unaccountable reason, his symptoms were especially severe in windy and stormy weather. I gave him a round of *Chamomilla* 1M, plus *Chamomilla* 30C as needed, and within a week his episodes were much shorter and milder, except for one that was very brief but memorably intense after his mother treated herself to a big bowl of ice cream. But this attack proved to be his last; by 8 weeks of age he was completely free of colic and continued to thrive and develop normally. . .

Colocynthis, tincture of the fruit pulp, *Cucumis colocynthis,* bitter cucumber.

Much as in the adult type, infantile colic that is relieved by *Colocynth.* usually presents as violent cramping that causes the child to double over or pull the knees up, and is relieved somewhat by heat, but especially by hard pressure. In many cases, it is helpful for the parents to lay the baby face down across their knees and rub or massage firmly. (See Chapter 6.)

> *Case 11.22.* A woman of 27 had her second baby at home after a short labor with no complications. By 3 weeks of age, the girl was colicky almost every evening, when she would scream and cry, throwing arms and legs out in all directions and loudly passing gas while straining at stool. Being rubbed hard and having a bowel movement were her sole relief, but she continued to nurse well and gain weight. After a few doses of *Colocynth.* 30, her complaints were gone by their 6-week visit and didn't return. . .

Nux Vomica.

Often overlooked in colic, *Nux vomica* should always be considered whenever constipation and straining at stool are prominent features, and the symptoms are relieved dramatically after a bowel movement.

Confirmatory symptoms, such as nervous overstimulation, wakefulness, irritability, startling, and hypersensitivity to noise and bright light, will usually be present as well. (See Chapter 6.)

> *Case 11.24.* After 7 years of trying, a woman of 27 finally conceived and had a home birth with no trouble. Although the girl was an avid nurser, in the first two weeks she developed abdominal pain and severe constipation, appeased somewhat by being carried about, but always associated with flatulence and straining at stool. Although *Chamomilla* 200 was helpful for a time, before long her constipation returned and continued to get worse, with the baby grunting mightily while attempting to pass a stool and breaking into a joyful smile whenever she succeeded. The mother also reported that she startled easily from noise and bright light. *Nux vomica* 200 was given, and within a week the child was well. . .

Lactation and Nursing.

If the woman is not nursing, or the baby dies or is given up for adoption, two remedies are well known for helping women to dry up the milk and minimize the pain and discomfort of engorgement, without the risk of side effects from hormonal suppression.

Pulsatilla.

With a special affinity for the hormonal regulation of nursing, Pulsatilla is the first remedy to think of, either to dry up the milk when necessary, to increase milk production when it is deficient, or to restore it when it has been suppressed by a breast infection. When indicated by the totality of symptoms, it is also splendid for swollen and tender breasts in the non-pregnant state, especially before the menstrual period.

If the woman is not planning to nurse, *Pulsatilla* may be given preventively and more or less routinely at the time of the birth, without waiting for more specific indications; it may also be given later as needed for the pain and discomfort of engorgement and letdown. (See Chapter 4.)

> *Case 11.25.* A single woman of 25 became pregnant and decided to put the baby up for adoption. The pregnancy and birth were healthy and trouble-free, but even with a hormone injection she remained painfully engorged on the fifth postpartum day. After a few doses of *Pulsatilla* 30, the pain and swelling were largely gone by the next morning, eliminating the need for more hormones or strapping. . .

When *Pulsatilla* has been tried without success, *Lac caninum,* made from bitches' milk, is similarly useful in preventing or minimizing the pain of engorgement, and may also be used semi-routinely without waiting for more specific indications. Like *Pulsatilla,* it is equally valuable for augmenting or restoring the milk.

Cracked and Sore Nipples.

Unequalled in their power to heal simple cuts and abrasions, preparations of *Calendula* -- marigold flowers -- should be included in routine breast care and hygiene before and after the birth, to help condition and toughen the nipples and areolae in preparation for nursing. Along with good nutrition, massaging the nipples regularly with *Calendula* lotion, cream, or ointment will significantly reduce the incidence and severity of cracks and soreness throughout the nursing period, and thus enhance the nursing experience as a whole.

When cracks and soreness actually develop, *Castor equi,* prepared from the rudimentary thumbnail of the horse, is reputed to be virtually specific for these complaints, particularly in nursing women, and is highly touted as healing them even in advanced or "hopeless" cases. Unfortunately, having learned of it only recently, I cannot yet report on it from my own experience. . .

Silica, triturate of silicon dioxide, flintstone or sand, SiO_2.

An important constituent of the earth's crust, and capable of deep, prolonged action, *Silica* is especially useful in slow processes, like promoting the extrusion of foreign bodies and the healing of fissures, abscesses, granulomas, fistulas, and other forms of chronic suppuration. With its cystic glands and elaborate duct system, in which unused, inspissated, or soured milk readily attracts the bacteria living nearby, the lactating breast can be an excellent culture medium for the slow ulcerative and suppurative processes that call for *Silica.*

In the early weeks of nursing, if the nipples are very sore and crack easily, *Silica* 6C may be given q.i.d. as needed to toughen them. When indicated, it is also an excellent remedy for the deeper cracks, lumps, and abscesses that can develop later. while its detailed chronic symptom-picture would far exceed the scope of this book, *Silica* can also be prescribed with confidence for those unforgettably sharp, splinter-like pains in the nipple when the child nurses, which often extend through the breast to the shoulder. In general, it is a chilly remedy, and patients needing it are often intolerant of and adversely affected by cold in any form.

> *Case 11.26.* After 3 miscarriages, a 36-year-old woman finally had her second child at home, worrying us a bit with slow labor and some meconium-stained amniotic fluid, but with normal fetal heart tones throughout. At her one-week visit, she complained of sharp, needle-like pains in her right nipple when the baby started to nurse that she felt all the way to the shoulder. Although they would lessen somewhat as the feeding continued, they were so intense that she would have to clench her teeth or pull away, and dreaded the sound of her own child each time he cried out for her. The breast nevertheless yielded an abundance of milk, with no lumps or fissures, and the nipple itself appeared normal except for a tiny spot of grayish matter covering the opening that we couldn't figure out how to remove. I gave her a round of *Silica* 200, followed by the 6C as needed; and about a week later she reported that the pain had first lessened for a few days, then became intolerable again during a feeding, and finally ended for good when the nipple discharged a ribbon of grayish, caseous material smelling like old ear-wax. The nursing was painless and trouble-free after that, and she remained in good health after that.

Breast Infections.

When one or more milk ducts are blocked by dried milk, the lactating breast can become vulnerable to colonization and superinfection by pus-forming organisms from the skin. The broad term "breast infection" covers a whole spectrum of clinical responses, ranging from acute mastitis with high fever to more localized chronic or relapsing phenomena, like abscesses, lumps, and fissures.

These events are best prevented by good nutrition, to boost the immune system and maintain the normal skin flora in healthy balance. A second precaution is to encourage the baby to empty both breasts at every feeding, to pump and save whatever remains, and thus not allow unused milk to accumulate, sour, and harden in the duct system.

Homeopathic remedies are useful at every stage, not only for treatment of acute mastitis, breast abscess, and their chronic sequelæ, but also preventively, when these problems appear imminent or threatening.

Belladonna, tincture of whole flowering plant, *Atropa belladonna,* deadly nightshade.

A leading remedy for acute mastitis, *Belladonna* is especially useful when a nursing mother suddenly develops a high fever, with violent throbbing or bursting pains in the breast and other signs of acute inflammation. The affected area is acutely swollen, bright-red or even shiny in appearance, and exquisitely tender and sensitive to the slightest jar, such as someone sitting down next to her on the bed. A throbbing or bursting headache, wild-eyed expression, extreme sensitivity to light and noise, and other typical features may also be present. (See Chapter 5.)

> *Case 11.28.* A woman of 25 had her second child at home after a surprisingly difficult labor, but everything went well until 4 months later, when she developed a fever of 104°, and her left breast felt "as if hit with a baseball bat" whenever she tried to move her arm or roll over. Originating in the lower half of the breast, the pain was worse from the least movement of any kind, and made her want to be left alone; but *Bryonia* 30 was of no value. By the next day, she had a pounding headache, and for the baby even to touch the breast made her "crazy." At this point, she got *Belladonna* 30 instead, and by the next morning there was no fever or sign of infection, and she remained in good health for the remainder of her nursing period.

Bryonia.

The other great remedy for acute mastitis, *Bryonia* is especially suitable when the illness develops a bit more slowly and, in spite of the soreness, the patient may lie on the painful side to shield the breast from the slightest movement. Other typical keynotes, such as extreme thirst, gruff or irritable mood, dazed sensorium, and aversion to sensory or mental stimulation of any kind, are also likely to be present.

> *Case 11.29.* After a difficult first pregnancy, a 21-year-old woman had a strong labor and successful home birth, with no complications except a fever and chills ten days later that subsided almost immediately after *Pyrogenium* 200. All went well until shortly after her 6-week visit, when her right breast became increasingly sore and tender to the touch, and she developed an unusual thirst and a fever that went up slowly during the day and reached 102° by evening. Because her breast hurt most with every step and from the slightest movement, she was forced to hold herself rigidly in place and to wear a tight

bra for support. After a few doses of *Bryonia* 30, her illness subsided over the next 36 hours and never came back.

Phytolacca, tincture of the ripe berries, *Phytolacca decandra,* poke root.

Widely praised in the herbal literature for the treatment of breast cancer, in homeopathy *Phytolacca* is used for a wide variety of breast ailments, and for tumors, abscesses, and inflammations of other lymphatic and glandular structures as well, particularly the throat and tonsils.

In my experience, at least three-fourths of my acute mastitis patients with high fever have benefited substantially from either *Belladonna* or *Bryonia,* or both; and almost that many recovered completely without requiring other remedies. *Phytolacca* has no peer in healing the assorted lumps, pains, and congestions that can easily lead to acute infection if not corrected, or are left over after the acute remedies have done their work. The breast that needs *Phytolacca* feels lumpy, hard, and tender in spots, and its pains frequently wander to other areas of the breast, elsewhere in the chest, or other parts of the body.

> *Case 11.30.* With a history of recurrent mastitis after each one of her previous births, a woman of 33 had her fifth child at home after a short labor with no problems of any kind. In less than 3 weeks, as if right on cue, she developed a fever of 102°, pain in the left breast from the least movement, and a reduction in the milk supply on that side. With *Bryonia* 30, the acute infection subsided quickly, but her milk production continued to dwindle and wasn't fully restored until *Pulsatilla* 30 was given q.i.d. for a whole week.
>
> Although her breasts remained lumpy and sore afterward, as they had throughout her extensive nursing career, she neglected to come back until her next acute episode a year later, this time with a raging fever, a hard, red lump in her left breast after a day in the hot sun, and the sensation that her breast was "burning up." Within a few hours after *Belladonna* 30, her fever spiked to 105.6°, and then plummeted sharply as she awoke from an out-of-body experience; but she continued to have a low fever with much sweating, and a big lump that was sore to the touch and reminded her of many others she had endured in the past. At this point I gave her Phytolacca 30, and the lump gradually became smaller and finally disappeared in 4 days, after which she was able to continue nursing without any further problems.

Silica.

In addition to its many uses for sore and cracked nipples, *Silia* when indicated can be valuable for promoting healing of old lumps, abscesses, or draining sinuses left over from chronic or recurrent mastitis that never fully resolved. In such cases, other typical keynotes such as caseous discharges, extreme chilliness, and sensitivity to cold air and drafts will ordinarily be present.

> *Case 11.32.* Late in her second pregnancy, a 33-year-old woman consulted me for painful lumps in her right breast. *Phytolacca* 30 was briefly helpful; but by 33 weeks both breasts were huge and pendulous, and the right one was a mass of hard, tender nodules, some of which had opened and were discharging fluid that reminded me of cream of tomato soup. Nevertheless, she managed to have a successful home birth with a local midwife, and began to nurse in spite of dire warnings from two specialists that these galactoceles would persist and become chronically infected until she weaned the baby. At this point the drainage was either yellow or milky, and she was complaining of frequent, sharp, needle-like pains here and there, while number of older lesions had developed indurated areas resembling scar tissue. After two rounds of *Silica* 30, one week apart, the cysts grew smaller and less painful, and finally they stopped draining. Best of all, she was able to continue nursing until she conceived again a year later; and this time her breasts looked and felt fine, and functioned normally for the whole period of her nursing.

Some Thoughts on the Beginnings of Life*

I want to make some basic observations about the beginning and end points of the gestational process, i.e., after conception, when the fertilized ovum implants within the mother's womb, and during labor and birth, when the new baby sets out on its career in the world at large.

Nausea of Pregnancy.

Typically dismissed as a simple hormone imbalance, this commonest of first-trimester complaints bears further investigation. My interest in it was piqued by the close correspondence between the symptom-picture of *Sepia,* the leading remedy for nausea in my home-birth practice, and what is known about the biology of implantation, which also adds a new dimension to the symptom itself. In particular, the embryo contains many foreign antigens, and the placenta literally invades and digests the uterine wall as it grows, which means that every woman who conceives must learn to overcome, ignore, or at least mitigate the basic programming of her immune system, to destroy and expel all foreign elements, and more generally to subordinate her personal needs and wants to those of the pregnancy, the child, the family, and indeed the species as a whole, an accommodation seldom achieved without some resistance. In this way I began to rethink nausea and vomiting as symptoms of normal placentation, and ultimately to follow the broader themes underlying them as they continue to develop later in pregnancy and in extrauterine life as well. Although still admittedly speculative, this embryological perspective could also explain why nausea recurs so often in the first trimester, even after successful treatment with remedies, as in the following typical case:

> A devoutly Catholic woman of 22 became pregnant on her honeymoon. With birth control and abortion out of the question for her, she was still far from eager to be a mother so soon. At six weeks she was intensely nauseated by the

---

* "Some Thoughts on the Beginnings of Life," *Spectrum of Homeopathy* (Germany), Spring 2013.

smell of food, and often vomited before breakfast, but felt better from eating a cracker or light snack. After work she felt carsick on the way home, and vomited when hungry and smelling her dinner. On *Sepia* 30 b.i.d., she was much better in a week; and when her symptoms came back full force at 10 weeks, the remedy acted beautifully once again. She had no further difficulties and gave birth successfully at home.

Sepia's trademark ambivalence may be seen in the character of the nausea, e.g., when intensified by the sight, smell, or thought of the foods usually preferred, and above all, by *not eating,* the classic pattern of "morning sickness," when the patient is repelled by food but feels even worse without it; and also emotionally, as a marked irritability or aversion to friends, loved ones, and indeed the pregnancy itself, whether it seems new and out of character, or an exaggeration of a prior state. In either case, the impression is of an organism confused and at war with itself, groping for a middle path between the extremes of total merging with the pregnancy and outright rejection of it as a foreign body.

To be sure, many other remedies are also useful for nausea, like *Pulsatilla, Nux vomica, Ignatia, Natrum mur., Cocculus, Colchicum, Phosphorus,* and *Ipecacuanha,* depending on the pattern of acute symptoms and the patient's underlying state; but *Sepia* merits special mention because of its peculiar, archetypal signature.

Since a fair number of women experience no nausea at all, my sense is that the symptom is simply one expression of the broader theme of bioenergetic ambivalence, and that this basic developmental issue continues to be important long after the nausea is gone, such that a *Sepia* state often resurfaces during the pregnancy, as well as in the postpartum period and beyond. At the six-week's check, for example, it has no equal in relieving the whole spectrum of typical postpartum complaints, ranging from bleeding, prolapse, backache, hemorrhoids, cystocele, and rectocele, to fatigue, depression, and "burnout," which are almost to be expected, since the modern nuclear family typically lacks sufficient physical and emotional resources to care for babies and small children around the clock without the help of grandparents, friends, and an extensive community support system that often no longer exists.

Dysfunctional Labor.

Although many remedies are useful in managing difficult labor, only *Caulophyllum* and *Cimicifuga* have been shown to produce painful uterine contractions at regular intervals. Introduced into homœopathy from American Indian medicine, both are still used primarily for complaints arising from the female reproductive cycle. With cramping pains suggestive of two common patterns of difficult labor, they provide useful standards against which other possible remedies can be measured, and may reasonably be tried when other more specific indications are lacking.

The muscle fibers of the mammalian uterus have the unique ability to relax isometrically at their contracted length, such that each contraction further reduces the volume of the organ. Centered in the fundus or upper segment, rhythmic contractions of this type accomplish the splendid athletic feats of normal labor: effacing the lower segment, dilating the cervix, and pushing the baby into, through, and out of the vagina. After labor, similar contractions expel the placenta and minimize further blood loss. The muscular work of childbirth thus involves both active and passive components acting in concert: the expulsive contractions of the fundus, and the exquisite suppleness of the lower segment, cervix, and vagina, which must dilate and stretch beyond imagining to receive and accommodate them.

Both *Caulophyllum* and *Cimicifuga* produce rhythmic but highly dysfunctional contractions of an easily recognizable type. Although typically very painful and distressing, they are centered mainly in the *lower* segment, and tend to be sharp or spasmodic in character, brief in duration, and extremely unstable, flitting or darting about here and there, or into the bladder, groins, or thighs. Above all, they fail to dilate the cervix, which remains thick and tightly closed, and to empty the uterus, which relaxes to its former length after each contraction, like any other muscle.

Contractions like these are typical of dysfunctional labor, when the intense pain and exhaustion are often misleading, the flabby tone of the upper segment is easily overlooked, and the vaginal exam reveals so little progress that the attendant feels embarrassed to break the news that the labor is not progressing.

With *Caulophyllum,* the problem is simply a hypotonic uterus, together with generalized weakness and exhaustion, as well as trembling, shivering, and nervous excitement; in these respects, it is very close to *Gelsemium.* In addition to abnormal labor, it is helpful in premature and false labor, after birth or miscarriage, and for retained placenta and hypotonic uterine bleeding. Many people also favor giving the 6C or 12C qd for the last 2-4 weeks of pregnancy to facilitate a speedier and more efficient labor. While it may be helpful in women with a history of such weakness in the past, I have never liked using it routinely in this way, even before the following case:

> A woman of 31 completed her first pregnancy and birth with no trouble until the placenta separated and an hour passed without the slightest contraction or urge to expel it. After 6 drops of *Caulophyllum* Ø, she cried out with painful contractions, her right arm began to shake, and she fell back exhausted into a dreamy, trance-like state -- but still no placenta. With everyone else out of the room, I spoke to her softly in a soothing voice, and the placenta slid out quietly and in one piece as the contractions subsided. Thus ended my experiments with *Caulophyllum* tincture.

While *Cimicifuga* resembles *Caulophyllum* in its dysfunctional contractions, as well as its neuralgias, rheumatic and arthritic complaints, trembling, nervous and emotional agitation, and a pervasive, bewildering changeability, with symptoms traveling from here to there or mutating into one another, its overall flavor and style are completely different, and indeed so distinctive as to be seldom mistaken for any other remedy. In the emotional sphere, there is often a certain moroseness, gloom, or dejection, perhaps indicated by a pessimistic outlook, or a presentiment of failure or misfortune about the pregnancy, the labor, or the parenting to follow, using phrases like "I can't do it," or "I can't go through with it," both of which are easily overlooked in difficult labor, when such sentiments are rarely absent:

> A woman of 28 was sailing through her first labor with no problems, except her oft-repeated conviction that she wouldn't be able to finish it. But with her cervix fully dilated, and the baby's head halfway down the vagina, her labor abruptly came to a complete stop, her oddball prophecy seemingly fulfilled.

With a single dose of *Cimicifuga* 30, the birth followed in a few minutes, as if nothing had happened.

At times the dejection feels almost tangible or palpable to the patient, who may speak of a "black cloud" enveloping her, or convey by her body language that an actual physical presence is meant. In fact, this kind of somatization, or alternation of mental states into physical symptoms and *vice versa,* is another hallmark of the remedy, in all its guises; the black-cloud sensation has been verified repeatedly in headache, depression, and many other situations.

But the patient may also harbor bizarre and disabling fears, often unvoiced and lurking beneath the depressive phenomena, that something terrible is going to happen to her, that she will die or be poisoned by the remedy you are offering her, or go off the deep end and never be the same again. Terrifying memories of a previous birth, miscarriage, or abortion may return to haunt her, but she may reveal little beyond a tangle of disjointed gestures, speech, and actions that spooks everyone around her. In my experience, the *Cimicifuga* state includes and indeed culminates in the threat or actuality of an acute mental breakdown, in which the common threads of experience are shattered into a jumble of fragmented thoughts and feelings, a truly pitiable state, justly to be feared by doctor and patient alike:

A woman of 29 became pregnant for the second time not long after her first ended in a miscarriage. After two episodes of first-trimester bleeding, she grew to term in stable condition, but at 42 weeks was still not in labor. At the prospect of a hospital birth, she admitted being frightened by memories of the miscarriage and D&C, and the premonition that the greater intensity of labor would push her over the edge once and for all. When she appeared at my office a few days later, she was already 6 cm. dilated, but wild-eyed and out of control, her speech fragmentary, her gestures disconnected and woeful. While remaining clinically psychotic the whole time, she progressed well in labor with a few doses of *Cimicifuga* 200, gave birth normally, and made a full recovery afterward.

An alarming and even prophetic fear of insanity, arising from an unbearably painful or terrifying memory of pregnancy, labor, miscarriage, abortion, or menstruation in the past, is thus a genuine keynote and theme of this remedy, repeatedly verified in my practice, and helpful in explaining other symptoms as well. But fear of insanity cuts so deep as to be well-guarded by most patients, and will seldom be volunteered or admitted readily:

> After giving birth to her second child at home, a woman of 28 developed severe, nauseating after-pains, which subsided promptly after a few doses of *Cimicifuga* 30. At six months of age the child developed fulminant acute leukemia and died after weeks of chemotherapy. In her grief the mother told me that she had always felt undeserving of the pregnancy and had frequent premonitions that the child would be taken away. Soon pregnant for the third time, she again gave birth normally, but developed a nasty, disabling arthritis of her right wrist that persisted for weeks, had few distinctive modalities to prescribe on, and didn't respond to the remedies I tried. Although neither of us found the words to talk about it, my own fears and prayers for her new baby led me to *Cimicifuga* 200, after which her wrist cleared up quickly and easily, as from a minor injury of which too much had been made.

* * *

> A woman of 36 consulted me for severe pain in her left ankle that had begun soon after the birth of her daughter by C-section five years earlier. Described as sharp and stabbing, "like a pinched nerve," the pain was connected with her learning of the baby's clubfoot, the mere mention of which evoked strange grimaces and ominous forebodings she couldn't or wouldn't identify. More symptoms uncannily reminiscent of her mother's stroke appeared when the latter was hospitalized and later committed suicide. Upbeat and optimistic as long as she avoided these unpleasant subjects, she became unnerved and disjointed whenever I returned to them. After a brief aggravation, her pains yielded to *Cimicifuga* 10M, as did the fears that rose up in their place. Six years later she phoned to report that she had been in good health ever since, and rarely needed to take the remedy again.

A similarly fragmented quality usually underlies the physical symptoms as well. While just as intense, the pains and other physical complaints of *Caulophyllum* are finely-textured, and tend to follow or change into one another quite easily, in the style of *Pulsatilla*, whereas those of *Cimicifuga* tend to be coarser, involving larger chunks or shards of experience that replace one another more abruptly, in a jumbled or random fashion. Thus a typical labor pain might begin well enough, with good focus and intensity, only to vanish before reaching its peak, or pass off into a disabling obturator neuralgia or sciatica, or alternate with pessimistic or psychotic ideation.

Similarly, although just as excitable as *Caulophyllum,* and as prone to trembling, convulsions, and the like, the involuntary movements of *Cimicifuga* are jerkier, often involving the basal ganglia and extrapyramidal system, as in chorea, athetosis, grimacing, etc. The remedy is also full of headaches and neuralgias, typically darting or lancinating, like "needles pricking" or "electric shocks here and there," which may likewise occur anywhere and change abruptly from one place to another without continuity or warning. Numbness, pain, and bruised soreness may be diffuse or localized to particular bones, muscles, or joints. Physically as well as mentally, the pattern of fragmenting and alternating of large segments of experience abruptly and at random makes the *Cimicifuga* picture not merely unstable, but freaky, both to the patient and to everyone near her. The basic style can be found at any stage of pregnancy, as well as around menstruation and menopause.

Trust the Process.

I have often noticed that well-chosen remedies tend to clarify an obscure or threatening situation, as in the following case:

> A 24-year-old woman had been in good health until 10 weeks into her second pregnancy, when her father died, leaving her in control of the family home and business, and arousing the resentment of her sister, who hadn't spoken to her since. At this point she began complaining of severe headaches that felt as if the top of her head would fly off, and made her dizzy, weak, and disinclined to do much except lying down to rest. Never prone to headaches in the past, she suspected that something was wrong with the baby, and soon noticed "weird" cramps low in the pelvis that would come and go quickly or alternate from side to side. With a round of *Cimicifuga* 200, and the 12C q2h as needed, she did indeed miscarry a week later, just as she had foreseen, but without needing a D&C or any other complications; and within 4 months she was pregnant again, this time carrying it through with ease and giving birth successfully at home.

Here is another example, this one dangerous to the mother, which resolved more quickly and easily than I thought possible, but again not in the way that I had hoped for:

A single woman was 5 months pregnant with her second child when she came in for bleeding. At three months she noted some spotting with a vaginal infection, but sought no treatment. By 4 months, it required tampons to control it, but still she chose not to tell anyone about it, and consulted me only a month later, when the flow was comparable to a light period. The blood was dark, with big clots, cramping pain in her back and hips when she passed them, and some mucus in her stools as well. Her past history included an episode of gonorrheal endometritis with an IUD in place. Weighing almost 200 pounds, she was powerfully built and visibly uncomfortable in the heat. Recommending strict bed rest, I gave her *Sabina* 200 4 times daily to control the bleeding, and sent her for an ultrasound, which confirmed the diagnosis of placenta previa. Within 48 hours she expelled a stillborn fetus of 22 weeks' gestation, once again alone and unattended, and required no further treatment, for all of which she thanked me profusely.

In a third case, a remedy helped me decide to go ahead with a home birth, in the face of convincing arguments against it:

33 weeks pregnant with her fourth child, a single woman with no prenatal care came to my office requesting a home birth. She was also in acute distress, pacing the floor, sighing deeply, fanning herself, and belching loudly to relieve herself. To top it all off, a brief exam showed that the baby was breech. Clearly the most immediate issue was her illness, which she ascribed to her past history of recurrent bronchitis and pneumonia, and the antibiotics she had been given for them, as well as a recent flare-up of indigestion from rich food and overeating. Needless to say, I gave her *Carbo veg.*, and within 2 days she was greatly improved, and I noticed that the baby had turned. At that point I agreed to a home birth, which went quite well, in spite of a transient postpartum fever that subsided quickly, and she remained in good health thereafter.

Based on the fact that remedies can act to elicit symptoms as well as relieve them, the homœopathic phenomenon means that the same remedy can bring about opposite results, depending on dosage and the sensitivity of the patient, and thus help a confused and troubled organism "decide" which way it really needs to go. This at times scary openness is beautifully illustrated by the remedy *Pulsatilla,* which is often used to sustain difficult pregnancies and prevent miscarriage, but also does good service when miscarriage is imminent or inevitable. One 19-year-old patient miscarried abruptly and completely within hours after a single dose of *Pulsatilla* 30X for vaginitis, without needing a D&C, a *fait accompli* that helped her realize and accept the general consensus that she wasn't yet ready for motherhood.

Another example is its well-known rôle in turning a breech presentation into the vertex or head-down position, which it will reliably accomplish in about 30% of the cases when used routinely, in the absence of strong indications, and after which the labor tends to follow quite soon and proceed smoothly. Conversely, when the baby didn't turn in spite of my best efforts, my admittedly unverifiable impression was that it delivered most quickly and easily in the abnormal position. In any case, as everyone knows, the best remedy for correcting a breech presentation is the one indicated by the totality of symptoms, as in my *Carbo veg.* patient.

Pulsatilla is also the leading remedy for drying up the milk when the baby is given for adoption, and for restoring the milk when it is lost in the wake of a breast infection. These linked mysteries are one good reason why I have faith in the homœopathic process to lead me and my patients to a satisfying result often enough that most of them will forgive me the mistakes I make along the way.

III. Writings on Vaccination:

"The Case Against Immunizations"

"Vaccination: a Sacrament of Modern Medicine"

"Hidden in Plain Sight: the Rôle of Vaccines in Chronic Disease"

The Case Against Immunizations**

For the past ten years or so, I have felt a deep and growing compunction against giving routine vaccinations to children. It began with the fundamental belief that people have the right to make that choice for themselves. But now I can no longer bring myself to give the shots, even when the parents wish me to. I have always believed that the attempt to eradicate entire microbial species from the biosphere must inevitably upset the balance of Nature in fundamental ways that we can as yet scarcely imagine. Such concerns loom ever larger as new vaccines continue to be developed, seemingly for no better reason than that we have the technical capacity to make them, and thereby to demonstrate our right and power as a civilization to manipulate the evolutionary process itself.

Purely from the viewpoint of our own species, even if we could be sure that the vaccines were harmless, the fact remains that they are *compulsory,* that all children are required to undergo them, without sensitivity to or proper regard for basic differences in individual susceptibility, to say nothing of the values and wishes of the parents and the children themselves. Most people can readily accept the fact that, from time to time, certain laws may be necessary for the public good that some of us strongly disagree with. But in this case the issue involves nothing less than the introduction of foreign proteins and live viruses into the bloodstream of entire populations. For that reason alone, the public is surely entitled to convincing proof, beyond any reasonable doubt, that vaccination is in fact a safe and effective procedure, in no way injurious to health, and that the threat of the corresponding natural diseases remains sufficiently clear and urgent to warrant the mass inoculation of everyone, even against their will if necessary.

Unfortunately, such proof has never been given; and even if it could be, continuing to employ vaccines against diseases that are no longer prevalent or dangerous hardly qualifies as an emergency. Finally, even if

** "The Case Against Immunizations," *Journal of the American Institute of Homeopathy* 76:7, 1983

there were such an emergency, and artificial immunization could be shown to be an appropriate response to it, the decision would remain at bottom a *political* one, involving issues of public health and safety that are far too important to be settled by any purely scientific or technical criteria, or indeed by *any* criteria less authoritative than the clearly articulated sense of the community about to be subjected to it.

For all of these reasons, I want to present the case against routine immunization as clearly and forcefully as I can. What I have to say is not quite a formal theory capable of rigorous proof or disproof. It is simply an attempt to explain my own experience, a nexus of interrelated facts, observations, reflections, and hypotheses, which taken together are more or less coherent and plausible and make intuitive sense to me. I offer them to the public in large part because the growing refusal of some parents to vaccinate their children is so seldom articulated or taken seriously. The fact is that we have been taught to accept vaccination as a kind of involuntary Communion, a sacrament of our participation in the unrestricted growth of scientific and industrial technology, utterly heedless of the long-term consequences to the health of our own species, let alone to the balance of Nature as a whole. For that reason alone, the other side of the case urgently needs to be heard.

1. Are the Vaccines Effective?

There is widespread agreement that the time period since the common vaccines were introduced has seen a remarkable decline in the corresponding natural infections; but the usual assumption that the decline is *attributable* to the vaccines remains unproven, and continues to be seriously questioned by eminent authorities in the field. The incidence and severity of whooping cough, for example, had already begun to decline precipitously long before the pertussis vaccine was introduced,[1] a fact which led the epidemiologist C. C. Dauer to remark, as far back as 1943,

> If the mortality [from pertussis] continues to decline at the same rate during the next 15 years, it will be extremely difficult to show statistically that [pertussis immunization] had any effect in reducing the mortality from whooping cough.[2]

Much the same is true not only of diphtheria and tetanus, but also of TB, cholera, typhus, typhoid, and other common scourges of a bygone era, which began to disappear toward the end of the Nineteenth Century, largely in response to improvements in public health and sanitation, but in any case long before antibiotics, vaccines, or any specific medical measures designed to eradicate them.[3] Reflections such as these led the great microbiologist René Dubos to observe that microbial diseases have their own natural history, independent of drugs and vaccines, in which asymptomatic infection and symbiosis are much more common than overt disease:

> It is barely recognized but nevertheless true that animals and plants, as well as men, can live peacefully with their most notorious microbial enemies. The world is obsessed by the fact that poliomyelitis can kill and maim several thousand unfortunate victims every year. But more extraordinary is the fact that millions upon millions of young people become infected by polio viruses, yet suffer no harm from the infection. The dramatic episodes of conflict between men and microbes are what strike the mind. What is less readily apprehended is the more common fact that infection can occur without producing disease.[4]

The principal evidence that the vaccines are effective actually dates from the more recent period, during which time the dreaded polio epidemics of the 1940's and 1950's have never reappeared, at least in the developed world, while measles, mumps, and rubella, which even a generation ago were among the commonest diseases of childhood, have become much less prevalent, at least in their classic acute forms, since the triple MMR vaccine was introduced into common use. Yet how the vaccines actually accomplish these changes is not nearly as well understood as most people like to think it is. The disturbing possibility that they act in some other way than by producing a genuine immunity is suggested by the fact that the corresponding natural diseases have continued to break out, even in highly immunized populations, and that in such cases the observed differences in incidence and severity between immunized and non-immunized populations have often been much less dramatic than expected, and in some cases not measurably significant at all.

In a recent British outbreak of whooping cough, for example, even fully-vaccinated children contracted the disease in large numbers, and their rates of serious complications and death were not reduced significantly.[5] In another recent outbreak, 46 of the 85 fully-vaccinated children studied eventually contracted the disease.[6] In 1977, 34 new cases of measles were reported on the UCLA campus, among a population that was supposedly 91% immune, according to careful serological testing.[7] In 1981, another 20 cases were reported in the area of Pecos, New Mexico within a few-month period, and 75% of them had been fully vaccinated, some quite recently.[8] A survey of sixth-graders in a well-immunized urban area similarly revealed that about 15% of this age group are still susceptible to rubella, a figure essentially identical with that of the pre-vaccine era.[9] Finally, while the incidence of measles has dropped sharply, from about 400,000 cases annually in the early 1960's to about 30,000 by 1974-76, the death rate has remained exactly the same,[10] while among adolescents and young adults, the group with the highest incidence at present, the risk of pneumonia and liver abnormalities has increased quite substantially, to well over 3% and 20%, respectively.[11]

The simplest explanation for these discrepancies would be to stipulate that vaccines confer at most partial and temporary immunity, which sounds reasonable enough, inasmuch as they consist of either live viruses, rendered less virulent by serial passage in tissue culture, or bacteria and bacterial products that have been killed by heat and chemical adjuvants, such that they can still elicit an antibody response without initiating a full-blown disease. In other words, the vaccine is a "trick," in the sense that it *simulates* the true or natural immunity developed in the course of recovering from the natural disease, and it is therefore reasonable to expect that such artificial immunity will in fact "wear off" in time, and even require additional "booster" doses at regular intervals throughout life to maintain peak effectiveness.

Such an explanation would be disturbing enough to most people. Indeed, the basic fallacy in it is already evident in the fact that there is no way to know how long this partial, temporary immunity will last in any given individual, or how often it will need to be re-stimulated, since the answers to these questions presumably depend on the same individual variables that would have determined whether and how severely the same person would have contracted the disease if they had not been vaccinated.

In any case, a number of other observations suggest equally strongly that this simple explanation cannot be the correct one. In the first place, one careful study has shown that when a person vaccinated against the measles again becomes susceptible to it, even repeated booster doses will have little or no long-lasting effect.[12] In the second place, the vaccines do not act merely by producing pale or mild copies of the original disease; they also commonly produce a variety of symptoms of their own, which in some cases may be more serious than the natural disease, involving deeper structures, more vital organs, and less of a tendency to resolve themselves spontaneously, as well as being more difficult to recognize.

Thus in a recent outbreak of mumps in supposedly immune schoolchildren, several developed atypical symptoms, such as anorexia, vomiting, and erythematous rashes, but no parotid involvement, and hence could not be diagnosed without extensive serological testing to rule out other concurrent diseases.[13] The syndrome of "atypical measles" can be equally difficult to diagnose, even when it is thought of,[14] which suggests that it may not seldom be overlooked entirely. In some cases, atypical measles can be much more severe than the regular kind, with pneumonia, petechiæ, edema, and severe pain,[15] and likewise often goes unsuspected.

In any case, it seems virtually certain that other vaccine-related syndromes will be described and identified, if only we take the trouble to look for them, and that the ones we are aware of so far represent only a very small part of the problem. But even these few make it less and less plausible to assume that vaccines produce a normal, healthy immunity that lasts for some time but then *wears off,* leaving the patient miraculously unharmed and unaffected by the experience.

2. Some Personal Experiences.

I will now present a few of my own vaccine cases, to give a sense of their variety, to show how difficult it can be to trace them, and also to begin to address the underlying question that is seldom asked, namely, how the vaccines actually *work,* i. e., how they do whatever it is that they do inside the body, and how they produce the results that we see clinically in the patient.

My first case was that of an 8-month-old girl with recurrent fevers of unknown origin. I first saw her in January 1977, a few weeks after her third such episode. These were brief, lasting 48 hours at most, but very intense, with the fever often reaching 105°. During the second episode she was hospitalized for diagnostic evaluation, but her pediatrician found nothing out of the ordinary. Apart from these episodes, the child appeared to be quite well, and growing and developing normally.

I could get no further information from the mother, except for the fact that the episodes had occurred almost exactly one month apart, and from consulting her calendar we learned that the first one had come almost exactly one month after the third of her DPT shots, which had also been given at monthly intervals. Then the mother remembered that the girl had had similar fever episodes immediately after each injection, but that the pediatrician had dismissed them as common reactions to the vaccine, as indeed they are. Purely on the strength of that history, I gave her a single dose of the ultradilute homeopathic DPT vaccine, and I am happy to report that she had no more such episodes, and has remained entirely well since.

This case illustrates how homeopathic "nosodes," medicines prepared from vaccines or their corresponding diseases, can be used for *diagnosis* as well as treatment of vaccine-related illness, which, no matter how strongly they are suspected, might otherwise be almost impossible to substantiate. Secondly, because fever is among the commonest reactions to the pertussis vaccine, and the child seemed perfectly well between the attacks, her response to it has to be regarded as a relatively strong and healthy one, disturbing because of its recurrence and periodicity, but also quite simple to cure, as indeed it proved. But I keep wondering what happens to the vaccine inside those tens and hundreds of millions of children who show no obvious response to it at all.

Since that time, I have seen at least half a dozen cases of babies and small children with recurrent fevers of unknown origin, some associated with a variety of other chronic complaints, like irritability, temper tantrums, and increased susceptibility to tonsillitis, pharyngitis, colds, and ear infections, which were similarly traceable to the pertussis vaccine, and which likewise responded beautifully to treatment with the homeopathic DPT nosode. Indeed on that basis I submit that the pertussis vaccine is an important cause of recurrent fevers of unknown origin in this age group.

My second case was that of a 9-month-old girl who presented acutely with a fever of 105°, and very few other symptoms. She had had two similar episodes previously, but at irregular intervals, and her parents, who were ambivalent about vaccinations to begin with, had given her only one dose of the DPT, but her first episode occurred a few weeks afterward.

I first saw her in June of 1978. The fever remained high and unremitting for 48 hours, despite the usual acute remedies and supportive measures. A CBC showed WBC's of 32,000 per cu. mm., with 43% lymphocytes, 11% monocytes, 25% neutrophils (many with toxic granulations), 20% band forms (also with toxic granulations), and 1% metamyelocytes and other immature forms. Without giving any history, I showed the slide to a pediatrician friend, and "pertussis" was his immediate reply. After a single dose of the homeopathic DPT vaccine, the fever came down abruptly, and the girl has remained well since.

This case was disturbing mainly because of the hematological abnormalities, which fell within the leukemoid range, together with the absence of any cough or illness with distinctive respiratory symptoms, all suggesting that introducing the vaccine directly into the blood may actually promote deeper or more systemic pathology than allowing the pertussis organism to set up typical symptoms of local inflammation at the normal portal of entry.

The third case was a 5-year-old boy with chronic lymphocytic leukemia, whom I saw in August of 1978, while visiting an old friend and teacher, a family physician with over 40 years' experience. Well out of earshot of the boy and his parents, he told me that the leukemia had first appeared following a DPT vaccination, that he had treated the child successfully with homeopathy on two previous occasions, when the blood picture improved dramatically, the liver and spleen shrank down to almost normal size, and that full relapse had occurred soon after each DPT booster.

It was disturbing enough to think that vaccinations might be implicated in some cases of childhood leukemia, but the idea also completed the line of reasoning opened up by the previous case. For leukemia is a cancerous transformation of the blood and blood-forming organs, the liver, the spleen, the lymph nodes, and the bone marrow, which are also the basic anatomical units of the immune system. Insofar as vaccines are capable of producing serious complications of any kind, the blood and immune organs would be the logical place to begin looking for them.

What shocked me even more was the fact that even my teacher's remarkable success in treating this boy did not dissuade his parents from revaccinating him at least two more times, and that the connection between the vaccine and the disease was not generally known to the public or seriously considered by the medical community. It was this case that convinced me of the need for frank and open discussion among doctors and patients alike, about our collective experience with vaccine-related illness. While careful scientific investigation of these matters will hopefully ensue, the level of public commitment required even to frame the question properly seems far away.

I will now present two cases from my limited experience with the MMR vaccine.

In December of 1980 I saw a three-year-old boy with loss of appetite, stomach ache, indigestion, and swollen glands for the past 4 weeks or so. The stomach pains were quite severe, and often accompanied by belching, flatulence, and explosive diarrhea. The nose was also congested, and the lower eyelids were quite red. The mother also reported some unusual behavior changes, extreme untidiness, wild and noisy playing, and waking at 2 a.m. to get in bed with her.

The physical examination was unremarkable except for some large, tender posterior auricular and suboccipital lymph nodes, and marked enlargement of the tonsils. That piqued my curiosity, and I learned that the boy had received his MMR vaccination in October, about 2 weeks before the onset of symptoms, with no apparent reaction to it at the time. I gave him a single dose of the highly-dilute homeopathic rubella vaccine, and the symptoms disappeared within 48 hours.

The following spring, the parents brought him back for a slight fever, and a 3-week history of intermittent pain in and behind the right ear, as well as a stuffy nose and other cold symptoms. On examination, the whole right side of the face appeared to be swollen, especially the cheek and angle of the jaw. He responded well to acute homeopathic remedies, without ever needing the mumps nosode, and has remained well since.

This boy exhibited some interesting features that I have learned to recognize in other MMR cases. At an interval of a few weeks after the vaccine, which is roughly the same as the incubation period for the corresponding diseases, a nondescript illness developed, which then became subacute and rather more severe than rubella in the same age group, with abdominal and joint pains and marked adenopathy, but no rash. The diagnosis was suspected because of enlargement of the posterior auricular and suboccipital nodes, for which rubella and a few other diseases have a marked affinity, and confirmed by a favorable response to the homeopathic rubella nosode. Furthermore, his second illness, and especially the parotid enlargement, may well have represented continuing activity of the mumps component of the vaccine, although it cleared up so promptly that I never needed to test my hypothesis by using the homeopathic mumps nosode. Either way, it strongly suggests the possibility that a variety of "mixed" or composite syndromes may occur, representing the patient's responses to two or perhaps all three of the vaccine components, either more or less simultaneously, or one by one over time, as the next case illustrates:

In April 1981 I saw a 4-year-old boy for chronic bilateral enlargement of the posterior auricular nodes, which were also somewhat tender at times. The mother had noticed the swelling for about a year, during which time he had also become more susceptible to various upper respiratory infections, none of them very severe. Over the same period of time, she had also observed recurrent parotid swelling at irregular intervals, which also began shortly after the MMR vaccine was given at the age of 3.

At his first visit, the boy was not ill, and the mother was about 2 months pregnant; so I decided to observe him but if possible do nothing further until the pregnancy was over. He did develop a mild laryngitis in her third trimester, but it responded well to bed rest and simple acute remedies. The following spring he came down with acute bronchitis, and I noticed that the posterior auricular glands were once again swollen and tender, so I decided to give him a dose of the homeopathic rubella nosode at that point. The cough promptly subsided, and the nodes regressed in size and were no longer tender. But two weeks later, he was back, this time with a hard, tender swelling on the outside of the cheek, near the angle of the jaw, and some pain on chewing or opening the mouth. One dose of the homeopathic mumps nosode was given, and the child has been well since.

What was particularly noteworthy about this case was its strong pattern of *chronicity,* with an increased susceptibility to weaker, low-grade responses, in contrast to the vigorous, *acute* responses typically associated with diseases like measles and mumps when acquired naturally.

3. How Do Vaccines Work?

It is dangerously misleading, if not the exact opposite of the truth, to claim that a vaccine renders us "immune" to or *protects* us against an acute disease, if in fact it only drives the disease deeper into the interior and causes us to harbor it *chronically* instead, with the result that our responses to it become progressively weaker, but show less and less of a tendency to heal or resolve themselves spontaneously. What I propose, then, is to investigate as thoroughly and objectively as I can how the vaccines actually *work* inside the human body, and to begin by simply paying attention to the implications of what we already know. Consider the process of falling ill with and recovering from a typical acute disease, such as the measles, in contrast with what we can observe following administration of the measles vaccine.

We all know that measles is primarily a virus of the upper respiratory tract, both because it is acquired by susceptible persons through inhalation of infected droplets in the air, and because these droplets are produced by the coughing and sneezing of a patient with the disease. Once inhaled by a susceptible individual, the virus undergoes a prolonged period of silent multiplication, first in the tonsils, adenoids, and accessory lymphoid aggregations of the nasopharynx; later in the regional lymph nodes of the head and neck; and eventually, several days later, it passes into the blood and enters the spleen, the liver, the thymus, and the bone marrow, the "visceral" organs of the immune system.[16] Throughout this "incubation" period, which lasts from 10 to 14 days, the patient typically feels quite well, and experiences few or no symptoms of any kind.[17]

By the time the first symptoms of measles appear, circulating antibodies are already detectable in the blood, and the height of the symptomatology coincides with the peak of the antibody response.[18] In other words, the "illness" that we call the measles is simply the definitive effort of the immune system to clear this virus from the blood. Notice also that this expulsion is accomplished by sneezing and coughing, i.e.,

79

via the same route through which it entered in the first place. From the above it is abundantly clear that the process of mounting and recovering from an acute illness like the measles involves a general mobilization of the immune system as a whole, including inflammation of the previously sensitized tissues at the portal(s) of entry, activation of leukocytes, macrophages, and the serum complement system, and a host of other mechanisms, of which the production of circulating antibodies is only one, and by no means the most important.

Such splendid outpourings indeed represent the decisive experiences in the normal physiological maturation of the immune system in the life of a healthy child. For recovery from the measles not only protects children from being susceptible to it again,[19] no matter how many more times they may be exposed to it, but also prepares them to respond promptly and effectively to any other infections they may encounter in the future. The ability to mount a vigorous acute response to infection must therefore be reckoned among the most fundamental requirements of health and well-being that we all share.

By contrast, the live but artificially attenuated measles-virus vaccine is injected directly into the blood, by-passing the normal port of entry, and sets up at most a brief inflammatory reaction at the injection site, or perhaps in the regional lymph nodes, with no local sensitization at the normal portal of entry, no "incubation period," no generalized inflammatory response, and no generalized outpouring. By "tricking" the body in this fashion, we have accomplished precisely what the entire immune system seems to have evolved to prevent: we have placed the virus directly into the blood, and given it free and immediate access to the major immune organs and tissues, without any obvious mechanism or route for getting rid of it.

The result is the production of circulating antibodies against the virus, which can in fact be measured in the blood; but this antibody response occurs as an isolated technical feat, without any overt illness to recover from, or any noticeable improvement in the general health of the recipient. Indeed I submit that exactly the opposite is true, that the price we have to pay for these antibodies is the persistence of viral elements in the blood for long periods of time, perhaps permanently, which in turn carries with it a systematic weakening of our capacity to mount an acute response, not only to the measles, but to other infections as well.

Far from producing a genuine immunity, then, my suspicion and my fear is that vaccines act by interfering with and even *suppressing* the immune response as a whole, in much the same way that radiation, chemotherapy, corticosteroids, and other anti-inflammatory drugs do. Artificial immunization focuses on *antibody production,* a single aspect of the immune process, disarticulates it, and allows it to stand for the whole, in much the same way as chemical suppression of an elevated blood pressure is accepted as a valid substitute for genuine healing or cure of the patient whose blood pressure has risen. It is the frosting on the cake, without the cake. The worst part of this counterfeiting is that it becomes more difficult, if not impossible, for vaccinated children to mount a normally acute and vigorous response to infection, by substituting for it a much weaker, essentially chronic response, with little or no tendency to heal itself spontaneously.

Furthermore, excellent models already exist for predicting and explaining what kinds of chronic disease are likely to result from long-term persistence of viral, bacterial, and other foreign proteins within the cells of the immune system. It has long been known that live viruses are capable of surviving for years within host cells in a latent form, without necessarily provoking acute disease, simply by attaching their own genetic material as an "episome" or extra particle to the genome of the host cell, and replicating along with it, allowing the latter to continue its normal functions for the most part, but adding new instructions for the synthesis of viral proteins as well.[20]

Latent viruses of this type have already been implicated in three distinct types of chronic disease, namely,

1) *recurrent or episodic acute diseases,* such as herpes simplex, shingles, warts, etc.;[21]

2) *"slow-virus" diseases,* whether subacute or chronic, progressive, and often fatal conditions, such as kuru, Creutzfeldt-Jakob disease, possibly Guillain-Barré syndrome, and subacute sclerosing panencephalitis (SSPE), a rare complication of measles;[22] and

3) *tumors,* both benign and malignant.[23]

In all of these varieties, the latent virus "survives" as a clearly foreign element within the cell, which means that the immune system must continue to try to make antibodies against it, insofar as it can still respond to it at all. But because the virus is now permanently incorporated within the genetic material of the cell, these antibodies will now have to be directed against the cell itself. The persistence of live viruses and other foreign antigens within the cells of the host thus cannot fail to provoke auto-immune phenomena, because attacking and destroying the infected cells is now the only possible way to remove this constant antigenic challenge from the body. Since universal compulsory vaccination introduces live viruses and other highly antigenic material into the blood of virtually every living person, it is not difficult to predict that a significant harvest of auto-immune diseases will automatically result.

Sir Macfarlane Burnet has observed that the various components of the immune system function as if they were collectively designed to help the organism to distinguish "self" from "non-self," i. e., to help us recognize and tolerate our own cells, and to identify and eliminate foreign or extraneous substances as completely as possible.[24] Lending further credence to this hypothesis are the acute response to infection, as we saw, and the rejection of transplanted tissues or organs from the same species, i. e., *homografts,* both of which accomplish complete and permanent removal of the offending substances from the body. If Burnet is correct, then latent viruses, auto-immune phenomena, and perhaps also cancer could be regarded as different aspects of the same basic reality, which the immune system can neither escape nor resolve. For they all entail a certain degree of *chronic immune failure,* a state in which it becomes increasingly difficult or impossible for the body either to recognize its own cells as unequivocally its own or to eliminate its parasites as wholly foreign.

In the case of the attenuated measles virus vaccine, introducing it directly into the blood might continue to provoke an antibody response for a considerable period of time, which of course is the whole point of giving the vaccine; but eventually, as the virus achieves a state of latency, that response would presumably wane, both because circulating antibodies normally cannot cross the cell membrane, and because they are also powerful immunosuppressive agents in their own right.[25] After that, the effect of circulating antibodies would be in effect to imprison the virus inside the cell, i. e., to continue to prevent any acute inflammatory response, until such time as, perhaps under circumstances of an emergency or cumulative stress, this precarious balance breaks down, antibodies begin to be produced in large numbers against the cells themselves, and frank auto-immune phenomena, including necrosis and tissue damage, are likely to appear. In this sense, latent viruses are like biological "time bombs," set to explode at an indeterminate time in the future.[26]

Auto-immune phenomena have always seemed obscure, aberrant, and bizarre to physicians, because it is not intuitively obvious why the body should suddenly begin to attack and destroy its own tissues. They make a lot more sense, and perhaps should even be regarded as "healthy," to the extent that destroying chronically infected cells is the only possible way to eliminate an even more serious threat to life, namely, the foreign antigenic challenge persisting within the cells of the host.

According to the same model, tumor formation could be understood as simply a more advanced stage of chronic immune failure, inasmuch as the longer the host is subjected to enormous and constant pressure to make antibodies against itself, the less effective that process will likely become. Eventually, under stress of this magnitude, the auto-immune mechanism itself could break down to the point that the chronically infected and genetically transformed cells, no longer clearly "self" or non-self," begin to free themselves from the normal restraints of "histocompatibility" within the architecture of the surrounding cells and tissues, and begin to multiply autonomously at their expense. A tumor could then be described as "benign," if the weakening of histocompatibility remains strictly localized to the tissue of origin, "malignant" if the process spills over into other cell types, tissues, and organs, even in more remote areas, and not necessarily rigidly or permanently one or the other, since they differ primarily in degree and therefore might or might not even change back and forth into each other in due course.

If what I am saying turns out to be true, then all we have achieved by artificial immunization is to have traded off our acute epidemic diseases of past centuries for the weaker and far less curable chronic diseases of the present, with their suffering and disability paid out little by little, rather than all at once, and amortized over the patient's lifetime. Perhaps even more, I fear that in doing so we have opened up limitless possibilities for new diseases in the future by *in vivo* genetic recombination within the cells of the race.

4. The Individual Vaccines Reconsidered.

I will now consider each of the vaccines individually, in relation to the natural diseases from which they are derived.

The triple MMR vaccine comprises attenuated, live measles, mumps, and rubella viruses, administered in a single intramuscular injection at about 15 months of age. Subsequent booster doses are no longer recommended, except for young women of childbearing age, in whom the risk of Congenital Rubella Syndrome (CRS) is thought to warrant it, even though the effectiveness of such boosters is at best questionable, as we saw.

Before the vaccine era, measles, mumps, and rubella were classified as "routine diseases of childhood," which most schoolchildren acquired before the age of puberty, and from which nearly all recovered, with lifelong immunity and no complications or sequelæ. But they were not always so harmless. Measles, in particular, is devastating when a population encounters it for the first time. Its importation from Spain undoubtedly contributed to Cortez' conquest of the mighty Aztec empire with only a handful of soldiers: whole villages were carried off by epidemics of measles and smallpox, leaving only a small remnant of cowed, superstitious warriors to face the bearded *conquistadores* from across the sea.[27] In more recent outbreaks among isolated, primitive peoples, the case fatality rate from measles averaged 20 to 30%.[28] In these so-called "virgin-soil" epidemics, not only measles, but also polio and many other epidemic diseases take their highest toll of death and serious complications among adolescents and young adults, seemingly healthy and vigorous people in the prime of life, and leave relatively unharmed the group of school-age children before the age of puberty.[29]

The evolution of a disease like the measles from a dreaded killer to a routine disease of childhood presupposes the development of non-specific or "herd" immunity in young children, such that when they are finally exposed to it, it activates defense mechanisms already in place to receive it, resulting in the prolonged incubation period and usually benign, self-limited course described above. Under these circumstances, the rationale

84

for vaccinating young children against it is limited to the fact that a very small number of deaths and serious complications have continued to occur, chiefly pneumonia, encephalitis, and the rare but dreaded subacute sclerosing panencephalitis (SSPE), a slow-virus disease with an incidence of 1 per 100,000 cases.[30] Pneumonia, by far the commonest of them, is also benign and self-limited in most cases, even without treatment,[31] and even in those rare cases when bacterial pneumonia supervenes, adequate treatment is currently available.

By all accounts, then, the death rate and risk of serious complications from measles are very low in the developed world, while the general benefit to the child who recovers from it, as well as his contacts and descendants, is very great. Even if the vaccine could be shown to lower the risk of death and serious morbidity still further, these small achievements would hardly justify the high probability of auto-immune diseases, cancer, and whatever else may result from the harboring and propagation of latent measles virus in human tissue culture for life.

Ironically, what the vaccine certainly *has* done is to reverse the historical or evolutionary process to the extent that measles is now once again a disease of adolescents and young adults,[32] with a correspondingly higher risk of complications, and a general tendency to produce more illness and disability than it does in grade-school children. As for the claim that it has helped to eliminate measles encephalitis, even in my own relatively small general practice I have already seen two children with major seizure disorders that the parents clearly traced to the measles vaccine, although they would never have been able to prove the connection in court, and never even considered the possibility of compensation. Such cases never make it into the official statistics, and are duly omitted from conventional surveys of the problem, in spite of the fact that injecting measles into the blood would naturally favor a higher incidence of visceral complications affecting the lungs, liver, and brain, organs for which the virus has a known affinity.

The case for immunizing against mumps and rubella seems *a fortiori* even more tenuous, for exactly the same reasons. Mumps is also essentially a benign, self-limited disease in children before the age of puberty, and recovery from a single attack likewise confers lifelong immunity. The major complication is meningo-encephalitis, mild or subclinical forms of which are relatively common, but the death rate is extremely low,[33] and sequelæ are rare. The mumps vaccine is prepared and administered in much the same way as the measles, almost always in the same injection, and the dangers associated with it are also comparable. It too is fast becoming a disease of adolescents and young adults,[34] age groups who tolerate it much less well. With them he main complication is epididymo-orchitis, which occurs in 30-40% of affected males past the age of puberty, and usually results in atrophy of the testicle on the affected side,[35] but it also shows a definite affinity for the ovary and pancreas, and may attack these organs as well.

For all of these reasons, the greatest favor we could do for our children would be to expose them to the measles and mumps when they reach school age, which would not only protect them from contracting more serious versions after puberty, but would also greatly enhance their immunological maturation with minimal risk, as was the rule before the vaccine was introduced.

The same discrepancy is evident for rubella or "German measles" as well, which in young children is a disease so mild that it frequently escapes detection,[36] but in adolescents and adults is much more likely to produce arthritis, purpura, and other systemic indications of greater severity.[37] The main impetus for marketing the vaccine was certainly the recognition of Congenital Rubella Syndrome (CRS), resulting from intrauterine damage to the embryo when the mother acquires the virus in her first trimester of pregnancy,[38] and the unusually high incidence of CRS during the rubella outbreak of 1964. Here again, we have an almost entirely benign, self-limited disease made over by the vaccine into a considerably less benign one of adolescents and young adults of reproductive age, precisely the group that most needs to be protected from it, while the easiest and most effective way to prevent it would likewise be to expose kids to the disease in elementary school. Re-infection does sometimes occur after recovery, but much less commonly than after vaccination.[39]

The equation looks rather different for the diphtheria and tetanus vaccines. First of all, both natural diseases are serious and sometimes fatal, even with the best treatment. This is especially true of tetanus, which still carries a mortality of at least 10-20%. Furthermore, these vaccines are not made of live organisms, but only of certain toxins elaborated by

86

them. These poisonous substances are responsible for all of the death and destruction wrought by these diseases, and remain highly antigenic even after being inactivated by heat. Diphtheria and tetanus "toxoids" thus do not protect against infection *per se,* but only against the systemic action of these poisons, in the absence of which both infections are of minor importance clinically. It is therefore easy to understand why parents might want their children protected against diphtheria and tetanus, if safe and effective protection were available; and both vaccines have been in use for a long time, with a very low incidence of serious complications reported, so that there has been very little public outcry against them.

On the other hand, both diseases are readily controlled by simple sanitary measures and careful attention to wound hygiene, and both have been steadily disappearing from the industrially developed countries since long before the toxoids were introduced. Diphtheria now occurs only sporadically in the United States, often in areas with significant reservoirs of unvaccinated children. But the claim that the vaccine is protective is belied by the fact that, when the disease does break out, the supposedly "susceptible" kids are no more likely to develop it than their fully-immunized contacts. In a 1969 outbreak in Chicago, for example, the Board of Health reported that 25% of the cases had been fully immunized; another 12% had received one or more doses and serologically were fully "immune;" and another 18% had been partly immunized, according to the same criteria.[40]

So once again we are faced with the likelihood that diphtheria toxoid has not produced a genuine immunity to diphtheria, but rather some sort of chronic immune *tolerance* to it, by harboring highly antigenic residues somewhere within the cells of the immune system, presumably with long-term suppressive effects on the immune mechanism generally. This suspicion earns further credence from the fact that all of the DPT vaccine components are alum-precipitated and preserved with Thimerosal, an organomercury derivative, to preserve them from being metabolized too rapidly, so that the antigenic challenge will continue for as long a time as possible. The fact is that we do not know or even seem to *care* what actually becomes of these foreign substances once they are inside our bodies and those of our children.

87

Exactly the same questions haunt the seemingly favorable record of the tetanus vaccine, which almost certainly has had some impact in reducing the incidence of tetanus in its classic acute form, yet presumably also persists for years or even decades as a potent foreign antigen within the cells of the immune system, with long-term effects on the immune mechanism that for the present are invisible and therefore impossible to calculate.

Much like diphtheria and tetanus, "whooping cough" began to decline as a serious epidemic threat, as we saw, long before the DPT vaccine was introduced. Moreover, the pertussis vaccine has not been particularly effective, even according to its proponents, and the incidence of known side-effects is disturbingly high. Its power to damage the central nervous system, for example, has received growing attention since Dr. Gordon Stewart and his colleagues in the UK reported an alarmingly high incidence of encephalopathy and severe convulsive disorders in British children that were traceable to the vaccine.[41] My own cases, a few of which were cited above, suggest that hematologic disturbances should also be investigated, and that the *known* complications represent at most a small fraction of the actual total.

In any case, the pertussis vaccine has become controversial even in the United States, where medical opinion remains almost unanimous in favor of vaccines generally, while several other countries, such as West Germany, have discontinued routine pertussis vaccination entirely.[42] The disease pertussis is also extremely variable clinically, ranging in severity from asymptomatic, mild, or inapparent infections, which are not uncommon, to very rare cases in young infants less than 6 months of age, where the mortality is claimed by some to reach 40%.[43] In children over a year old, however, the disease is rarely fatal, or even that serious a threat of future difficulty, despite its intensity, while antibiotics play a very small part in the outcome.[44]

Most of the pressure to immunize at present thus seems attributable to the higher death rate in very young infants, which has led to what to me seems like a terrifying practice of giving this most clearly dangerous of the vaccines to tiny infants, beginning at 2 months of age, when their mothers' milk would normally protect them from all infections about as well as can ever be done for this age group,[45] and its effect on the still-developing blood and nervous systems is most apt to be catastrophic. For all of these reasons, routine pertussis immunization should be discontinued until more studies are done to assess and defray the cost of whatever damage it has already done.

Poliomyelitis and the polio vaccines present an entirely different situation. The standard Sabin vaccine is trivalent, consisting of attenuated live polioviruses of each of the three strains known to produce paralytic disease, and administered orally, the same way the infection is acquired in Nature. Thus allowing the recipient to develop something resembling a natural immunity, by sensitizing cells of the digestive tract at the normal portal of entry, could represent a considerable safety factor. On the other hand, wild-type polio viruses produce no symptoms whatsoever in well over 90% of the people who contact them, even under epidemic conditions;[46] and of those who do become ill, the vast majority suffer nothing worse than a typical gastroenteritis that is more or less indistinguishable from any other of the common summer diarrheas in children. Only 1 or 2% of them ever progress to the full-blown picture of paralytic "poliomyelitis," with its typical lesions in the motor neurons of the spinal cord and medulla oblongata.[47] Poliomyelitis thus also requires peculiar and unusual conditions of susceptibility in the host, indeed an *anatomical* susceptibility, since the virulence of the poliovirus is so low for most people, even under epidemic conditions, and the number of cases resulting in death or permanent disability was always comparatively so small.[48]

Given the fact that polio viruses were ubiquitous before the vaccine was introduced, and could be found routinely in samples of city sewage wherever it was looked for,[49] it is evident that effective natural immunity to them was already as close to being universal as it could ever be, and *a fortiori* that no artificial substitute could ever equal or even approximate that record. Since the virus was of such low virulence to begin with, it is difficult to imagine what else further attenuation of it could possibly accomplish, other than perhaps to abate the full vigor of the natural immune response to it. For the fact remains that even the attenuated virus is still alive, and that the people who were anatomically susceptible to it before are still susceptible to it now. This means that at least some of these same people will develop paralytic polio from the vaccine,[50] and that all or most of the others may still be harboring the virus in latent form, perhaps within these same target cells.

The only advantage of giving the vaccine, then, would be to expose the population to the virus when its virulence is lowest,[51] i. e., when they are still infants, but this benefit might be more than offset by weakening the immune response, as we have seen. In any case, the whole matter is clearly one of considerable complexity, and also illustrates the hidden dangers and miscalculations inherent in the almost irresistible temptation to try to beat Nature at her own game, to eliminate a problem that cannot be eliminated, the susceptibility to disease itself.

So even in the case of the polio vaccine, which appears to be about as safe as a vaccine ever can be, the same basic dilemma remains. Perhaps the day will come when we will be ready to face the consequences of deliberately feeding live polio viruses to every living infant, and admit that we should have left well enough alone, and addressed ourselves to the art of healing the sick when we have to, rather than the technology of eradicating the *possibility* of sickness, when we don't have to and can't possibly succeed in any case.

5. Vaccination and the path of Medical Technology.

In conclusion, I want to go back to the beginning, to the essentially political aspects of vaccination, that oblige us to reason and deliberate together about matters of common concern, and to reach a clear decision about how we choose to live. I have stated my own views regarding the safety and effectiveness of vaccines, and I hope that others of differing views will do the same. But I am deeply troubled by the atmosphere of fanaticism that surrounds the subject, whereby vaccines are forcibly imposed on the public in the absence of any public health emergency, often against their will, and serious discussion of them is ridiculed, stifled, and ignored by the medical authorities as if the question had been settled definitively and for all time. Here is a the classic triumphalist view, from the great scientist Macfarlane Burnet, whom we have met before:

> It is our pride that in a civilized country the only infectious diseases which anyone is likely to suffer are either trivial or easily cured by available drugs. The diseases that killed in the past have been rendered impotent, and in the

process general principles of control have been developed which should be applicable to any unexpected outbreak in the future.[52]

Quite apart from the truth or untruth of these claims, they exemplify the smug self-righteousness of a profession and a society that worships its own ability to manipulate and control the processes of Nature itself. That is why, as Robert Mendelsohn has said, "we are quick to pull the trigger, but slow to examine the consequences of our actions."[53] Indeed, *methodically* slow, one would have to say. In 1978, for example, the American Academy of Pediatrics was commissioned by Congress to formulate guidelines for Federal compensation of "vaccine-related injuries," and included the following eligibility restrictions in its report:

1) Such a reaction should have been previously recognized as a possible consequence of the vaccine given.

2) Such a reaction should have occurred no more than 30 days following the immunization.[54]

These restrictions would automatically exclude all of the chronic diseases, and indeed everything else except the very few adverse reactions that have so far been identified, which clearly represent no more than a tiny fraction of the problem. Still less can either the government or the medical establishment be considered ignorant of the threat that haunts every parent, that vaccines can cause cancer and other chronic diseases. Precisely that possibility was raised by Prof. Robert Simpson of Rutgers in a 1976 seminar for science writers sponsored by the American Cancer Society:

Immunization programs against flu, measles, mumps, polio, and so forth, may actually be seeding humans with RNA to form latent proviruses in cells throughout the body. These could be molecules in search of diseases: when activated under proper conditions, they could cause a variety of diseases, including rheumatoid arthritis, MS, systemic lupus erythematosus, Parkinson's disease, and perhaps cancer.[55]

Unfortunately, this is just the sort of warning that few people are ready, willing, or able to hear, least of all the American Cancer Society or the American Academy of Pediatrics. All of us still want to believe in the "miracle," as Dubos calls it, regardless of the evidence:

> Faith in the magical power of drugs often blunts the critical senses, and comes close at times to a mass hysteria, involving scientists and laymen alike. Men want miracles as much today as in the past. If they do not join one of the newer cults, they satisfy this need by worshiping at the altar of modern science. This faith in the magical power of drugs is not new. It helped to give medicine the authority of a priesthood, and to recreate the glamour of ancient mysteries.[56]

The idea of eradicating measles or polio has come to seem attractive to us, simply because the power of medical science makes it seem technically *possible:* we worship every victory of technology over Nature, just as the bullfight celebrates the triumph of human intelligence over the brute beast. That is why we do not begrudge the drug companies their enormous profits, and gladly volunteer our own bodies and those of our children for their latest experiments. Vaccination is essentially a religious sacrament of our own participation in the miracle, a veritable *auto-da-fé* in the name of civilization itself.

Nobody in his right mind would seriously entertain the idea that if we could somehow eliminate, one by one, measles and polio and all the known diseases of mankind, we would be any the healthier for it, or that other quite possibly even more serious diseases would not arise and quickly take their place. Still less would a rational being suppose that the illnesses he or she suffered from were "entities" somehow separable from the patients who suffer them, and that with the appropriate chemical or surgical sacrament such a removal can literally be carried out. Yet these are precisely the miracles we are taught to believe in, and the idolatries to which we aspire, forgetting the older and simpler truths that the liability to disease is deeply rooted in our biological nature, and that the phenomena of illness are the expression of our own life energy, trying to overcome whatever it is trying to overcome, trying, in short, to heal itself.

The myth that we can find purely technical solutions to all human ailments seems attractive at first, because it bypasses the problem of healing, which is a genuine miracle in the sense that it can always *fail* to occur. We are all authentically at risk of illness and death at every moment: no amount of technology can change that. Yet the quixotic mission of technomedicine is precisely to change that: to stand at all times in the front line against disease, to attack and destroy it whenever and wherever it shows itself.

That is why, with all due respect, I cannot have faith in the miracles or accept the sacraments of Merck, Sharp, and Dohme and the Centers for Disease Control. I prefer to stay with the miracle of life itself, which has given us illness and disease, to be sure, but also the arts of medicine and healing, through which we can acknowledge and experience our pain and vulnerability, and sometimes, with the grace of God and the help of our friends and neighbors, an awareness of health and well-being that knows no boundaries. *That* is my religion; and while I would willingly share it, I would not *force* it on anyone.

NOTES.

1. Mortimer, E., "Pertussis Immunization," *Hospital Practice,* October 1980, p. 103.
2. Quoted in ibid.., p. 105.
3. Dubos, R., *Mirage of Health,* Harper, 1959, p. 73.
4. Ibid., pp. 74-75.
5. Stewart, G., "Vaccination Against Whooping Cough: Efficiency vs. Risks," *Lancet,* 1977, p. 234.
6. *Medical Tribune,* January 10, 1979, p. 1.
7. Cherry, J., "The New Epidemiology of Measles and Rubella," *Hospital Practice,* July 1980, pp. 52-54.
8. Unpublished data from the New Mexico Health Department.
9. Lawless, M., et al., "Rubella Susceptibility in Sixth-Graders," *Pediatrics* 65:1086, June 1980.
10. Cherry, op. cit., p. 49.
11. *Infectious Diseases,* January 1982, p. 21.
12. Cherry, op. cit., p. 52.
13. *Family Practice News,* July 15, 1980, p. 1.
14. Ferrante, J., "Atypical Symptoms? It Could Still Be Measles," *Modern Medicine,* September 30, 1980, p. 76.
15. Cherry, op. cit., p. 53.
16. Phillips, C., "Measles," in Vaughan, V., et al., Eds., *Nelson's Textbook of Pediatrics,* 11th Ed., Saunders, 1979, p. 857.

17. Davis, B., et al., *Microbiology*, 2nd Ed., Harper, 1973, p. 1346.

18. Ibid., p. 1346.

19. Ibid., p. 1342.

20. Ibid., p. 1418.

21. Hayflick, L., "Slow Viruses," *Executive Health Report*, February 1981, p. 4.

22. Ibid., pp. 1-4.

23. Davis, op. cit., pp. 1418-1449.

24. Burnet, M., *The Integrity of the Body*, Atheneum, 1966, p. 68.

25. Talal, "Auto-Immunity," in Fudenberg, H., et al., *Basic and Clinical Immunology*, 3rd Ed., Lange, 1980, p. 22.

26. Hayflick, op. cit., p. 4.

27. McNeill, W., *Plagues and Peoples*, Anchor, 1976, p. 184.

28. Burnet, M., and White, D., *The Natural History of Infectious Disease*, Cambridge, 1972, p. 16.

29. Ibid., pp. 90, 121, and *passim*.

30. Steigman, A., "Slow Virus Infections," in Vaughan, op. cit., p. 937.

31. Phillips, op. cit., p. 860.

32. *Infectious Diseases*, April 1979, p. 26.

33. Phillips, "Mumps," in Vaughan, op. cit., p. 891.

34. Hayden, G., et al., "Mumps and Mumps Vaccine in the U. S.," *Continuing Education*, September 1979, p. 97.

35. Phillips, "Mumps," op. cit., p. 892.

36. Phillips, "Rubella," in Vaughan, op. cit., p. 863.

37. Ibid., p. 862.

38. Glasgow, L., and Overall, J., "Congenital Rubella Syndrome," in Vaughan, op. cit., p. 483.

39. Phillips, "Rubella," op. cit., p. 865.

40. Cited in Mendelsohn, R., "The Truth About Immunizations," *The People's Doctor*, April 1978, p. 1.

41. Stewart, op. cit., p. 234.

42. Mortimer, op. cit., p. 111.

43. Feigin, R., "Pertussis," in Vaughan, op. cit., p. 769.

44. Ibid.

45. Barness, L., "Breast Feeding," in Vaughan, op. cit., p. 191.

46. Burnet and White, op. cit., p. 91ff.

47. Davis, op. cit., p. 1290ff.

48. Ibid., p. 1280.

49. Burnet and White, op. cit., p. 95.

50. Fulginiti, V., "Problems of Poliovirus Immunization," *Hospital Practice*, August 1980, pp. 61-62.

51. Burnet and White, op. cit., p. 95.

52. Burnet, op. cit., p. 128.

53. Mendelsohn, op. cit., p. 3.

54. Quoted in Wehrle, P., "Vaccines, Risks, and Compensations," *Infectious Diseases,* February1982, p. 16.
55. Quoted in Mendelsohn, op. cit., p. 1.
56. Dubos, op. cit., p. 157.

*Vaccination: A Sacrament of Modern Medicine**

I am honored by your invitation to participate in this Conference, and deeply moved by the fraternal spirit, youthful vitality, and sincere dedication to homeopathy everywhere in evidence here. Homeopaths in all lands and of every stripe would do well to follow your example. Andrew Tyler of the London *Evening Standard* recently told me that the National Health Service pays a substantial bonus to physicians with documented vaccination rates over 70%, and a still higher increment if the figure tops 90%.[1] His drift seemed to be that you overly civilized Brits need only informal pressures and inducements to obey authority, while we more rebellious, outspoken Yanks have to be coerced with laws and penalties. If that is true, I can understand why you wanted to fetch somebody from America, and I shall try my best not to disappoint you.

My interest in vaccinations arose out of a "gut" feeling not to do them that I have devoted a considerable part of my career trying to clarify. In this as in so many other ways, the study of homeopathy has helped me articulate what my heart and soul already seemed to know. To recognize the living organism as a "totality of symptoms" already implies that any more narrowly-defined standard of vaccine safety or effectiveness cannot possibly be adequate. Other equally troubling inconsistencies include imposing mandatory vaccination laws in the absence of any public health emergency, and waiving the established rules of scientific investigation in their honor. These special privileges give some measure of the reverence accorded to vaccines and vaccination in what can only be called the "religion" of modern medicine.[2] Its theology was admirably summarized by the French physiologist Claude Bernard well over a century ago:

> What we call the immediate cause of a phenomenon is nothing but the physical and material conditions in which it exists or appears. The object of the experimental method and the limit of every scientific research is therefore

* "Vaccination: a Sacrament of Modern Medicine," *Journal of the American Institute of Homeopathy* 84:96, December 1991

the same for living as for inanimate bodies. It consists in finding the relations which connect every phenomenon with its immediate cause, or putting it differently, which define the conditions necessary for its appearance. When the experimenter succeeds in learning the necessary causes of a phenomenon, he is in some sense its *master:* he can predict its course and appearance; he can promote or prevent it at will.

As a corollary to the above, neither physiologists nor physicians must imagine it their task to seek the cause of life or the essence of disease: that would be entirely wasting one's time in pursuing a phantom. The words "life," "death," "health," and "disease" have no objective reality. Only the vital phenomenon exists, with its material conditions. That is the one thing that they can study and know.[3]

Precisely as Bernard foresaw, the search for identifiable components of human structure and function, and for powerful technologies to control them, has obscured both the need for and the possibility of any unifying concept of life or health against which to judge them. Thus to be considered effective by present standards, vaccines need satisfy only two very minimal statistical criteria, i. e., reducing the incidence of the corresponding natural diseases substantially, and demonstrating measurable blood levels of specific antibodies to them for long periods of time. They have become sacraments of our faith in biotechnology in the sense that their safety and efficacy are widely seen as self-evident, and requiring no further proof; that they are given automatically to everyone, by force if necessary, and always in the name of the public good; and that they ritually initiate our loyal participation in the medical enterprise as a whole.

In short, they celebrate our right and our power as a civilization, to manipulate biological processes, for profit and more or less at will, without undue concern for or even an explicit concept of the total health of the populations about to be subjected to them. For that reason, I want to re-examine and update the major concerns of my previous article[4] from this quasi-theological standpoint. Now as then, I have mostly a lot of *questions* to offer, questions so thorny and difficult that years and even decades of careful investigation and painstaking research will be needed to disentangle them. But they seem so basic and important that it would be reckless indeed to require vaccination of every newborn child without adequate measures being taken to address them. Until then, my position remains simply to make the vaccines *optional* and freely available to all at the discretion of their parents, as is now the rule in the UK and other European countries.

A Brief History of the Measles Vaccine.

I want to begin with the dramatic career of the measles vaccine, which highlights a great many issues that are pertinent to the others as well. In its natural state, the measles virus enters the body of a susceptible person through the nose and mouth, and incubates silently for about 14 days, first in the tonsils and lymphoid tissues of the nasopharynx, then in the regional lymph nodes of the head and neck, and finally in the liver, spleen, bone marrow, and the lymphocytes and macrophages of the peripheral blood. The illness known as "the measles" is the process by which the virus is expelled from the blood, through the same orifices by which it entered, and involves a massive and concerted effort of the entire immune system. Once specific antibodies have succeeded in targeting the virus, the ability to synthesize them on short notice remains as a coded "memory" of the whole experience, and a virtual guarantee that those who have recovered from the measles will never get it again, no matter how many times they are re-exposed.

In addition to conferring this *specific* immunity, the process of mounting and recovering from a major illness like the measles also "primes" the immune system non-specifically, to respond promptly and efficiently to other microbial infections in the future. A crucial step in the maturation of a healthy immune system, the ability to mount a vigorous, acute response to infection unquestionably represents a fundamental ingredient of optimal health and well-being in general.

Finally, measles is about 20% fatal in populations exposed to it for the first time. It has required many centuries of adaptation for us to convert it into an ordinary disease of childhood, such that, when I first encountered it at the age of six, non-specific mechanisms were already in place to help me deal with it effectively. In that larger sense, the lifelong specific and nonspecific immunity each of us acquires from mounting and recovering from the natural disease represents an absolute and substantial net gain for the total health of the race as well.

However the vaccines may act inside the human body, true natural immunity in both these senses cannot be ascribed to them: their effectiveness is merely a statistic, and the resulting "immunity" a narrowly-defined technicality. In contrast with the natural disease, the attenuated vaccine virus is designed to produce no local sensitization at the portal of entry, no massive outpouring of the immune system as a whole, and no acute disease of any kind. It can elicit long-term antibody production solely by surviving in latent form within the lymphocytes, macrophages, and plasma cells of the peripheral blood and blood-forming organs. The considerable technical feat of providing these antibodies thus becomes a memory of the *chronic* infection, and the price we must pay for them is simply that we have no way of getting rid of them. Nobody would be foolish enough to argue that vaccines render us "immune" to viruses if in fact they merely weakened our ability to expel them, and forced us to harbor them chronically instead. On the contrary, such a long-term carrier state would also tend to compromise our ability to respond to *other* infections as well, and would have to be regarded as *immunosuppressive* to that extent.

The laws mandating vaccination against the measles were enacted in the 1960's, when the disease was limited almost entirely to children in elementary school, and deaths and serious complications had already reached an all-time low. The decision appears to have been made purely as a matter of *policy,* as soon as the vaccine became available; and with very little public debate, and very few people requesting exemptions, the compliance rate averaged well over 95%. From an average of over 400,00 cases annually in the pre-vaccine era, the incidence of measles in the United States dropped to less than 5000 by the early 1980's,[4,5] and it looked as though the disease would soon be eliminated.

In the 1980's, however, this comforting scenario began to unravel, as measles began to reappear even in fully-vaccinated populations, and public health authorities grappled with the mysterious phenomenon of "vaccine failure." In 1984, for example, 27 cases were reported at a high school in Waltham, Mass., where more than 98% of the students had been vaccinated.[6] Over a 3-month period in 1985, 157 cases were reported in Corpus Christi and the surrounding Nueces County, Texas, notwithstanding a vaccination rate of over 99% and supposedly "immune" antibody titers in over 95%.[7] In 1989, a High School in Illinois with documented vaccination records for 99.7% of the students nevertheless reported 69 cases over a 3-week period.[8] In all three outbreaks, the authors concentrated on the documented vaccination rates, and curiously neglected to mention the number of actual cases that had *not* been vaccinated. But they convincingly refuted the conventional assumption of a "reservoir" of the disease in the unvaccinated, an argument still popular with pediatricians and health departments alike for browbeating wavering parents into compliance.

As the data were collected and analyzed, tentative generalizations were made, and new strategies formulated. A survey of over 15,000 Canadian cases in 1985-86 indicated that 60% of the patients had documented vaccination records, 285 were "unvaccinated," and 12% were listed as "unknown,"[9] which presumably refers to those who claimed to have been vaccinated but were unable to prove it. A comparable American survey of over 9000 cases in 152 separate outbreaks in the same 2-year period yielded similar results:

1) a large majority (69%) were children in school, 5 to 19 years of age;

2) of these school-age kids, 60% had been "appropriately vaccinated" at 15 months or older, the schedule then in vogue, and another 20% had been vaccinated "inappropriately, " at 12 to 14 months, the schedule approved before 1979, with the exact number of unvaccinated children again oddly omitted; and

3) a significant minority of the total cases (26%) were children less than 5 years of age, mostly unvaccinated and belonging to black, Hispanic, and other indigent minorities in urban ghettoes.[10]

These data indicated a partial resurgence of the disease, mainly in older children and adolescents of high-school and college age, groups with much higher rates of serious complications. The favored explanation was simply that vaccine-mediated immunity was temporary, and "wore off" with increasing age, presumably leaving the child otherwise unaffected, and susceptible as before, an assumption which also, although rarely stated as such, provided the main rationale for re-vaccinating at a later date.

Unfortunately, this assumption had already been disproved by an earlier study, which demonstrated quite conclusively that previously vaccinated children with declining antibody titers responded only minimally and for an unacceptably short time to booster doses of the measles vaccine.[11] Another refutation came from a sustained outbreak of 235 cases in Dane County, Wisconsin, over a 9-month period in 1986. Along the same lines as in earlier studies, the authors found that the majority of cases were in children of school age (5 to 19), but that only 6% of these had not been vaccinated.[12] They were even more surprised by the sizeable number who developed "mild measles," with a typical measles rash, but little or no fever or systemic symptoms, a syndrome that was much commoner in vaccinated kids who lacked measles antibodies than in those who were unvaccinated, or those who had antibody titers that were read as "immune," both of whom were far more likely to develop the typical acute disease. Although the authors themselves failed to draw the inference, this paradoxical result suggested some kind of inapparent or latent activity of the vaccine virus that had not been suspected before, and that serological testing failed to detect.

Despite these warnings, none of these investigators seems to have taken seriously the possibility that the immunity conferred by the vaccines might not be genuine. Like the repeated bouts of chemotherapy for advanced cancer patients after the preceding rounds have failed, the purely quantitative redefinition of immunity cleared the way for simple escalation of force as needed, to approximate the desired goal. In the past three years, the policy of revaccination has carried the day, despite all the logical, scientific, and ethical considerations against it, and justified to some extent by the recent spread of the disease among unvaccinated minority infants in low-income urban neighborhoods.

In 1988, for example, over 500 cases were reported in Los Angeles County, more than 17% of the total nationwide, of whom about 65% were under 5 years old, 77% were Hispanic, and 38% were less than 16 months old,[13] the date at which the vaccine is usually given! These data have been used effectively to bully state legislatures into allocating more funds, and local officials into tighter enforcement of vaccination laws in minority districts. In such relatively higher-incidence areas, even lowering the vaccination age to 9 months has been recommended, an idea that brings us back full-circle to the pre-1979 era, when large numbers of kids were "inappropriately vaccinated" according to similar guidelines, as we saw.

Finally, although these considerations apply solely to the measles vaccine, both the medical and public health authorities are presently advocating revaccination against mumps and rubella vaccine as well, for no better reason than that the triple MMR vaccine is the only one still commonly available, but are not yet in agreement as to the proper age, leaving state legislatures to decide for themselves. Thus the American Academy of Family Practice currently advocates a second MMR booster at 4 to 6 years of age,[14] while a bill before the Ohio legislature mandates documented proof of revaccination before entering the seventh grade.[15] The obvious implication is that the extra dose can't possibly hurt, so there's no reason not to throw in the mumps and rubella vaccines as well.

The DPT Story.

The DPT vaccine was the first to be developed and marketed on a large scale, and still remains the major battlefront of the vaccine controversy in the United States, as well as the area in which most of my own experience with vaccine-related illness has so far been concentrated. Thanks largely to parent organizations like Dissatisfied Parents Together (DPT), and books like *A Shot in the Dark,* by Harris Coulter and Barbara Loe Fisher,[16] the plight of vaccine-injured children and their families is at last being recognized and taken seriously by the general public.

In 1986, despite intensive lobbying efforts by the vaccine manufacturers, the American Academy of Pediatrics, and other medical and public health authorities, Congress enacted the National Childhood Vaccine Injury Act, which directs the Public Health Service to investigate all reports of vaccine injury, and to formulate guidelines for compensation.[17] Unfortunately, both the PHS and the Centers for Disease Control, its subsidiary agency, are funded mainly to advocate and enforce the same mandates that the Act charges them to investigate, and can therefore be expected and indeed relied upon to minimize the risks.

The official compensation guidelines accordingly rule out every condition other than the few already identified, namely, "collapse," anaphylaxis, and encephalopathy, or "brain damage," as well as everything of a persistent or chronic nature, unless it appears in less than 7 days after the vaccination.[18] Even these massive exclusions are insufficient for many leading vaccine proponents, who still adamantly refuse to accept any connection at all between even the most egregious cases of encephalopathy and the DPT.[19,20]

Since these guidelines were published and put into effect, the unit cost of the DPT has skyrocketed, as have the number and size of personal injury awards against the vaccine manufacturers, with the result that many pediatricians are privately willing to give the DT alone if the parents insist. Meanwhile, whooping cough itself has made a bit of a comeback in recent years, the CDC reporting 10,500 cases in the years 1986-88,[21] and once again, as with measles, the bureaucratic language effectively conceals the true demographics. Thus, of the cases with known vaccination status, 63% had been "inappropriately immunized," and 34% had not been vaccinated at all. From these figures, we are meant to infer that the vaccine is highly effective, with very few cases in the vaccinated group.

Only by reading the fine print do we learn that those whose vaccination status was "unknown," a whopping 7700 cases, actually comprised more than 70% of the total. With even its chief proponents conceding the DPT to be among the least effective of all the vaccines, it is a safe bet that "inappropriately vaccinated" means simply having received 1 to 4 doses, but not the full 5 required for entrance to kindergarten, while "status unknown" once again refers to those claiming to have been fully vaccinated but lacking documentary proof. Indeed, after reporting several cases in infants less than 2 months old, a Philadelphia pediatrician recently advocated that the vaccine be given even earlier, ideally "as soon after birth as possible."[22] The sacramental status of vaccines is thus widely interpreted by public health authorities as blanket authorization for vaccinating almost anyone against anything at any time.

Other Vaccines.

The same generic faith continues to bless the pharmaceutical industry in its hugely profitable quest for more and more new vaccines, often for no more compelling reason than its technical capacity to make them. Thus in the late 1980's, a vaccine was introduced against *Hæmophilus influenzæ B,* an organism associated with scattered outbreaks of bacterial meningitis in overcrowded day-care facilities. At first purely optional for pre-schoolers from 2 to 4 years old, it was eventually made compulsory for *all* infants, even those who never need day care, and is presently given at or before 18 months, in some cases before the first birthday.

Always primarily a disease of adults using IV drugs, hepatitis B inevitably found its way into blood banks, and thus became a more or less institutionalized risk of hospitalized patients requiring transfusions of whole blood, plasma, and other blood products. While the Hep B vaccine was actually developed in the 1970's, the medical authorities have never figured out how to target the IV drug subculture in a selective fashion. So when the disease began propagating through the blood banks, the favored solution, as always, is simply to vaccinate *everybody*. In the past few months, the American Academy of Pediatrics and the CDC have accordingly decided to mandate Hep B vaccination for all newborn babies,[23] and are still trying to decide whether to give it at birth, or with the DPT at 2 months of age. It remains to be seen if the American public, already increasingly upset over the vaccination issue, will simply acquiesce in this latest baptism of the newly born, explicitly intended as their very first immunological experience.

While still theoretically optional, comparable transubstantiations are also available at the other end of life. Originally intended and still widely promoted for reducing the risk of pneumonia and death among the elderly, especially in nursing homes and extended-care facilities, the influenza and pneumococcus vaccines have not been very popular with that demographic, and a number of studies have shown them to be ineffective as well.[24,25] In 1978, the dreaded swine flue epidemic never materialized, large numbers of vaccinees developed the crippling Guillain-Barré polyneuritis, and the American public began to question the *concept* of vaccination openly for the first time. Yet the elderly and infirm continue to be pressured heavily to accept these rejects on a yearly basis, as a form of extreme unction against both diseases.

Thus the search goes on, seemingly without limit, now indissolubly linked to the biotechnology industry. Currently in the works are vaccines against Group A streptococci, the common cold, and bronchiolitis, all of which are being bred into the gene pool of mice, rats, baboons, and other experimental animals, without any discernible caution, restraint, or regulation. Not far off, a fitting *dénouement* is the AIDS vaccine, which is monstrous even in principle, inasmuch as those at risk are already seriously immunocompromised, so that a suppressive vaccine would not only increase *their* chances of getting it, but would also help to soften up the general population as well.

Some Vaccine Cases.

With that as background, I want to speak about some of my own patients, with illnesses traceable to the DPT vaccine, the one I am most familiar with. Because the link is often far from easy to document, and indeed may not even be suspected until long after the fact, I have no doubt that other vaccines will prove to be equally important clinically, once we learn better how to recognize and look for them.

By no means least of what homeopathic medicine has to teach is the reaffirmation of the individual patient as the bearer of what the physician needs to know. Whereas modern medicine seeks to define itself quantitatively, as a series of technologies powerful enough to manipulate and control antibody levels and other key variables, the homeopathic vision is essentially *qualitative,* matching the unique ensemble of signs and symptoms in each patient with the equally characteristic totality of the medicine that most closely resembles it. I offer the following cases as evidence for the speculations and hypotheses I have so far proposed, because they are the ultimate source of them as well.

Although the DPT has already been implicated in brain damage and a variety of other neuropathic syndromes, as we saw, which are themselves amenable to homeopathic treatment to some extent, today I want to concentrate on illnesses that are less serious, but also much commoner, easier to understand, and more representative of the problem as a whole. Both involving high fevers of unknown origin that were cured by a single dose of the vaccine nosode, my very first DPT cases illustrate the thought process whereby various symptoms may be added to the clinical picture of any given vaccine. Although ideally the history must also show that the child has never been well since one or more DPT injections, this connection may not be obvious or even suspected, unless specific questions are asked to elicit it.

In some cases, an abnormal white count and differential may give independent pathological confirmation, while other examples include tender or enlarged posterior auricular and suboccipital nodes for rubella, parotid swellings for mumps, and the like. Naturally, acute symptoms like fever, that seem aberrant or unusual to the parents, are more suspicious and easier to trace. But only a curative response to the corresponding nosode suffices to prove that the illness in question was specifically related to the vaccine.

> **Case 1.** A baby girl of 8 months had had 3 episodes of high fever, typically 105° or more, but lasting 48 hours at most. During the second episode, she was hospitalized for tests, but her pediatrician found nothing. Each time she felt well afterwards, and appeared to be growing and developing normally. The only other inormation I was able to elicit from the mother was that the episodes had occurred exactly one month apart, and that the first episode had come just one month after the last of her DPT shots, which had likewise been given at one-month intervals. Recognizing this coincidence further helped her to recall that similar episodes had also occurred after each injection, but the pediatrician had advised her to ignore them, since fever is the most common reaction to the vaccine. I therefore gave the girl one dose of the homeopathic remedy *DPT* 10M, prepared from the vaccine, and the child never had another episode.

> **Case 2.** A 9-month-old baby girl was brought in with a fever of 105° and very few other symptoms. Two previous episodes had occurred at irregular intervals, and the parents, who already felt ambivalent about vaccinations in general, had given her only one DPT shot, especially since the first episode came less than 2 weeks after it. For the next 48 hours, I tried several acute remedies without success, and finally ordered a CBC. With a white count of 32,000, the differential showed 43% lymphs, 11% monos. 25% neutrophils, many with toxic granulations, and 20% immature band forms. A pediatrician friend who looked at the slide immediately identified it as pertussis. After *DPT* 10M, the fever came down in 2 hours, and the girl has been entirely well since.

These cases are noteworthy for two reasons: first, because they both exhibited a characteristic symptom or keynote of the DPT vaccine, namely, high fever; and second, because their responses were strong and healthy, such that their illnesses, while recurrent, quickly resolved without sequelæ. But, like the brain-damaged cases, they are also the exception, rather than the rule, and instructive mainly in contrast to the others, which are less specific and therefore more difficult to trace.

In all the remaining cases, the vaccine appeared to act *nonspecifically,* either by exacerbating an already established chronic condition, or by casting a long shadow over the background of a chronic condition that did not materialize until later. Because excellent results were obtained with the usual constitutional or miasmatic remedies employed in such conditions, the specific nosode was often not needed, so the vaccine connection could not always be proved. In other cases, the nosode was useful later, in removing a "block," i.e., when seemingly well-indicated remedies didn't work, or failed to hold or act deeply.

In general, these cases are reminiscent of the way that grief, physical injury, or some other stress simply exacerbates the pre-existing "miasmatic" or chronic disease structure, rather than substituting the specific picture of *Ignatia, Arnica,* or other remedies illustrating a "never well since" pattern. In another subgroup, those symptoms specific to the vaccine and those already latent or pre-existing in the patient come all mixed up together, and begin to disentangle only as the treatment develops. But far from being restricted to any particular category, vaccine-related illnesses encompass the full range of chronic diseases seen in children, from asthma, allergies, and otitis media, far and away the commonest in my practice, to learning disabilities and emotional and behavior problems.

Case 3. A girl of 6 was brought in for being "sick all the time," especially with ear infections, which she had had repeatedly since the age of 5 months, when she was given antibiotics continuously for 4 months. Especially vulnerable in the fall, and with abrupt changes in the weather, she would often become "grumpy" when ill, and lost her appetite, but rarely had fever or earache. Although showing no obvious reaction to her regular DPT shots at 2, 4, 6, and 18 months, she had had another ear infection for 4 months straight soon after her last one, just before entering first grade. Over the next 18 months, she did beautifully on *Sulphur, Pulsatilla,* and *Mercurius,* coming down with colds and acute illnesses at times,but responding well to these remedies, never needing antibiotics, and seeming entirely well in between. Three years later, her mother called to report that she had not missed a day of school since, and required no further treatment.

Case 4. A 5-year-old girl was brought in for treatment of seasonal asthma, which had begun the previous spring, did not respond very well to the usual drugs, and worried the parents in view of their own allergic histories. Soon after weaning at 13 months, her health problems began in earnest, with protracted ear infections, often associated with teething, and always requiring antibiotics.

While her first series of vaccinations provoked no obvious reaction, she had recently developed pneumonia with a high fever two weeks after her 5-year DPT booster, followed by the return of her asthma, for the first time in the dead of winter. After two years of treatment with *Arsenicum album, Phosphorus,* and *Lachesis,* her health steadily improved, to the point that she no longer needed drugs or remedies, and the nosode was never given.

Case 5. A 2-year-old boy was brought in for treatment of recurrent ear infections that tended to drag on for months, and responded only temporarily to antibiotics. His first one followed a URI at 6 months of age, and was picked up at a routine office visit with no symptoms whatsoever, although he often complained of earache at other times. But his worst illnesses had been acute episodes of high fever and prolonged screaming soon after his first two DPT shots, because of which he was given the DT only, with no obvious reaction. While his ear infections quickly subsided with infrequent doses of *Calcarea sulph.* and *Tuberculinum,* he developed intense jealousy and extreme tantrums around the birth of his baby sister a year later, and was finally given *DPT* 10M when the seemingly well-indicated remedies failed to help. Now 4 years old, he is healthy, free of ear infections, and continues to grow and develop normally.

Case 6. A baby girl of 10 months was brought in with acute otitis media, high fever, earache, and screaming, her 4th such attack since the age of 2 months, each one beginning soon after stopping the antibiotics from the one before. Weaned at 2 months, when her mother returned to work, she could not tolerate her milk-based formula, but did well on soy milk. When cranky behavior developed soon after her first DPT shot, and the first ear infection followed close behind, she was given only the DT thereafter, and didn't seem to react to it, but the ear infections went on as before. These stopped readily enough after *Chamomilla* and *Calcarea carbonica,* but recurred 8 months later, when her parents separated, and she received the MMR while visiting her father. Again she did beautifully on remedies, mainly *Lycopodium* and *Sulphur,* despite occasional relapses, like the one that followed soon after a DPT booster that her father insisted on, which ended only after the DPT nosode was given. Over the past 4 years, I have continued to see her after further relapses that coincided with visits to her father, who plied her with dairy, vaccines, and antibiotics. Yet she remains fundamentally healthy, with longer and longer intervals in between.

Case 7. After 5 episodes of otitis media, all treated with antibiotics, a 16-month-old boy was referred to me for constitutional treatment. Colicky for the first three months, he developed acute otitis with fever at six months, but all the subsequent episodes were afebrile. He also reacted violently to his first DPT shot, with vomiting and "hard crying," somewhat less so to the second, with general malaise and "sad crying," and not at all to the third, or the MMR, which had just been given the week before I saw him. I gave him one dose of *Sulphur* 10M, and within 3 days he ran a high fever with diarrhea, from which he soon recovered. Next he was given *Calcarea carb.* 10M, 1 dose, and *Calcarea sulph.* 12C, to be used p. r. n. for a threatened or actual cold, and he had no more ear infections and no more remedies for well over a year. I then repeated the *Sulphur,* and he has been well for the past 3 years. The nosode was never needed.

Case 8. A boy of 3 had never reacted to any vaccination, and appeared to be in good health until about 8 months before seeing me, when he contracted a flu-like illness, followed by otitis media, for which antibiotics were prescribed. According to his mother, he seemed lethargic and "not himself" while taking them, with outbursts of stuttering and a foul diarrhea, from which *Giardia lamblia* was isolated. At this point no gamma-globulins could be found in his serum, and he had to be given transfusions on a regular basis. Over the next 6 months he was given *Influenzinum, Stramonium, Cuprum,* and then *Sulphur* the following year. Within a few weeks of starting the treatment, his serum proteins rose dramatically, the stuttering subsided, and he continued to improve steadily after that. The transfusions were discontinued after a year, and he has remained well since. No one vaccine was clearly implicated, and no nosodes were needed, but total unresponsiveness to vaccines and general immune collapse are two similar paths whereby any vaccine could act non-specifically to weaken the immune system of a sensitive individual.

Case 9. A girl of 15 months was brought in for repeated ear infections and courses of antibiotics since her first episode at 4 months of age. Associated with typical URI symptoms, ear involvement was often accompanied by pain, but she had never had a fever in her life. An hour after her first DPT shot, she awoke from a nap screaming, and soon developed her first cold. The same thing happened after the second dose, with her first earache 2 days later, which coincided with her mother going back to work and putting her on a milk-based formula. A similar episode followed her third DPT, and this time the eardrums did not improve from antibiotic treatment, but the mother tried homeopathy only when myringotomy was proposed 8 months later. Responding almost miraculously to *Calcarea carbonica,* the girl cut 3 teeth almost immediately, and her ears cleared up, but she later developed persistent diarrhea after a bottle of cow's milk. At this point I gave her the DPT nosode, and within an hour she developed a high fever, the first in her life, the diarrhea was gone the next day, and her health has continued to improve ever since, with no ear infetctions and no other remedies needed for the past 5 years.

As documented in many of these cases, the evolution and natural history of otitis media in recent years exactly parallels the theoretical concerns we discussed above. As a medical student in the early 1960's, I saw acute ear infections daily in the Emergency Room, with high fever and violent earache. Almost always, they responded to penicillin at levels of 100,000 units daily, or less. If the eardrum had already burst, as often happened, the children recovered promptly and completely without any treatment at all.

Today, although such cases are still seen occasionally, otitis media is predominantly a chronic or relapsing illness, with significantly less fever and pain than in the past. In a surprisingly large number of cases, there are no symptoms whatsoever, and the diagnosis is made solely by otoscope at the time of a routine examination. For no doubt the same reasons, it is also much less likely either to heal spontaneously or to respond favorably to antibiotics, has a much greater tendency to relapse after the drugs are stopped, and is more often associated with residual symptoms, such as behavior problems, learning disabilities, swollen tonsils, and hearing loss. Recent studies also indicate that myringotomy tubes inserted to facilitate drainage, the most advanced technology yet available, are themselves an important cause of permanent hearing loss, the same risk that is always invoked to justify them.[26]

To be sure, many immunosuppressive factors other than vaccines must also be considered, such as the widespread use of antibiotics, the inevitable development of resistant organisms, urban and industrial pollution, and doubtless many more. But my fear is that any other chronic disease of children will tell the same tale. In addition to their specific effects, only a very few of which have so far been identified, I suspect that every vaccine probably has non-specific effects of an auto-immune or immunosuppressive type, which would look quite different for each individual patient, but would all involve favoring *chronic* responses at the expense of acute ones, i. e., having to do with "style," rather than specific *content*. Certainly for the DPT vaccine, and I daresay for the others as well, the net will have to be widened to include enuresis, asthma, eczema, allergies, sinusitis, nervous and mental diseases, auto-immune phenomena, cancer, and indeed the entire spectrum of pediatric and adult medicine.

Research.

In conclusion, I want to address the most important and difficult problem of all, namely, the research that will have to be done in the future, and the political will that will be required to carry it out. Both of these aspects are inseparably connected, and both will need radically new models to succeed. Since current studies ignore the chronic dimension entirely, and therefore *preclude* any concept of the total health picture of an individual over the lifetime, they cannot provide unambiguous information about how vaccines act. At the same time, well-controlled scientific investigations of vaccines, based on the totality of signs and symptoms that they produce, will obviously require a large population of unvaccinated kids, precisely what the existing laws are designed to prevent. To those parents who decide *not* to vaccinate we therefore owe a considerable debt of gratitude.

Moreover, the standard accusation that unvaccinated children help to propagate the corresponding natural diseases and thus threaten the rest of the population cuts both ways. For if that argument were true, it would also mean that the vaccines are ineffective by their own test; and conversely, if the "immunity" they conferred were genuine and long-lasting, then the unvaccinated kids would pose a threat only to themselves.

Furthermore, it will not be possible to study each vaccine independently unless we legally authorize parents to choose some vaccines, but not others. At present, even the most liberal states allow parents to refuse *all* vaccines, on religious or philosophical grounds, but not to make informed medical decisions for their children. Once vaccines are made totally optional, as in the UK and various other countries, the experimental and control groups can become purely self-selecting for each vaccine, with those receiving it matched as closely as possible to those exempted. Once these groups are in place, it will be necessary to follow them prospectively for at least a generation, if not a whole lifetime. For the present, pilot studies could also be done retrospectively, using kids with known vaccination histories.

But by far the most difficult and important questions are the theoretical one of *what* to measure, and the technical one of *how* to measure it, which are of course thoroughly interconnected. As homeopathic clinicians, we already have a reasonably good sense of how to ascertain a

107

working totality of symptoms that is tailored to our individual patients, and how to follow them over extended periods of time. In studying large populations, we will need to identify a few key variables that are broad and inclusive enough to reflect the most fundamental aspects of human functioning, yet also flexible enough to accommodate the infinite richness and diversity of real people. Which ones we choose will then further determine and be determined by the techniques with sufficient detail and precision for measuring them. Probably this means that we won't really know what we need to measure without first following a much smaller pilot group very closely for a shorter period of time, perhaps 4 or 5 years, and just see what happens to them. In any case, what I shall call the homeopathic *agenda,* ascertaining the total health picture of the individual over time, is still the best available methodology for such an investigation, and any progress that we can make toward achieving it will also inevitably contribute to a more fruitful design in biomedicine generally.

How, then, are we to investigate the total health picture of large populations over extended periods of time? Clearly, to begin with, we need to follow the outline of a standard medical history, regarding the incidence and severity of both usual and unusual acute and chronic diseases. Regular physical and laboratory examinations might also reveal persistent or subclinical changes of a more "constitutional" or chronic variety, analogous to the swollen nodes of rubella, inflamed parotids for mumps, abnormal WBC and differential counts for pertussis, and so forth, as well as global and nonspecific developmental criteria (height, weight, dentition, nursing behavior, gross and fine motor co-ordination, vision, hearing, etc. Other important variables lying to some extent outside the medical history *per se* would include intelligence testing, language development, family and school socialization, and other demographic, socioeconomic, and psychological factors (poverty, race, learning disabilities, mood, behavior, and temperament, and school attendance and performance).

At the other extreme, pilot studies of the pneumococcal and influenza vaccines might require only a few simple variables, since they are given primarily to elderly people at high risk or in nursing homes, when their chronic disease structure is already more or less firmly established.

Under these circumstances, a reasonable first approximation of how these vaccines act might be simply to measure their effect on the *life span,* the sheer ability to survive, compared to that of their unvaccinated friends, neighbors, and peer group.

Finally, I want to say a few words about why, in spite of the very real and present dangers I have been discussing, and many others that could as well be mentioned, I remain strangely optimistic about the future of the healing arts, and indeed of homeopathy in particular. The chief reason has to do with the growing awareness of ordinary people taking more responsibility for their health, including their transactions with the medical system as a whole. In the United States, the vast and growing movement for free choice in health care now includes not only groups critical of mandatory vaccination, like DPT, but also supporters of midwifery, home birth, homeopathy, and other forms of "alternative" or complementary medicine, and the right to die with dignity and self-determination. Within the last 10 years or so, these groups have already helped bring about substantial changes in the doctor-patient relationship. With even the vaunted American economy manifestly unable to afford the top-heavy medical system now in place, no matter how it is financed, it is virtually certain that these changes will continue to accelerate, and that organized medicine will face still more bruising reversals, until it accepts them.

In the meantime, lest you suppose that I am opposed to religious concepts of any kind in medicine, I propose the following three aphorisms of Paracelsus, the great Renaissance physician and alchemist, as a practical and ecumenical theology of healing that health professionals and lay people of every persuasion can accept and live by, without having to ram them down anybody's throat:

> The art of healing comes from Nature, not the physician . . .
> Every illness has its own remedy within itself . . .
> A man could not be born alive and healthy were there not already a
> Physician hidden in him.[27]

Taken together, these sayings encompass most of what the present medical system has tended to leave out, and I interpret them roughly as follows:

1. Healing implies wholeness.

The verb "to heal" comes from the same Anglo-Saxon root as "whole." Meaning simply to make whole [again], "healing" is a basic attribute of all living systems, and is evident not only in wound healing and spontaneous recovery from illness, but in effective medical and surgical treatment as well. As a concerted response of the entire organism, it implies a living totality, a qualitative integration on a deeper level than can be defined by any assemblage of parts, or approximated by any purely quantitative measurement.

2. All healing is self-healing.

As a fundamental property of all biological systems, healing proceeds continuously throughout life, and often completes itself spontaneously, with or without outside help. This means that all healing is ultimately self-healing; that the role of physicians and other professional or designated "healers" is essentially to assist and enhance the natural process that is already under way, not to interfere with it; and that the mechanical correction of abnormalities, while still legitimate and useful under certain circumstances, earns that legitimacy by virtue of this prior standard.

3. Healing pertains solely to individuals.

Always possible, but also problematic, even risky, healing applies only to individuals in unique, here-and-now situations, rather than to abstract "diseases," principles, or categories. In other words, it is inescapably an art, and can (and should) never be reduced to a mere technique or procedure, however scientific its formulation.

To these I would add a fourth of my own devising, which is not exactly theological, but feels like a political and legal right, in the spirit of Magna Carta and the American Bill of Rights:

Health, illness, birth, and death are inalienable life experiences belonging wholly to the people undergoing them, which nobody else has the right to manipulate or control without their explicit request, or that of somebody duly authorized by them to act on their behalf.

My concluding principle was contributed by Lao-Tse, and provides an appropriate "bottom-line" criterion:

A leader is best when people hardly know he exists,
Not so good when they obey and acclaim him,
And worst when they despise him.
Of a good leader, when his work is done and his aim fulfilled,
The people will say, "We did this ourselves."[28]

NOTES.

1. Tyler, A., *London Evening Standard* Magazine, September, 1991, p. 74.
2. Mendelsohn, R., *Confessions of a Medical Heretic,* Contemporary, Chicago, 1979, p. xiv.
3. Bernard, C., *An Introduction to the Study of Experimental Medicine,* Dover, New York, 1957, pp. 65-67, *passim.*
4. Cherry, J., "The New Epidemiology of Measles and Rubella," *Hospital Practice,* July 1980.
5. Markowitz, L., et al., "Patterns of Transmission in Measles Outbreaks in the U. S.," *New England Journal of Medicine* 320:77, 12 January 1989.
6. Nkowane, B., et al., *American Journal of Public Health* 77:434, 1987.
7. Gustafson, T., et al., "Measles Outbreak in a Fully-Immunized Secondary-School Population," *New England Journal of Medicine* 316:771, 26 March 1987.
8. Chen, R., et al., *American Journal of Epidemiology* 129:173, 1989.
9. *Medical Tribune,* 26 August 1987, p. 2.
10. Markowitz, *op. cit.,* pp. 75-81.
11. Cherry, *op. cit.,* p. 52.
12. Edmondson, M., et al., "Mild Measles and Secondary Vaccine Failure During a Sustained Outbreak in a Highly-Vaccinated Population," *Journal of the AMA* 262:2467, 9 May 1990.
13. "Measles: Los Angeles County, 1988," MMWR Report, *Journal of the AMA* 261:1111, 24 February 1989.
14. *Family Practice News,* 1 April 1990, p. 3.
15. LSC 119 0411-1, Sub. H. B. 168, Ohio General Assembly, 1991-92.
16. Coulter, H., and Fisher, B. L., *A Shot in the Dark,* Harcourt Brace Jovanovich, 1985.
17. "Vaccine Adverse Event Reporting System (VAERS)," Public Health Service, 1986.
18. "Reportable Events Following Vaccination," VAERS, *op. cit.*
19. Griffin, R., et al., "The Risk of Seizures and Encephalopathy after Immunization with the DPT Vaccine," *Journal of the AMA* 263:1641, 23 March 1990.

20. Cherry, J., "Pertussis Vaccine Encephalopathy: It's Time to Recognize It as the Myth That It Is," Editorial, *Journal of the AMA* 263: 1679, 23 March 1990.
21. "Pertussis Surveillance: United States, 1986-88, MMWR Report, *Journal of the AMA* 263: 1058, 23 February 1990.
22. *Family Practice News,* 15 November 1990, p. 6.
23. *Boston Globe,* 11 June 1991, p. 1.
24. *Medical World News,* 14 April 1986, p. 53.
25. Simberkoff, M., et al., "Efficacy of Pneumococcal Vaccine in High-Risk Patients," *New England Journal of Medicine* 313:1318, 20 November 1986.
26. *Family Practice News,* 15 December 1990, p. 1.
27. *Selected Writings of Paracelsus,* Pantheon, New York, 1958, pp. 50, 76.
28. Lao Tzu, *The Way of Life,* trans. W. Bynner, Perigee, New York, p. 46.

Hidden in Plain Sight:
The Rôle of Vaccines in Chronic Disease*

Introduction.

Thirty-five years of medical practice have convinced me that all vaccines carry an important risk of chronic disease that is inherent in the vaccination process and indeed central to how they work. Yet the growing concerns of parents and legislators and media reports about them rarely if ever elicit anything beyond automatic denials by medical and public health authorities alike. Reflecting on this glaring discrepancy is the main focus of this essay. Writing these lines has also helped me appreciate how much the invisibility heightens the risk and how intimately these phenomena are connected, like mirror-images of the same reality, which makes it imperative to study them together.

Since I am mainly a clinician, I will begin with a story. It concerns a 12-year-old boy whom I know of solely from his mother's letter, but her words are so heartfelt and so congruent with the rest of my experience that I cannot doubt their veracity:

> My son Adam was healthy until his first MMR at 15 months. Within 2 weeks he had flu and cold symptoms, which persisted for 6 weeks, his eyes became puffy, and he was hospitalized with nephrotic syndrome. A renal biopsy showed "focal sclerosing glomerulonephritis," but he didn't respond to steroids. I asked if it could be related to the vaccine, but they told me it couldn't, and we accepted that. Over the next 4 years he was hospitalized repeatedly but finally went into remission, seeming normal and healthy, and stayed off all medications for 5 years.
>
> When he turned 10, his pediatrician recommended a booster, saying that a rise in measles cases made it dangerous for him not to be protected. I checked the PDR and other sources but found no warning for kidney disease and no listing of it as an adverse reaction, so I agreed to it. In less than 2 weeks he relapsed, with 4+ proteinuria, swelling, and weight gain, signs that we recognized at once. He

* "Hidden in Plain Sight: the Rôle of Vaccines in Chronic Disease," *American Journal of Homeopathic Medicine* 98:15, Spring 2005.

was admitted in hypertensive crisis, with blood in the urine, fluid in the lungs, and massive weight gain. On Cytoxan, massive doses of Prednisone, and three other drugs he slowly improved, but missed another 7 months of school.

It's been 2 years since that horrible episode, and he still needs Captopril for high blood pressure and spills 4+ protein every day. The doctor says he sustained major kidney damage, will always need medication to control his blood pressure, and will worsen as he grows, necessitating a transplant eventually. This time I was convinced that his condition was related to the vaccine, but still the doctors didn't take me seriously and told me it was a coincidence.

I searched for information and even contacted the manufacturer of the vaccine. Finally they sent me two case reports of nephrotic syndrome following the MMR vaccine. It's very difficult for lay people to get information or even ask questions, since we don't use correct medical terms and feel stupid. Please tell me if my ideas are reasonable. I don't think my son could tolerate another episode, and I think he'd have normal blood pressure and kidney function if not for that second shot. I also have great concern for other children who develop nephrotic syndrome some weeks after receiving MMR and whose doctors never make the connection. They could all be at great risk if revaccinated. I realize that this letter has taken up a lot of your time, and I'd appreciate any help you can give me. Thank you.[1]

Like many others who seek my help, this woman honestly believed that her son had been crippled for life by the MMR vaccine, yet had no intention of suing the drug company who manufactured it, the doctors who administered it, or the Federal Vaccine Injury Compensation program, as she was legally entitled to do. Whether she didn't think she could win, a conclusion my experience would certainly justify, or simply was not a litigious person, as seems more relevant in her case, the absence of such motive only lends further credence to her story. She was writing to me simply to find a physician to hear and validate the truth of her experience, which neither the pediatrician who gave the shots, nor the specialists who treated Adam in the hospital, nor any of the other doctors she spoke to were willing to do. Although I had very little else to offer her, it was more than enough to earn her gratitude.

To those inclined to discredit such tales, I reply that the confidences our patients entrust to us represent the truth as they live it. Yet when vaccines are involved, such stories are routinely dismissed out of hand, as if they couldn't possibly be true or worthy of serious consideration. That was the reaction of every doctor involved in Adam's care, despite compelling evidence to the contrary, even after case reports were supplied by the drug company itself. Whether a canny strategy to defeat possible litigation or simply the instinctive shielding of a cherished world-view from the threat of change, this defensive and hostile stance is so pervasive in the medical profession as to merit careful study in itself.

Richard Horton, Editor of *The Lancet,* felt the sting of censorship himself after publishing an article linking cases of infantile autism and colitis to the MMR vaccine:

> Today vaccines are largely an untouchable subject, their benefits too obvious to be questioned. Any hint of dissent concerning their clinical effectiveness and overall social value is met with bitter rebuttal and resentment. A former President of the UK Academy of Medical Science actually threatened to get me sacked for publishing work that raised questions about the MMR vaccine, while at a dinner party years later, the partner of a government vaccine specialist asked, "Will you *ever* be forgiven?" Forgiven for *what,* I wondered?[2]

Dr. Horton himself neither believed in the research nor endorsed its conclusions. His only "mistake," if mistake it was, lay in permitting the author, a well-known British gastroenterologist, to publish his findings without regard for their political correctness. Needless to say, the snubs and threats he faced for rocking the boat were less serious than the reprisals exacted against the author, whose work was officially repudiated without testing it, and whose career at a London teaching hospital was abruptly terminated.[3]

Finally, Adam's misfortune obliges us to ask about the process by which "glomerulonephritis," "autism," "encephalopathy," or any other ailment is identified as a *bona fide* complication of a vaccine, such that the victim becomes eligible to receive damages in court. In spite of two reports of MMR nephritis documented by the manufacturer, renal failure is still not recognized as an adverse effect of the vaccine, an omission that undoubtedly helped Adam's doctors to frustrate his mother's inquiries.

Exactly similar editing characterizes the Federal guidelines for compensation of vaccine-injured patients, which would never have been enacted in the first place without the repeated insistence of their parents, and which continue to be pared down even further by the determined opposition of the vaccine manufacturers, the American Academy of Pediatrics, and other authoritative and influential pro-vaccine groups. As reflected in the official compensation guidelines, research studies of vaccine-related injuries are limited to a few extreme reactions to particular vaccines, because these alone occur often enough to attain statistical significance in large populations. Such a policy automatically disqualifies two much larger and partly overlapping classes of phenomena that my own experience and research have uncovered: 1) exacerbation of the ordinary chronic diseases of childhood, according to individual susceptibility, often representing 2) a nonspecific effect of the vaccination process in general, for which any vaccine will do.

Restricting the issue of vaccine safety to specific effects of specific vaccines is a major reason why the true extent of vaccine-related illness has always been invisible and will likely remain so until the question is reframed in a more comprehensive way.

An equally troubling problem with the approved list of vaccine-related injuries is their restriction in *time* to acute events occurring within a few days afterward,[4] i.e., soon enough for the vaccine to be regarded as the necessary and sufficient cause of the reaction, as if independently of any prior susceptibility. In Adam's case as in many others, vague, nondescript symptoms appeared soon after vaccination, but the full picture of nephritis did not emerge and could not be diagnosed until six weeks after the first shot and two weeks after the second, by which time it was no longer an acute or fixed injury, but already a chronic, self-sustaining *illness* that continued to develop and worsen over the years, so that a claim on his behalf would have doubtless been rejected even if it had been filed.

In what follows I will consider five aspects of the vaccine issue:

1) specific effects of specific vaccines, as described in the literature;

2) nonspecific effects of the vaccination process *per se,* based on cases from my own practice;

3) how vaccines actually work inside the human body;

4) several individual vaccines; and

5) implications for vaccine and health policy.

1. Specific Effects of Specific Vaccines.

The vaccination literature contains no mention of adverse effects of the process itself, but only a few documented effects of specific vaccines, such as encephalopathy, autism, anaphylaxis, and so forth, most still hotly contested by authorities in the field. Even those officially recognized as legitimate grounds for compensation under the Federal guidelines are actually vague, generic terms that are applicable to more than one vaccine. Anaphylaxis, for example, is compensable not only for DPT and its components but also for MMR, and will undoubtedly implicate some or all of the newer vaccines in the future.

DPT Encephalopathy.

This all-purpose diagnostic category was the first adverse reaction to be identified and made compensable under the Vaccine Injury Compensation Act of 1986, which it also helped bring about, and is by far the most extensively documented. Here is the story of a 3-year-old girl whose mother wrote to me for support of her mother's pending litigation against the child's doctors and the Canadian government:

> Our daughter was damaged by her 18-month vaccination, which consisted of the DPT, HiB, and oral polio vaccines. One week later she had a bizarre screaming episode, and is now labeled "autistic." An MRI showed brain inflammation and demyelination. She had 25 words at 18 months and was ahead in some developmental milestones as well as being quite social. After her screaming episode she stopped talking, ignored the neighborhood kids, made no eye contact, and developed hand-flapping and other repetitive behaviors. Her pediatrician agreed that she was autistic, and we told the specialist that she changed abruptly after the vaccine, and showed him a video of her as an infant and toddler, in which she seemed totally normal. From photos taken before and after, the damage is obvious: her eyes have lost their gleam, and she looks sad and alone, but the doctors dismissed it as coincidence, and no mention of any vaccine was ever included in their reports.[5]

Leaving aside the extremity of her misfortune and the refusal of her doctors to accept any responsibility for it, I call attention to her *diagnoses,* "encephalopathy," a synonym for "brain damage," and the equally vague

117

term "autism," which today is linked more commonly with the MMR vaccine. Both her sad tale and the necessity of fixing a label to it indicate that these are merely broad, generic, and often interchangeable categories, referring to conditions that can result from several different vaccines, rather than being characteristic of any particular one.

Here is another case, from the lawyer who represented him, a 3-year-old boy who reacted badly to his first DPT and suffered permanent brain damage after the second:

> Our firm represents a child who was born normal and healthy in every way. After the first DPT at 6 weeks, he began falling off growth charts, exhhibited multiple developmental delays, and was diagnosed as "failure to thrive," but then slowly began to recover. At 5 months he received a second DPT, and his delays became much more extreme. He has never recovered. He is now 3 years old, with the mental capacity of an infant of a year and a half. I am convinced that his problems came about as a result of the DPT. In view of what happened after the first shot, he should not have had the second, or at least the pertussis component of it.[6]

This tragic pattern of a warning ignored, of a lesser version of the same illness with eventual recovery, followed by death or irreversible brain damage after a repeat vaccination, formed a major subtext of the exposé *DPT: A Shot in the Dark,* in which medical historian Harris Coulter and Barbara Loe Fisher, the mother of such a child, collected the stories of over 100 little victims.[7]

The outcry over DPT encouraged Ms. Fisher and a friend to found the National Vaccine Information Center, a support and advocacy group for families and friends of vaccine-injured children. NVIC still hosts conferences, provides educational materials, and maintains a database and network of local chapters all over the country. It has kept vaccine issues in the public eye, lobbied and testified before Congress, and helped to write the Vaccine Injury Compensation Act of 1986, which created a program for no-fault compensation of vaccine injuries as an alternative to litigation.

Yet Coulter and Fisher's book was withdrawn by the publisher soon after its release, while an influential group of pediatricians still refuses to accept even these most egregious cases as having any connection with the vaccine. In 1990, Dr. Edward Mortimer et al. published a review in the *Journal of the AMA* which claimed that

> No child who was previously normal without a prior history of seizures had a seizure in the three days following a DPT vaccine that marked the onset of epilepsy or other neurological or developmental abnormality. Our negative findings reinforce those of previous investigators that serious neurological events are rarely if ever caused by DPT.[8]

In the lead editorial of the same issue, Dr. James Cherry, another leading vaccine advocate, cited these data as conclusive proof that DPT encephalopathy is a "myth," or coincidence, which should be erased once and for all from the ever-shrinking list of "genuine" adverse reactions providing an acceptable basis for compensation:

> In recent months three controlled studies examine the risk of seizures and other acute neurological illnesses after DPT, involving 230,000 children and 713,000 vaccinations. These studies found no evidence of a causal link between the DPT and permanent neurological illness. It is not surprising that physicians tended to blame the vaccine for these events. But these recent studies show that the major problem has been our failure to separate sequences from consequences. It is late in the 20th century, and it's time for the myth of "DPT encephalopathy" to end.[9]

His words also tally closely with the official report of the Advisory Committee on Immunization Practices, which acknowledged the opposing claims of parents but then muddled them up into a tangled skein of evasions, equivocations, and government bureaucratese:

> Rare but serious acute neurological illnesses, including encephalitis, encephalopathy, and convulsions, have been reported following the whole-cell DPT. The National Childhood Encephalopathy Study provides evidence that DPT can cause encephalopathy. This occurs rarely, but detailed follow-up indicates that children who had a serious neurological illness after DPT were significantly more likely than children in the control group to have chronic CNS dysfunction 10 years later and to have been given the DPT within 7 days of its onset.

The ACIP proposed 3 possible explanations for this association: 1) the dysfunction could have been caused by DPT; 2) the DPT could trigger events in children with brain or metabolic abnormalities who might also experience them if other stimuli such as fever or infection are present; and 3) the DPT might cause the event in children with underlying abnormalities who would have become dysfunctional even without it.

The data do not support any one explanation over the others. The evidence was consistent with a causal relationship, but insufficient to determine whether DPT increases the overall risk 10 years later.[10]

But even an innate predisposition to develop such complications by no means excludes the possibility of a vaccine reaction, since all illness requires both external morbid influences and an individual receptive to them. This is the ultimate riddle of all medical practice, which the emphasis on specific effects for specific vaccines blithely glosses over.

It is intuitively obvious to me, as to most parents, that a family history of serious adverse reactions, especially in parents or siblings, places children in a much higher risk pool and therefore provides valid grounds for exempting them from vaccinations. Yet even affidavits from Board-certified pediatricians don't always suffice:

I am writing about our 3-year-old son, for whom we seek medical exemption from the DPT, MMR, and HiB. Two older siblings had severe reactions to these shots, with fever of 105,° sleeplessness, and swelling at the injection site. Until age 6 both kids had recurrent ear infections, for which tonsillectomy was proposed, while our youngest has not been immunized, and has no ear infections. We tried oral polio vaccine as an infant, which was followed by extreme irritability and insomnia that lasted for weeks. 6 months ago we repeated it, with the same result. Our pediatrician has written that he is at high risk for reacting adversely, but the judge ignored her. By State law, a letter from a licensed doctor stating medical reasons why he should not be vaccinated for is sufficient. But the city guidelines give the Health Department final say, so we've ended up in court.[11]

Before their hearing, the mother obtained a second letter from another pediatrician, which the City Health Department similarly rejected:

The family history indicates epilepsy in the father and extensive allergies in the mother. The child displays a pattern of nervous system hyperactivity in response to foods, and was also sick for weeks after oral polio both as an infant and again recently. I strongly recommend against any further immunizations for this child, the risks of which outweigh any potential benefits for him or the general public.[12]

Since my testimony was never required, I surmise that the parents eventually won; but their ordeal attests to the draconian spirit in which vaccination laws are often enforced.

DPT and SIDS.

For decades the leading cause of death in infants less than one year old, Sudden Infant Death Syndrome has always baffled pediatricians. Yet pertinent research on SIDS continues to be ignored in this country because its conclusions are unpalatable to the small coterie of doctors who conduct vaccine research, journal editors who publish it, and manufacturers who fund it.

In 1985, Dr. Viera Scheibner, a research scientist investigating SIDS in Australia, and her partner, Leif Karlsson, an engineer, developed an electronic monitor that made it possible to follow breathing patterns of young infants from an adjoining room.[13] Designed to sound the alarm if breathing fell below a minimum rate or amplitude, the device immediately produced surprising results:

Soon parents were reporting alarms while their babies were deeply asleep, often in clusters of 5 to7 within a 15-minute period. These occurred after the babies were exposed to stress, or a day or before they developed a cold or cut a tooth. In most cases, the babies were only breathing shallowly and soon resumed normal patterns.

Without intending to, we also noted their breathing patterns before and after vaccination, and the results were extremely significant. We didn't know that its merits were being hotly debated at the time. We saw flare-ups of shallow breathing or apnea for 45-60 days after the DPT. When we showed our findings to pediatricians, they pointed to the arrow when the shot was given, saying "This is the cause!" and to the abnormal breathing pattern, saying "This is the effect!" But when we told them our interpretation of these data, we realized that we had touched on a very sensitive area.[14]

121

In Australia the medical community greeted these findings with a stony silence, which continues to this day, while the American literature has never published a single study to try to validate or refute it. An equally wet blanket has been thrown over the few epidemiological studies connecting SIDS to the vaccine. In 1979 the Tennessee Health Department reported 4 cases occurring within 24 hours of the first DPT,[15] while in a study of 70 cases prompted by them, Dr. William Torch found that

> 6.5% occurred in less than 12 hours after a DPT shot,
> 13% within 24 hours,
> 26% within 3 days,
> 37% within 7 days,
> 61% within 14 days, and
> 70% within 21 days.[16]

He concluded,

> DPT may be a major unrecognized cause of sudden infant death, and the risks may outweigh the benefits. Re-evaluation and possible modification of current policy is indicated by this study.[17]

Further confirmation came from Japan, where 57 encephalopathic cases and 37 deaths between 1970 and 1974, followed by two dramatic SIDS deaths in 1975, raised a storm of protest that persuaded the government to postpone all DPT vaccinations until two years of age,[18] and to promote the development of a safer acellular vaccine. As Dr. Cherry and his colleagues later conceded, the result of this policy was that "SIDS disappeared when whole-cell and acellular pertussis vaccinations were delayed until 24 months of age."[19]

Yet these same experts never contemplated such a strategy for our own country, even when the acellular vaccine failed to lower the risk of brain damage to an appreciable extent.[20] Today the United States is the only industrialized country that requires the DPT vaccine for all young infants, despite all the evidence against it and the nearly unanimous opinion of Western European, Japanese, and other foreign medical sources.

MMR and Autism.

First described by the American psychiatrist Leo Kanner in 1943, the neurological condition he called "autism" has never been satisfactorily explained. Just as it could have been mere coincidence that his first case appeared very soon after the DPT vaccine was introduced in 1942, no strong evidence for a vaccine link emerged until the late 1990's.

In 1995 Dr. Andrew Wakefield, a British gastroenterologist, compared 3550 adults vaccinated against the measles as infants with 11,400 peers who had not been, and found that the vaccinated group were three times more likely than their unvaccinated controls to develop Crohn's disease later in life, and twice more likely to develop ulcerative colitis.[21] These oddities led Wakefield to study children who reacted adversely to the MMR, many of whom developed normally during the first year but then regressed to an autistic state following the vaccine, and suffered from digestive symptoms and food and environmental allergies, or both.[22] Detailed comparison of these children with age-matched controls revealed

1) inflammatory lesions in the small intestines of autistic children that microscopically resembled those of Crohn's disease and ulcerative colitis;

2) circulating antibodies in the blood of the autistic children that were specific to measles, but not to mumps and rubella, the other MMR components;

3) measles antigens in the lymphoid aggregations of the small intestine, but none from mumps or rubella; and

4) no antigens of any kind in the intestines of normal, unvaccinated children.[23]

These findings have since been replicated by Japanese investigators,[24] and the identical combination of autistic symptoms, enterocolitis, and environmental and food allergies following MMR vaccination has been reported by parents in the US, the UK, Canada, Australia, Western Europe, and parts of Asia.[25] Further support for Wakefield's MMR hypothesis has come from the circumstance that the UK, which uses the same diagnostic criteria for autism as we do, experienced a similarly dramatic increase in autism cases at the time when the MMR was introduced in Britain,[26] and from the experience of holistic physicians in Europe and America that alleviating the food and environmental allergies is proportionately beneficial for the autistic symptoms as well.[27]

Yet no proof has ever convinced the pro-vaccination forces, who maintain a seemingly unbreakable stranglehold over American health policy. A few years ago, Rep. Dan Burton chaired Congressional hearings on the issue when his grandson became seriously ill after his MMR and was diagnosed with autism. Disregarding the NIH's own estimate of the incidence of autism at about 1 in 500 in 1996, an increase of over 400% since the 1960's,[28] Dr. Colleen Boyle of the CDC reaffirmed the official line that "current scientific evidence does not support a link between vaccination and autism or any other behavior disorder."[29] Similar denials by Dr. Paul Offit of ACIP led Burton to respond that Offit's consultations for Merck, the vaccine manufacturer, amounted to a conflict of interest that should have disqualified him from serving on the Committee:

> Even if they exclude themselves from voting, people who sit on advisory panels and are paid by pharmaceutical companies, influence other members. Are we letting pharmaceutical companies have too great an influence on decisions that affect the health of our nation?[30]

Even if it is finally recognized as a *bona fide* complication of MMR, "autism" as a diagnostic category is as vague as "encephalopathy," is also applicable to DPT cases, as we saw, and will undoubtedly become so to Hep B, HiB, and other vaccines as well.

Hepatitis B and Auto-Immune Diseases.

The official ACIP verdict on the Hep B vaccine makes it sound like one of the safest currently available:

> Hepatitis B vaccines are safe to administer to adults and children. More than 10 million adults and 2 million infants and children have been vaccinated in the US and over 12 million children worldwide. Pain at the injection site and fever have been among the most frequently reported side-effects, but no more so than in the controls receiving placebo or DPT. The incidence of anaphylaxis is low. Large-scale programs in Alaska, New Zealand, and Taiwan have not established an association with other adverse events. Any presumed risk that might be causally associated must be balanced against the expected risk of hepatitis B liver disease.[31]

124

In my experience, however, the vaccine carries a major risk of auto-immune diseases of every type, including lupus, thyroiditis, and major blood dyscrasias, which is also confirmed by a large volume of anecdotal case reports, and by warnings listed in the PDR by the manufacturers themselves. As we saw, the main value of the ACIP whitewash is to guarantee that nearly all private lawsuits and no-fault claims will fail.

Here is a case from my own practice, an 18-year-old college student who became ill soon after his second Hep B vaccination at the age of 10:

> He remained in good health and developed normally until the age of 10, when two doses of Hep B vaccine were given, with no ill effects from the first. One week after the second dose, a swollen lymph node appeared in his neck, with fever, malaise, joint pains, and other flu-like symptoms, from which he has never fully recovered. Losing 20% of his body weight, he developed large subcutaneous nodules near major joints, and.a very high sedimentation rate.

> Diagnosing an auto-immune "mixed connective-tissue disease," a rheumatologist kept him on nonsteroidal anti-inflammatory drugs and Prednisone for 6 years, as a result of which his growth and sexual maturation were seriously retarded. When I saw him, he had taken no drugs for 6 months, but his face and eyes were still swollen, his cheeks were covered by a diffuse, bright-red rash, and his muscular and sexual development were those of a puny 12-year-old. Over the past two years, he has improved a lot under homeopathic treatment, but continues to be chronically ill, seriously handicapped, and likely to remain so.

> His parents are certain that Hep B vaccine was the main cause of his illness, but his medical records contain no written statement to that effect.[32]

Here are two claims of Hep B vaccine injury whose medical records I have studied thoroughly enough to write detailed reports to their Federal hearing officer. While quite different in the organs and tissues affected, they resemble each other in their overall flavor and style:

> An adolescent girl with type 1 juvenile diabetes was in good health and stable condition before receiving the vaccine. Within a few days of her first dose, she developed fatigue and malaise, itched intensely from hives all over her body, and her skin grew puffy and swollen. In a few weeks she developed joint pains, and the hives made her scratch to the point of bleeding. Medications gave temporary relief. Her high sed rate and anti-nuclear antibody titer indicated an auto-immune llness resembling lupus, but vigorous treatment did not

help, and she developed allergic reactions to chemicals and food additives that had not bothered her before, while her diabetes, which had been stable for years, went seriously out of control.

Finally her mother broke off the treatment, saying, "Before the shot she was active, full of life, and not allergic to anything. Now she has to analyze everything she eats, avoids the sun, and has to take EpiPen wherever she goes. She is allergic to preservatives and food colorings, but has no idea what else will trigger hives and rashes." After four years, her claim is still pending.[33]

* * *

A previously healthy 31-year-old lab tech developed auto-immune thyroiditis soon after her second round of Hep B vaccinations. At 24 her doctor gave her two shots two months apart, as required for her training. 3 months after the second dose, she developed a cough that lasted for weeks and cleared up on antibiotics, after which she took the third dose. With no antibody titer 4 years later, she was thought to be still susceptible; so her new employer insisted that she be receive a second round. Within a few days after the first dose, she developed a sore throat and cold symptoms, followed by weakness, fatigue, hoarseness, and weight gain that persisted for months.

She took a second dose and grew much worse, with a more intense version of the cough she had had in the past, causing palpitations and anxiety at night. Finding her TSH to be twice normal, her doctor gave her thyroid, followed by her third dose of Hep B, and her symptoms and elevated TSH lasted for months with no improvement. When thyroid antibodies were found, she continued to worsen, despite ever-higher doses of hormone and normal tests. She has since developed a nodular goiter, difficulty swallowing, and esophageal reflux. In short, this previously healthy young woman will remain chronically ill for the rest of her life, needing regular supervision and strong medication. The most clear-cut of any that I've reviewed, her claim was dismissed without a hearing, based on current Federal guidelines.[34]

These cases are also recognizably similar to other reports of auto-immune diseases from Hep B vaccination in the literature, e. g., cryoglobulinemia,[35] lupus and rheumatoid arthritis,[36] Guillain-Barré syndrome,[37] optic neuritis and MS,[38] chronic fatigue syndrome,[39] vasculitis,[40] and diabetes.[41] As with DPT and MMR, many of the same old diagnoses, such as seizures, autism, and demyelinating diseases, keep popping up after Hep B as well. As I will presently show, the term

126

"auto-immune disease" encompasses the whole gamut of non-specific reactions to the vaccination process *per se.*

As for SIDS, it could follow *any* vaccine given early enough, especially Hep B, which is given soon after birth, as this father learned too late to save his newborn son:

> For 12 days, Nicholas ate and slept well, like any other baby. On the 13th day he was given a Hep B. When I got home from work, he was crying a lot more than usual, even screaming at times, but we'd just taken him for a checkup and they told us he was big and healthy. We didn't know that vaccines can cause problems. He cried on and off for most of the night. When I went to work the next day, he was still crying, and he continued most of the day and evening. The next morning my wife found him dead in his crib, looking as if he'd been dead for several hours. An autopsy showed that Nicholas had died of SIDS. The pediatrician said he was one of the healthiest babies he'd ever seen.[42]

2. Nonspecific Effects of the Vaccination Process in General.

Having questioned the specificity of four well-documented reactions to particular vaccines, around which all of the debate has so far been framed, I will now consider the far more prevalent adverse reactions that I have witnessed in my practice. For the most part, these represent simple intensification of underlying tendencies that were already present, and encompass the full range of common ailments encountered in any pediatric practice, like ear infections, eczema, asthma, and behavioral and developmental issues.

Although the details of their treatment are irrelevant, it is significant that these children responded to the same medicines, homeopathic or otherwise, that would be given in such cases, whether vaccinated or not. From these strange circumstances, I conclude that the small number of adverse reactions reported in the literature make up no more than the tip of an enormous iceberg, the remainder of which lies hidden, unseen, and invisible, because it blends into the mainstream of clinical medicine, and because vaccines play a major but by no means exclusive role in causing them.

Making the Connection: Childhood Ear Infections.

As we saw, causal connections between vaccines and chronic illness are obscured by the usual time lag of two weeks before their symptoms become diagnosable. Parents and doctors are equally unlikely to suspect a vaccine if the illness is an aggravated version of what the child already has and what his or her friends and classmates are also coming down with.

My first definite cases were *specific* reactions that I managed to identify from characteristic signs of a particular vaccine or component, and at times to confirm by the curative effect of homeopathic medicines prepared from the natural disease. In one such case, I noticed that in addition to its specific action on the parotid gland and the posterior auricular lymph nodes, the MMR also had a nonspecific effect on the immune system as a whole, making the boy more susceptible to other ailments going around the neighborhood:

> I saw a 4-year-old boy for bilateral soreness and enlargement of the posterior auricular nodes for the previous year, when he also became more prone to upper-respiratory infections. Over the same period, his mother also noticed recurrent swelling of the parotids, beginning soon after his MMR vaccine at the age of three. Because she was pregnant, I decided not to treat him until after the birth. A year later, he developed acute bronchitis, and again the nodes were swollen and tender; so I gave him the homeopathic rubella vaccine. The cough soon subsided, and the nodes regressed in size. Two weeks later he was back, with a hard, tender swelling in the cheek and pain on chewing or opening the mouth. After one dose of homeopathic mumps vaccine, these symptoms also subsided, and he remained well.[43]

As in other cases, the specific reaction to a vaccine helped me to recognize it, but the reaction as a whole was vague and nondescript, suggesting an underlying tendency that most children do not have. The rapidly increasing prevalence of childhood ear infections during those years soon taught me that such nonspecific reactions are the rule rather than the exception, and provided a large body of evidence that was ready to hand. Here is a typical example, a 19-month-old girl whose MMR vaccination was soon followed by ear infections and a flare-up of allergies and eczema, which she had had only mildly before:

At 19 months of age she had already suffered 5 ear infections and 5 rounds of antibiotics since her MMR 4 months earlier, with eczema and allergic rhinitis as well. Although her allergies began soon after birth, they were mild, while the eczema was confined to a few small patches on the face. With no obvious reaction to her DPT's, she did fine until the MMR, after which her ears flared up repeatedly, often with high fever, earache, and listless, clingy behavior, and never cleared up despite 5 rounds of antibiotics, while her allergies became intense and unrelenting, and the eczema spread over her entire body. Advising the parents not to use antibiotics if she got sick and not to vaccinate her for a while, I gave her homeopathic medicine, and the ears healed promptly, but her eczema and nasal congestion took a bit longer. Now 12, she has had no more shots, and enjoys excellent health and normal hearing.[44]

Occasioned by the MMR more than the DPT or other vaccines, and not included on any official list, this girl's reaction consisted mainly of ear infections, one of the commonest illnesses of her age group, as well as a recurrence and intensification of the same allergies and eczema she had had in the past. Here is another typical variant, a girl of 15 months who had had 11 ear infections and 11 full courses of antibiotics by the time I first saw her:

Otherwise in good health, a chubby girl of 15 months was brought in for recurrent ear infections, which had never cleared up despite 11 rounds of antibiotics. After a healthy pregnancy and labor, her mother didn't nurse, and her first ear infection came with a fever of 103° at 2 months of age, soon after her first DPT, HiB, and polio combination. All later episodes were afebrile, with fretting, screaming, and pulling at the ear, and were relieved by being carried about. Twice she seemed fine, but her doctor found some fluid, and the drugs caused persistent diarrhea both times.

Asking the parents to stop vaccinating her, I gave homeopathic medicines, and in 2 weeks she developed a replica of her first episode, with fever of 102° and intense screaming. With the aid of homeopathic remedies, she came through it in a day or so and has been entirely well since, once catching a cold without ear involvement for the first time. By then she was thriving, growing, and gaining weight, with good appetite, sleep, and energy. That was 3 years ago. Since then she's had no ear infections and no vaccines.[45]

In spite of the clear link between her first episode and the combined vaccines, this girl's condition became so chronic that later shots made no difference, except for her last episode, which presented with fever, just like her first. From such cases I have learned to regard acute illness as a good prognostic sign, indicating strong vitality and an immune system that is developing normally, and to worry about children who are unable to mount a fever or acute response to infection, as the immune system is programmed to do. My sense is that all vaccines, whatever their specific effects, tend to reprogram the organism to react more chronically in general, whatever the illness, as shown by my next case, a girl with recurrent ear infections of the same type following several different vaccines:

A baby girl of 10 months was brought in for otitis media with high fever, intense earache, and loud screaming, her 5th episode since two months of age, each beginning soon after finishing the antibiotic from the one before. The cycle began when her mother weaned her to go back to work, and she became fussy, as well as developing a rash on milk-based formula. All symptoms were intensified after her first DPT, HiB, and polio combination, culminating two weeks later with high fever and violent earache, as with all later episodes. After that, she was given the DT, which she didn't react to in any way, except that her ear infections continued as before.

With homeopathic medicines, they stopped soon enough; but they came back with a vengeance when her parents separated 6 months later, and her father insisted on taking her for the MMR. Three acute ear infections and three rounds of antibiotics followed in rapid succession. Again she responded well to homeopathic treatment, and remained in very good health overall, despite a tendency to relapse whenever she visited her father, who indulged her with dairy and took her to the doctor for her quota of vaccines and antibiotics. Now a freshman in college, she still gets sick at times, but her ear infections are gone, and her robust immune system has helped her respond acutely and vigorously and recover quickly.[46]

This girl's almost identical reaction to two different vaccines indicated a definite predisposition to fall ill in a certain way that was recognizably her own and already in place when the vaccines were given, the obvious contribution of vaccines being simply to reactivate and intensify it.

Making Worse What's Already There: the Common Diseases of Childhood.

From this viewpoint, I began to notice a similar causal link between childhood vaccines and the usual chronic pediatric illnesses, such as asthma, eczema, sinusitis, behavioral problems, and the like. As with ear infections, if the condition was already symptomatic prior to vaccination, a dramatic intensification was observed not long afterward, while if quiescent it was often reactivated. As before, many children reacted in a similar way to two or more different vaccines, indicating a peculiar characteristic of the individual rather than a specific effect of the vaccine, and often linked with a family history or past history of the same kind. At times the reaction occurred too long afterward for anyone to suspect a vaccine until the same pattern was observed from a later dose or a different vaccine. Moreover, these reactions similarly encompassed the usual range of ailments seen in any pediatric practice, vaccinated or not, and were curable by the same group of medicines, whether homeopathic or otherwise. Unlike the specific effects of specific vaccines, which are narrowly defined to be as serious and as rare as possible, these nonspecific reactions are common enough to be the rule, not the exception, though by no means necessarily minor or trivial:

A 15-month-old boy was brought in for croup, recurrent colds, swollen glands, and developmental issues. Born to a diabetic mother, he weighed 8 pounds at birth and spent weeks on a respirator in the Newborn ICU for "undeveloped lungs," with cyanosis and unstable blood sugars. In the early months he was colicky and had a severe diarrhea that stopped when his mother eliminated wheat from her diet. At 3 months, soon after his first DPT, HiB, and polio, he became very restless, with swollen glands and a sickly pallor that lasted for months and culminated in a prolonged attack of croup, high fever, and sunken chest that required hospitalization and IV corticosteroids for relief. When the cough persisted, his mother put off the second round of shots for months, but even so the croupy cough came right back, as did the swollen glands and exactly the same symptoms as before.

With a marked fear of strangers, the boy appeared subnormal, drooling profusely with his mouth hanging open, and hiding behind his mother. Once I found a good homeopathic medicine that fit his symptom-picture, the illness cleared up in a few days and never came back. A month later, his mother was ecstatic. For the first time, in the dead of winter, he had no croup or swollen

131

glands, slept well, and seemed more alert, more interested in his surroundings, and less fearful around strangers. That was 6 years ago, and I've not seen him since; but his mother called recently to say that he is still thriving and developing normally, "like other children his age."[47]

In another case, a boy with severe asthma accomplished a sustained remission with homeopathic treatment, but relapsed almost immediately after a DPT booster:

Asthmatic since age two and testing positive for a broad spectrum of allergens, a 4-year-old boy was brought in because a regimen of bronchodilators and inhaled steroids all year round had not prevented major flare-ups the previous fall and winter, several of them requiring oral prednisone and antibiotics as well. During the first 6 weeks of homeopathic treatment, he cut his inhaled steroids by half, maintained higher peak flows of 150 or more, and got through a cold for the first time without developing asthma or requiring any drugs. Emotionally, too, he was calmer and less wild, even expressing remorse after a fit of rage, which he had never done before.

The following spring and summer, at the peak of his allergy season, he was still doing well on half-doses of inhaler, and remained healthy and energetic, with peak flows at record levels of 160-175. That fall he got his DPT booster before entering kindergarten and quickly came down with bronchitis, for which he was given antibiotics, and his allergies also returned in full force. Again he responded to the same homeopathic medicine as before, and has continued to improve over the past 2 years, without needing to come back or take it again.[48]

His mother's narrative leaves little doubt that DPT reactivated and intensified his pre-existing condition, which had been in almost complete remission for many months. Although it is certainly possible that the DPT and other vaccines may have played a role in the *origin* of his asthma as well, an underlying predisposition would have been an important contributing factor in any case. What matters is that he was well on his way to being cured until a DPT booster set him back a lot and for a long time.

Nonspecific Reactions: any Vaccine Will Do.

As with ear infections, additional evidence of nonspecific reactions was provided by children who responded in the same way to two or more different vaccinations. The following case of environmental sensitivity was so severe and its exacerbation by each vaccine so obvious that even the allergist recognized it and agreed to withhold further doses:

A 2-year-old boy came in for asthma and allergies. Severely allergic herself, his mother reluctantly agreed to give him Hep B at birth and a second dose at two weeks. After his first DPT, HiB, and polio at two months he erupted with eczema all over his body, which she knew had been caused by the vaccines; but the pediatrician ridiculed the idea. After the second round, his stools became green and watery for 6 weeks, and she weaned him; but Similac led to apnea, cyanosis, vomiting, and giant hives everywhere. Finding him highly sensitive to dairy, eggs, peanuts, and animals, the allergist agreed he should not be vaccinated again, but the family doctor insisted on an HiB booster at 18 months, and in two weeks his asthma was back for real. When I saw him he needed Albuterol daily, all year round. He too has responded well to homeopathic medicines and is now rarely asthmatic, although still avoiding vaccines and careful with animals and foods.[49]

3. How Vaccines Work: A Preliminary Hypothesis..

In spite of their importance in medicine and public health and an abundance of detailed knowledge about how the immune system works, a vaccine need satisfy only two minimal criteria to be considered effective: 1) that the incidence of the corresponding natural disease decline significantly after administering it, and 2) that measurable titers of specific antibodies be found in the serum of vaccinated individuals for extended periods of time. These standards are analogous to those of the of the drug industry as a whole, which expects vaccines and drugs to act mainly as they are intended to, in that everything else they do is relegated to the fine print as "side" effects, and often simply forgotten. In short, the medical system does not seek or even seem to want any broader conception of how medicines affect the organism as a whole. In search of a more comprehensive view, I will reflect on how we come down with and recover from an acute disease such as the measles, and contrast it with what happens after the corresponding vaccine is administered.

Natural Immunity: Absolute, Qualitative, and Lifelong.

With its affinity for the respiratory mucosa, the measles virus is dispersed through the air by the sneezing and coughing of infected droplets, and inhaled by susceptible persons on contact with them. For 10 to 14 days, the virus multiplies, first in the tonsils, adenoids, and accessory lymphoid tissues of the pharynx, then in the regional lymph nodes of the head and neck, and finally in the blood, spleen, liver, thymus, and bone marrow, the major organs of the immune system. Throughout this prolonged "incubation" period the patient usually feels quite well and experiences few or no symptoms of any kind.[50]

With the first signs of illness, circulating antibodies are already detectable in the blood, in concentrations roughly proportional to the severity of the disease.[51] In other words, the illness we know as the measles is simply the concerted effort of the immune system to clear the virus from the blood, largely via sneezing and coughing, the same routes through which it entered in the first place. This mighty exploit involves a general mobilization that includes inflammation of already sensitized tissues at the portal of entry, activation of B- and T-lymphocytes, macrophages, and the serum complement system, and a host of other mechanisms, of which the production of specific antibodies is only one, and depends for its effectiveness upon its collaboration with the system as a whole.

Such a magnificent effort leaves no doubt that coming down with and recovering from acute illnesses of this kind are decisive experiences in the healthy maturation of the immune system. The immunity resulting from it is *specific*, to be sure, in that those who recover from the measles will never again be susceptible to it, no matter how many times they are re-exposed in the future. But it is also *non-specific*, in the equally important sense of priming the system to respond rapidly and effectively to other infections it may encounter in the future.

The natural immunity acquired through recovering from acute diseases thus represents an enormous net gain for the health of individuals and their descendants, and thereby also of the community and the race as a whole. The measles virus has a fatality rate of 20% in populations exposed to it for the first time, and centuries of adaptation were required for our own ancestors to convert it into a routine disease of childhood, such that when I caught it at the age of six, nonspecific mechanisms were already in place to help me recover from it with no complications or sequelae, an achievement that I credit in no small part for the good health I enjoy today. The ability to respond acutely and vigorously to infection ranks among the most basic and fundamental requirements of general health and well-being, a truth so obvious and elementary that even having to reaffirm it will attest to how far we have strayed from a saner and more wholesome conception of life.

Artificial or Vaccine-Induced Immunity: Relative, Partial, and Temporary.

When the live, attenuated vaccine virus is injected into the blood, at most a brief inflammatory reaction may be noted at the injection site, with no local sensitization at the portal of entry, no incubation period, no acute illness, and no massive outpouring. Like a conjuror's trick, vaccination yields measurable titers of specific antibodies in the blood, but without any overt illness or inflammatory response, and without any significant improvement in the general health of the recipients, apart from reducing their statistical risk of developing the acute disease as we know it. But where the virus *goes,* how it persuades the immune system to continue producing antibodies against it for years at a time, and what price we have to pay for the counterfeit immunity that they represent, are questions that are rarely asked.

Vaccines seem tailor-made to accomplish through deception what the immune system seems to have evolved to prevent, giving viruses, bacteria, and other foreign antigens free and immediate access to the organs of the immune system without any easy or obvious way of getting rid of them. No mere side effect, the continuing production of specific antibodies over the long term requires the physical presence of live viruses and other highly antigenic substances inside the cells of the immune system on a more or less permanent basis.

In the case of measles and other live-virus vaccines, excellent models already exist for imagining how this chronicity might occur and predicting the pathologies that are likely to follow from it. Many viruses are known for their capacity to survive in latent form indefinitely within the cells of the immune system without provoking acute disease, by attaching their own DNA or RNA as extra particles or "episomes" to the genome of the host cell and replicating along with it, allowing the cell to perform its normal functions but adding instructions for the synthesis of viral proteins as well.[52] Residing as foreign elements within the cells of the host, latent viruses of this type would automatically pose a significant threat to the immune mechanism as a whole, which is programmed to destroy and remove them by every available means. Once viral elements are incorporated into the genetic material of the host, such attacks no longer have any possible target but the infected cells themselves. Chronic intracellular parasitism by latent viruses could thus virtually guarantee a rich harvest of auto-immune phenomena, which would even have to be redefined as "healthy," now that removing the transformed cells is the only way to be rid of the foreign material they contain.

In short, my fear is that vaccinating children against measles and other live viruses simply reprograms their immune systems to respond chronically and weakly rather than acutely and vigorously to other infections, and indeed to antigenic challenges of any kind, a conclusion amply borne out by the clinical evidence already presented of alarming and as yet unexplained increases in the chronicity of ear infections, asthma, eczema, autism, and other common diseases of children and adults alike. It is dangerously misleading, if not the exact opposite of the truth, to claim that measles vaccine "protects" us against the disease by obliging us to harbor the virus chronically instead, so that our immune systems are less capable of responding acutely, not only to the measles, but to everything else as well.

If that is true, the principal achievement of mandatory vaccination would amount to exchanging a few epidemic diseases of the past for the vastly more prevalent, diverse, and less curable chronic diseases of the present, with the suffering and disability they bring amortized at a high rate of interest over the rest of the patient's lifetime. It is difficult to imagine that most parents would accept such a devil's bargain if they were told the truth about it, to say nothing of opening a veritable Pandora's box of new diseases and mutations for the future, through *in vivo* genetic recombination within the cells of the race.

Vaccine Adjuvants.

Made from killed bacteria, inactivated toxoids, tissue extracts, and genetically recombinant viruses, the non-living vaccines are also designed to remain inside the cells of the host and to continue to provoke antibody responses over long periods of time. Although how they do it is poorly understood, something in their method of preparation and preservation

136

must promote similar long-term carrier states within the antibody-producing cells, presumably by conjugation with host-cell proteins, which would allow these non-living vaccines to remain highly antigenic for as long as possible.

At least three kinds of chemical additives are implicated in and indeed deliberately used for such purposes. First, vaccines prepared from toxoids and cellular extracts are precipitated onto adsorbents, usually aluminum hydroxide, to preserve them and enhance their antigenicity.[53] There is reliable evidence that vaccines prepared without them are much less toxic, as in recent studies of an aluminum-free pertussis vaccine.[54] Also used in cookware and other products, metallic aluminum and its salts have been implicated in a broad array of auto-immune, allergic, and neuropathic states, including Alzheimer's disease and encephalopathy[55]

Second, some vaccines prepared from live microorganisms or their toxins are first killed or inactivated with formaldehyde, which also fixes and preserves them in that form, much as in embalming the dead. Well-known as an efficient carcinogen,[56] even in minute amounts,[57] formaldehyde is among the very last things we would want injected into the bloodstream of our children, let alone to trap already dangerous vaccines inside them.

Third, several other vaccines are sterilized, denatured, and preserved with Thimerosal, an inorganic sulphur-mercury salt which prevents bacterial overgrowth. Already linked to a broad range of toxic and auto-immune reactions, from allergies to renal failure and dementia,[58] mercury salts and Thimerosal in particular have been studied and publicized so widely in recent years that the vaccine manufacturers themselves have been scrambling to develop or discover alternatives to it.

Clinical and Epidemiological Studies of Vaccine Efficacy.

The best evidence that vaccines really work dates from the introduction of the Salk polio vaccine in the 1950's and the measles vaccine in the 1960's, after which the dreaded polio epidemics began disappearing from the developed world, while the annual incidence of measles plummeted from over 400,000 to less than 10,000 cases in the United States.[59] Yet the disturbing possibility that vaccines act in some other way than by producing a genuine immunity is implicit in

137

the circumstance that measles, like other such diseases, has continued to break out even in heavily vaccinated populations, while in such cases the observed differences in incidence and severity between the vaccinated and unvaccinated children have been much less dramatic than expected.

In 1985, 157 cases of measles were reported in Corpus Christi and nearby Nueces County, Texas, over a 3-month period, notwithstanding a vaccination rate of over 99% and supposedly "immune" antibody titers in more than 95%.[60] In 1989, one Illinois high school similarly reported 69 cases in 3 weeks in spite of verified records of MMR vaccination for 99.7% of the students.[61] Although both reports oddly omitted the actual numbers of vaccinated and unvaccinated cases, they effectively discredited the common prejudice that unvaccinated children, assumed to be the main reservoir of the disease, pose a threat to their vaccinated classmates, a fear widely exploited by health departments to shame reluctant parents into compliance. In fact these outbreaks suggested quite the opposite, that if the immunity conferred by the vaccine were genuine, the unvaccinated kids would pose a threat to nobody but themselves.

These inconvenient facts were dismissed easily enough by the official explanation that artificial or vaccine-mediated immunity is only partial and temporary, and wears off with increasing age, leaving the child presumably unaffected and just as susceptible as before. Indeed, this assumption is the main rationale for revaccinating with "booster" doses at a later date.

But other studies indicate pretty conclusively that this assumption is false. In 1980, when the measles seemed to have been virtually eradicated in the United States, Dr. James Cherry, the well-known vaccine advocate whom we've met before, discovered that children previously vaccinated against the measles whose specific antibody titers had fallen below supposedly immune levels responded to a booster dose only minimally and for an unacceptably short time:

> In the booster vaccinees, there was only a modest initial rise in titer, and after a year the level was almost back to where it had been before the booster. In addition, we noted a lack of "take" in 14 other children, most of whom had probably been immunologically stimulated before. In short, the data suggested that another booster dose might not have any lasting effect on waning immunity.[62]

138

Both the outbreaks of measles in supposedly highly immune populations and the failure of Cherry's simple booster shot to remain effective for a long time cast doubt on the conventional wisdom that immunity is a purely quantitative variable, that the specific antibody titer accurately measures it, and that by applying sufficient chemical force it can be ratcheted up more or less at will. Nevertheless, within a very few years, when major outbreaks like those just cited generated intense pressure to do something about them, Cherry's suddenly inconvenient research was discreetly forgotten, and the MMR booster was duly mandated for all children and remains in force to this day.[63]

An even more suggestive finding emerged from a sustained outbreak of 235 measles cases reported in Dane County, Wisconsin, over a nine-month period in 1986.[64] In addition to the usual cases, only 6% of whom were unvaccinated,[65] the authors identified a large subset of cases with so-called "mild measles," consisting of a paler rash, no fever, and minimal discomfort or systemic involvement.[66] To their considerable surprise, they discovered that this syndrome was much commoner in previously vaccinated kids *without* specific antibodies than in either unvaccinated kids or those with high levels of antibody, both of whom were more likely to develop the full-blown disease:

> 36 of the 37 unvaccinated patients, or 97%, had illnesses with rash that met the CDC clinical definition of measles, but 29 of the 198 vaccinated patients, or 15%, did not, primarily because of low-grade or absent fever. Of 122 patients with seroconfirmed measles, 10 patients, all previously vaccinated, had no detectable measles-specific IgM antibodies and significantly milder illness than either vaccinated or unvaccinated patients with IgM-positive serum.[67]

This paradoxical result suggested a variety of latent viral activity that was undetected and indeed belied by routine serological testing, echoing Dr. Wakefield's original finding that children receiving the MMR vaccine were much more likely to develop inflammatory bowel disease later in life than their unvaccinated controls. The obvious inference is that artificial, vaccine-mediated immunity is not only counterfeit, but dangerous, culminating in a broad range of auto-immune diseases, as we have seen.

4. Some Individual Vaccines.

With the above as background, I want to re-examine a number of individual vaccines, all of which illustrate the basic issues that have already been discussed, yet differ widely in the seriousness and impact of the corresponding natural diseases. Since I have already written about DPT, MMR, and polio in the past,[68,69] I will focus on vaccines of more recent vintage.

Hæmophilus Influenzæ B (HiB).

Originally developed against outbreaks of bacterial meningitis in infants and preschool children in large day-care centers, the HiB vaccine has been adapted to a broader and more ambitious agenda in a sequence that has become typical in the industry and raises pertinent economic and political issues that I have referred to only in passing. The first vaccine to be prepared against an organism that resides in the healthy throat, HiB was directed against the mutant B strain of *Hæmophilus influenzæ,* which has at times been associated with serious invasive diseases, such as otitis media, sinusitis, meningitis, pneumonia, laryngitis, epiglottitis, and endocarditis. Since bacterial meningitis can be fatal or leave permanent brain damage in spite of the most vigorous antibiotic treatment, the vaccine establishment saw no downside in attempting to prevent these outbreaks by vaccinating children of two years and older who were being cared for in crowded public facilities. After a small pilot project of this kind, the vaccine was eventually mandated for all children at 18 months, and is now administered together with the DPT at 2, 4, 6, and 18 months, often in the same preparation.

Since it began in the late 1980's, the campaign to promote HiB was accepted by nearly all pediatricians without a murmur, and has in fact succeeded in producing moderate decreases in the incidence and severity of all systemic diseases involving this organism,[70] including ear infections,[71] which by then had become an intractable problem in its own right. Yet this seemingly glorious triumph for the vaccination concept has upstaged the obvious risk of new, less friendly species occupying the vacancy it left behind, or otherwise altering the normal ecological balance of the pharynx as a whole, possibilities that do not seem to bother or even have occurred to these experts.

In addition to its documented side effects, such as Guillain-Barré syndrome,[72] thrombocytopenic purpura,[73] and invasive HiB disease in the first two weeks after vaccination, associated with very low levels of specific antibody,[74] this reckless tampering with complex, well-established homeostatic mechanisms to achieve limited, short-term goals gives ample grounds for advocating a moratorium on HiB vaccination until more comprehensive studies are carried out.

Hepatitis B.

Introduced in the early 1990's, the Hep B vaccine raises a different set of issues. Widespread but only infrequently fatal, the disease hepatitis B presents acutely, chronically, or both, and occasionally leads to irreversible liver damage and cirrhosis, which carry high risks of liver cancer and death. Transmitted primarily through contaminated blood and to a lesser extent by sexual contact, the disease has long been an important source of ill health among IV drug users. In the 1980's, the medical system belatedly took notice when Hepatitis B and C, AIDS, and other blood-borne diseases began to appear as contaminants in donated blood, a scandal that pressured the blood banks into more rigorous screening procedures.[75]

Because the clandestine subculture of IV drug use has always remained beyond the reach of the medical system, campaigns of selective Hep B vaccination aimed at these high-risk groups have never been effective. In 1991 mandatory vaccination was finally introduced as a last resort for exerting some degree of leverage over this more and more intractable problem. The desperate and improbable strategy adopted was to vaccinate all newborns in the hospital, so that those who become drug addicts in their teens and twenties would be somewhat less likely to get the disease, while the blood supply would also be protected to that extent at least. Sound far-fetched? Most pediatricians thought so at first:

> "I don't see what the rush is," said one pediatrician at a UCSF conference, and neither did his audience. Only about a third of the 400 attendees said they were giving the vaccine routinely to infants. "We're trying to prevent a disease 25-30 years from now," he added. Others felt that children receive too many vaccines in the first year, and that each injection is a disagreeable experience which may adversely affect compliance.[76]

Letters of protest began pouring in, many of them dubious that the vaccine would last long enough to do any good, and predicting that boosters would also be needed later:

> The patient handout falsely assures parents that that the protective effects will last throughout the child's life, while the article admits that antibody levels decline over time, and booster shots may be needed. Since adolescence begins the period of greatest exposure, immunizing them might be more effective, and compliance would be higher.[77]

Nevertheless, most pediatricians remained strongly committed to vaccination as a general strategy for fighting disease; and by the mid-1990's the majority were actively on board with the Hep B campaign, just as reports of adverse auto-immune reactions began to appear in large numbers, and as usual it became their task to launder and sanitize them.

Among the first of its kind, the Hep B vaccine is a product of bio-engineering, a genetically recombinant form of the virus that is allegedly no longer capable of replicating itself and to that extent no longer "alive." Ignoring the ultramicroscopic realm of episomes and intracellular viral fragments, this purely semantic rationale is widely invoked to defeat compensation claims for Hep-B-related auto-immune diseases, as I have said. While such word games may have postponed another major scandal for a time, even the polite objections of ten years ago will suffice to predict a noisy failure for this hare-brained scheme of vaccinating all newborns against a disease of drug addicts that very few of them will ever come into contact with.

Rotavirus.

While quickly smoothed over and all-too-easily forgotten, this mini-disaster and the peculiar mentality that engendered it should be kept under glass as a specimen of what undoubtedly lies ahead. In 1996, the *AMA Journal* published a CDC report which advocated mass vaccination against rotavirus, a major source of infectious diarrhea:

> Rotavirus is the most common cause of severe diarrhea among young children in the US. Of children up to five years old, approximately 70% will become ill with rotavirus, of whom 1 in 8 will see a doctor and 1 in 80 will be hospitalized. Though it causes few deaths in this country, it causes 50,000 hospitalizations

and $550 million in direct medical costs annually. Safe live oral vaccines have been developed that will prevent 50-60% of the diarrhea and 70-100% of the severest cases. The decision to implement a national vaccination program will be based on the expected reduction in severe outcomes and cost-effectiveness. A previous study found it would yield net savings of $80 million in health care costs and $465 million in social costs, based on a price of $20 per dose.[78]

By their own math, however, the authors calculated a saving of only $300 million in social costs and a net *increase* of $100 million in health care costs that could only be offset by lowering the price of the vaccine to the break-even point of $9 per dose.[79] Entitled "When Is Too Much Too Much?" an editorial in the *New England Journal of Medicine* took up the same issue and concluded that the program would be extremely effective in the developing world, where rotavirus and other infectious diarrheas pose an enormous and urgent public health problem, but affordable and profitable only in affluent countries like our own:

> Diarrhea is no longer a serious threat in the United States. It remains common, but its severity has diminished to about 300 deaths per year. On the other hand, the vaccine is safe and can prevent nearly half of all infections, 80% of the severe episodes, and virtually all of the dehydration. An effective program of vaccination would significantly reduce mortality, hospitalization, and other medical costs, estimated at $500-600 million annually, as well as the indirect costs, including lost wages for parents and the cost of child care. When is too much too much? *One hundred preventable deaths per year are too many, and $500 million in direct health care costs is too high.* Hence a safe and effective vaccine, even at $30 per dose, can be recommended for routine use in the US and developed countries.[80]

Recommended by ACIP, the vaccine was mandated in 1998 for all infants, even though 5 cases of intussusception, a life-threatening form of intestinal obstruction, had already been reported in the trial population of 10,000 children, a risk of about 0.05%.[81] In the first eight months of the program, many new cases were discovered, and the vaccine was quietly withdrawn pending further investigation, which did establish "a strong, temporal, and specific causal association" between the vaccine and this dangerous complication that was much more prevalent than the trials had indicated.[82] The vaccine was then hastily recalled and the whole affair hushed up as if it had never happened.

For the moment I will leave aside the narrow callousness of the cost-benefit calculation, which ignores the possibility of chronic, non-specific effects like those I've described, and the fascinating process by which vaccines are rubber-stamped for general use with at most nominal regulation and oversight. The rotavirus fiasco could not have happened without the zealous, crusading attitude, usually left in the background but here made explicit, that even the smallest number of preventable deaths are unacceptable, and that mass vaccination of everybody is always an appropriate strategy to consider for eliminating them.

In a land so notoriously ruled by dollars and cents, these plainly and indeed supremely un-economical ideas both assume 1) that vaccination is inherently safe, and indeed an unmixed blessing for the health of individuals and nations alike, and 2) that whatever adverse effects an individual vaccine or batch may have, there is never anything cumulative about them, so that it is perfectly OK and indeed of great benefit to pile on as many as we wish. Even in the absence of other reasons, the enormous bulk of nonspecific reactions I have described are already sufficient to prove both assumptions false. With the new biotechnology companies now capable of manufacturing vaccines against viruses and bacteria almost as fast as they can identify them, the obvious unwisdom of giving away our public health and welfare to private, for-profit enterprises is an issue that is already ubiquitous and becomes ever more threatening with each new campaign.

Chickenpox.

Many of the same issues are illustrated even more pointedly in the history of the chickenpox or varicella vaccine, which although first developed by Merck in the 1960's, was never used on a large scale until the Clinton years, when government enthusiasm for all vaccination programs attained such dizzying heights that a plausible rationale could at last be invented for marketing it. Even then it was not an easy sell, since chickenpox is an illness so innocuous that the AMA *Encyclopedia of Medicine* described it as "a common, mild infectious disease" to which "all healthy children should be exposed at an age when it is no more than an inconvenience.[83] Even the American Academy of Pediatrics, which yields to no one in its righteous enthusiasm for vaccines of every stripe, affirmed in a 1996 brochure that

> Most children who get chickenpox and are otherwise healthy experience no complications from it. When adults get it, the disease usually lasts longer and is more severe, often developing into pneumonia. Adults are almost 10 times more likely than children under 14 to need hospitalization for the disease and more than 20 times more likely to die from it.[84]

Bucking these traditional, common-sense attitudes, the manufacturers' successful campaign to win a government mandate for universal vaccination represents a brilliant coup for them and the industry, clinched by exclusive "sweetheart" contracts with state health departments and Federal agencies guaranteeing millions of doses at their own chosen price. How did they pull it off?

Although nobody claimed that the disease was serious or even required medical attention in most cases, the Clinton Administration's oft-repeated boasts about the cost-effectiveness of vaccination as a favored health strategy enabled manufacturers to argue that the huge savings in social costs, chiefly in lost wages and extra day care, would make the vaccine a bargain for *parents,* as alleged in this handout from the American Academy of Family Physicians, to be distributed to parents as their kids were offered up:

> **Why is a vaccine needed?** Chickenpox is usually a mild illness, but can cause problems like brain swelling, pneumonia, and skin infections. It may be very serious in infants and adults. Because it is so contagious, children shouldn't go to school or day care until all the sores have dried or crusted. Many parents miss work during the illness, because of which the lost pay can be a significant cost to them.[85]

As with Hep B, many physicians were lukewarm to the program in the beginning, and compliance was very low. Here is a letter from 1997, expressing the worries that had already materialized in the case of MMR, the waning immunity in adolescents and young adults, associated with more severe illness and a higher risk of complications:

145

Chickenpox has been a benign disease of preschool- and school-aged children. Although immunization is supposedly axiomatic for public health, vaccinating all kids against chickenpox is a bad idea. It is unknown whether long-term immunity arises from an attack of the disease, or from the virus repeatedly boosting it in our communities, or how long immunity will last after the vaccination. Over time, mass vaccination will eradicate most naturally occurring varicella and its booster effect. If the immunity of vaccinated kids wanes with age, and unvaccinated kids escape disease because contagion is rarer, life-threatening outbreaks may occur as these kids grow older. Since morbidity and mortality are increased in fetuses and after childhood, an ever- expanding population of adults with unboosted or waning immunity, including pregnant women, may be created.[86]

As expected, these hesitations and warnings were drowned out by special pleading from the vaccination establishment. In a *JAMA* editorial entitled "Just Do It!" two Yale pediatricians concluded their pep talk with the following exhortation:

Do the benefits of universal immunization outweigh the risks? Many studies show the risk of complications from varicella in normal children, and there is evidence that they have been underestimated. Others show that the vaccine is cost-effective. Why would we deny children protection from this unpleasant rite of passage when the evidence is so favorable? Time to stop procrastinating, and JUST DO IT![87]

Pneumococcus.

Similar in many ways to HiB, the Pneumococcus vaccine raises many of the same issues. A mutant and sometimes pathogenic strain of Strep, the "pneumococcus," or *Streptococcus pneumoniæ,* shares capsular polysaccharide antigens with *Hæmophilus influenzæ,* which are also the basis of its virulence and the source of the vaccine. The organism also occupies a similar niche in the normal flora of the pharynx and has been implicated in the same diseases: otitis media, sinusitis, pneumonia, meningitis, and endocarditis. Long before HiB, the pneumococcal vaccine was introduced during the 1970's to prevent bacterial pneumonia in the elderly, especially in overcrowded nursing homes and residential facilities, where pneumococci were the species most frequently isolated. But the vaccine proved only marginally effective in this already debilitated population, as in this study of ambulatory but high-risk middle-aged and elderly patients in the VA system:

> We conducted a randomized, double-blind, placebo-controlled trial to test the efficacy of a pneumococcal polysaccharide vaccine in 2295 high-risk patients with one or more of the following: age over 55, diabetes, alcoholism, chronic cardiac, pulmonary, hepatic, or renal disease. We were unable to prove any efficacy of the vaccine in preventing either pneumonia or bronchitis in this population.[88]

As a result of such studies, the vaccine was not very popular with either the target population or their doctors, who continued to use it without enthusiasm. So matters stood until the Clinton years, when the war on childhood ear infections reached its climax and the conventional strategy of aggressive antibiotic treatment was exposed as a dismal failure. In the late 1990's, the vaccine was recycled for pediatric use when it was found to be moderately effective in preventing otitis media, in which the pneumococcus plays a major role.[89] Here at last was the marketing strategy that the establishment had been waiting for; and today the vaccine is being promoted aggressively not only for young children, but also for adolescents, young adults, mature adults, and even middle-aged fifty-somethings of the AARP set,[90] as if it might eventually qualify as a panacea for everyone and ideally need to be repeated throughout life.

Yet a sizeable number of pediatricians and have continued to resist this steam-roller. In 2001 the Finnish Otitis Media Study reported that the new vaccine was effective in preventing ear infections, but several letters quickly punched gaping holes in it:

> The vaccine manufacturer concludes that the new vaccine is effective for prevention. But the data do not support this conclusion. As the authors admit, the treated group could have had more episodes than the controls. In 1999 these same data were presented to the FDA, which rejected the use of this vaccine in otitis media. But the most interesting results are ecological. In a short time the predicted serotype replacement, as observed with other bacterial vaccines, was realized. With this clear warning sign, it is ecologically perilous to push this vaccine.[91]

The most telling criticism of all came from a pediatrician in Holland, where ear infections are very common but rarely medicated or even considered a major public health problem:

> According to the protocol, all infants received 4 vaccinations, which led to the prevention of only 6% of cases. More could be gained by changing our *attitude* toward acute otitis media, which in the Netherlands is seen as a self-limiting disease. Often parents do not take their children to the doctor for it, and antibiotics are only moderately effective anyway. As has been shown, educating parents and doctors will lead to a decrease in antibiotic prescriptions.[92]

Yet in spite of considerable evidence that it is ineffective and unsafe, the pneumococcus vaccine continues to be promoted aggressively, and I have no doubt that it will eventually be mandated, at least for children, once these technical scruples are swept aside.

Influenza.

Prepared from live influenza viruses that are attenuated in a medium of chick embryo cells, the influenza vaccine is inactivated by formalin, split by hydrocarbon ethers into antigenic fractions, and preserved with ThimerosaL Its unique challenge and profitability lie in the fact that annual flu epidemics involve different subtypes of this extremely mutable virus, which cannot be known with certainty in advance, so that it has to be recreated and marketed anew every year, *before* the epidemic, based on extrapolation from possible animal reservoirs, i. e., on *guesswork,* and is apt to be only partially effective, despite some degree of cross-reactivity between various strains.

Like the pneumococcus, influenza vaccines were originally designed to prevent pneumonia in the elderly, especially debilitated patients in nursing homes, assisted living, rehab, and extended-care facilities. But studies of these high-risk populations have yielded at best mixed results and at times no results at all,[93] and major adverse reactions, like the dreaded Guillain-Barré polyneuritis, have been reported with some frequency. In the 1978-79 season, the highly-touted "swine flu" epidemic never materialized, but over 40,000,000 people were given the vaccine, and several hundred cases of this life-threatening syndrome were officially confirmed within 10 weeks of receiving it, representing a five- or six-fold increase over its baseline prevalence in the unvaccinated,[94] while unofficial reports suggested a rate much higher than that. As ever, authoritative studies quickly materialized to discredit any causal link, but a large volume of legal claims were settled on the quiet by the manufacturer.

The annual flu shot nevertheless remained a popular ritual with many doctors and their elderly patients and was heavily promoted; but as with the pneumococcus, the "hard sell" for mandating it had to wait until the Clinton years, when vaccination came to be seen as the strategy of last resort against health problems that seemed intractable and unresponsive to other solutions, like otitis media, flu epidemics, and AIDS. Building on the example of the chickenpox vaccine and its narrowly economic rationale, the respected and influential American Academy of Family Practice took the lead by recommending that annual flu shots be offered to all adults aged 50 or older.[95]

In *Family Practice News*, Dr. H. F. Young, Director of Scientific Affairs, emphasized the major economic benefit of preventing absenteeism from work,[96] while Dr. Gregory Poland of the National Coalition for Adult Immunization cited the increased probability of complicating risk factors like heart disease, asthma, emphysema, cancer, and diabetes in this age group.[97] Once again, the economic argument was marshalled to advocate vaccinating all schoolchildren on a yearly basis, which a 1999 study claimed would save hundreds of millions of dollars in lost wages and eliminate the major reservoir of the disease.[98] Facing no real opposition, the same argument was applied to healthy young adults in the work force,[99] and eventually even to pregnant women, in order to protect their newborns from the risk of RSV and bronchiolitis, according to one imaginative CDC scientist.[100] As with pneumococcus, the influenza vaccine is clearly being groomed for routine and perhaps mandatory use on a yearly basis, with no recognition of even the possibility of a serious downside to the idea.

Anthrax and Bioterrorism.

Mandated for all U. S. military personnel serving in the Middle East from the time of the first Gulf War in 1991,the anthrax vaccine has been controversial from the start. First, there was speculation about its possible role in "Gulf War syndrome," an assortment of still unexplained diseases reported by many returning veterans and downplayed or covered up by officials of the Clinton and Bush Administrations. As reported in the *Boston Globe,* this account of one such veteran was typical of many:

> Sgt. Frank Landry's chest has been hurting a lot. He can't ride a bike, climb stairs, or play with his children. He wheezes even with medication, sleeps propped up on three pillows, and suffers from diarrhea and stomach pain. The worst of it is, he doesn't know what's wrong. He left in perfect health two years ago, to serve in the Gulf War as a specialist in nuclear, chemical, and biological weapons, and he returned coughing up phlegm and too short of breath to resume his job, as well as dropping from 150 to 128 pounds.

> Landry is one of many Gulf War veterans who report a variety of mysterious ailments, such as joint pain, hair loss, skin lesions, bleeding gums, asthma, and digestive disturbances. They don't know what causes them, but Landry's best guess is a reaction to the anthrax vaccine. He'd never had lung problems before, and within an hour of receiving it he began to wheeze, and felt as if his chest were filled with water. He's never been well since.

> He can't work and accepts $1000 a month in food stamps and Aid to Dependent Children, because he has two kids, his wife has a bad back, and they've sold off most of their possessions. Meanwhile the Government denies that his problems are service-related and has reclassified him as fit for duty. In spite of what happened, he's not bitter about the Army. He volunteered knowing the risks: "they gave me a life and education. I was illiterate and got my GED because I couldn't be promoted without it." No diagnosis has been made. All he knows is that he can't breathe, can't work, and can't support his family. And he's only 29 years old.[101]

A recent survey reported that over 230,000 of the 600,000 troops serving in the Gulf War have sought medical care, and that 185,000 have filed disability claims as a result of their ailments, a shockingly high percentage, while almost 10,000 have died, and no official explanation of their illnesses has ever been offered.[102] In the late 1990's, its enthusiasm for vaccines led the Clinton Administration to require all military personnel to receive the anthrax vaccine, whether on active duty or not, and the vaunted discipline of the Armed Forces began to crack. By 1999 several hundred officers and enlisted men from all branches had accepted dishonorable discharges rather than submit to the shots, as the Army reluctantly admitted in a *Boston Globe* cover story:

In Maine, where he grew up, Zack Johnson didn't have a reputation for civil disobedience. He was so law-abiding and laid back that his parents called him "Mr. Light 'n' Easy." But the 22-year-old Naval airman faces a court-martial because no threat of biological weapons, or a jail sentence, or even the loss of the GI Bill he planned to use for college could persuade him to take the anthrax vaccine. Ten Marines were court-martialed in California last month for the same reason.

An Army spokesperson says that over 300,000 military personnel have had at least one shot, and 175 to 200 people have refused, too few to affect battle-readiness. But Mark Zaid, an attorney representing the 10 Marines, said, "Some Air National Guard units have lost a third of their flight crews and can't be deployed any more." He estimates the number of refusals at 300 to 500.[103]

In a related story from the *New York Times,* the Surgeon-General of the Army acknowledged the seriousness of the problem:

The happy military career of Jeffrey Bettendorf ended abruptly Wednesday. A senior airman with an untarnished record, Bettendorf was dishonorably discharged for refusing to take the anthrax vaccine, because he believed that the Pentagon had never proved its safety or effectiveness. Facing rebellion from a growing number of cases, the Pentagon dismissed them as insignificant, but stopped counting how many had refused. "It speaks to an undercurrent of distrust of the Government and the military," said Lt. General Ronald Blanck, Surgeon-General of the Army, which oversees the anthrax program. "We have a credibility problem."

The Marine Corps in particular has been hit hard. Resisters note that there is no way to test the vaccine against the anthrax used in weapons, and criticize the lack of follow-up research on those who did receive it during the Gulf War. They also point to two FDA reports critical of the manufacturer, Michigan Biologic, a state agency which was sold last year to Bioport, a private company. One month later, Bioport was awarded a $29 million contract to produce the vaccine for the Pentagon, which insists that the program is safe and effective.

But reassurances are not enough for Marine Lance Cpl. Jason Austin, who read that the vaccine can cause sterility and refused to take it with four others in his antitank missile platoon and now faces a court-martial. While their numbers are small, they can upset the readiness of their units, notably in the Reserve and National Guard, whose members can resign more easily than those on active duty. In January, nine A-10 pilots with the Connecticut Air National Guard, a quarter of the squadron, quit rather than be vaccinated. At Travis

151

AFB in California, where Airman Bettendorf served, 11 of 40 Reserve pilots in his Squadron refused to take the vaccine, leaving them short-handed just before heading to the Persian Gulf.[104]

As news of these refusals and disciplinary actions spread, high-ranking officers began taking seriously the concerns of the men and women under their command. As Commander of an F-16 Fighter Squadron, Lt. Colonel Thomas Heemstra, a decorated combat veteran of 20 years' experience, decided to investigate the vaccine independently, and was outraged by what many personnel had endured, including disrespect, ridicule, and inadequate medical care. As told in his book, Col. Heemstra invited Dr. Meryl Nass, a government consultant who had raised serious doubts about the vaccine, to address his pilots.[105] Including first-hand accounts by three Michigan National Guardsmen who were disabled by the vaccine and treated harshly by their superiors, her lecture persuaded all twenty pilots who attended to refuse the vaccine, as a result of which they were cashiered, including the Colonel himself.[106] The same fate befell Major Sonnie Bates, another highly decorated combat pilot of long experience who later testified before Congress on a wide variety of auto-immune complaints observed in military personnel after taking the shot.[107]

As the scandal spread through the ranks, investigators discovered that many Gulf War syndrome patients who developed auto-immune diseases after the anthrax vaccine showed antibodies to squalene, a fat-soluble substance that was still being used by BioPort as an experimental adjuvant in the vaccine, despite strong FDA warnings in the past and solemn assurances by the Pentagon that they had abandoned the practice.[108] In part to counter the bad press, Admiral William Crowe, ex-Chairman of the Joint Chiefs of Staff, was named to BioPort's Board of Directors and given a 13% stake in the company in return for blessing the anthrax venture.[109] Ironically, he had previously brokered the sale of weapons-grade anthrax to Saddam Hussein by Donald Rumsfeld, President Reagan's special emissary, for later use against the Iranians and Kurds.[110]

Only a few weeks after the attacks of September 11, 2001 and the official Bush Administration "Declaration of War" against Terrorism, spores of weapons-grade anthrax made their way through the Postal Service to the offices of Democratic Congressional leaders and CBS

Television News, resulting in 22 cases of cutaneous and pulmonary anthrax and five deaths. Although the perpetrators of these crimes have not been identified and the results of an extensive Federal investigation have never been made public, it leaked out that the material had been manufactured in the U.S. Army Biological Warfare Laboratories, as the country trembled with the realization that even such minute amounts were enough to infect and kill people, and that the Government is essentially powerless to stop a large-scale biological attack by a determined enemy. These fears were assiduously cultivated by the Administration to win support for the public health agenda of the Patriot Act and the vast Homeland Security bureaucracy created to administer it, but fantasies of vaccinating the general population brought back the aftertaste of the military's incestuous relationship with BioPort, not to mention the ominous signs of its complicity in the Gulf War syndrome, and the plan never got off the ground.

After September 11, the equally abortive campaign to vaccinate everyone against smallpox was even more revealing. Amid the tragedy, confusion, and heroism displayed at Ground Zero, the whole country began taking seriously the possibility and indeed the likelihood of nuclear, chemical, and biological attacks in the future. Because anthrax cannot be transmitted from person to person, each intended victim must be targeted individually and be brought into direct physical contact with the spores, whose range is therefore limited to the environs of a large city. Smallpox, on the other hand, evokes deep mythic and historic fears of plague and pestilence, because it is highly contagious and capable of propagating itself from person to person, and thus to populations far beyond the target area, so that many authorities entertained the idea of reintroducing vaccinia, or cowpox, the original vaccine that had been used for 200 years and had in fact eliminated smallpox from the world.

Yet when the Administration attempted to obtain large quantities of it, and President Bush made a photo-op of rolling up his own sleeve to receive it, the public remained surprisingly cool to the idea. Even when a scaled-down plan was made optional and offered to doctors, nurses, firemen, and other first-responders and emergency personnel, very few of them actually took it,[111] and the predicted adverse reactions were widely publicized.[112]

153

Given the almost universal propensity to ignore or overlook the adverse effects of vaccinating not only our children but indeed everyone else against a host of other diseases both great and small, this sudden show of solicitude and cold feet regarding a vaccine that had seemed so familiar and effective is utterly fascinating to me. How these same people can then resume taking their annual flu shots and bringing in their babies for one disease after another without a murmur has to rank with the great unsolved mysteries of our time.

In any case, there is plenty of good sense in it, for it means either that the actual threat of the vaccine is perceived to be greater than the hypothetical threat of the disease, or that the public simply does not believe that any vaccine can reliably stop a determined enemy from doing us harm. In my view, both reservations are well taken. Larry Brilliant, M. D., a veteran epidemiologist formerly with WHO, said it better than anyone:

> If Saddam has smallpox, he might use it if he were about to be killed, but he also has the capacity to alter the virus to make it vaccine-proof. Why would he use a virus that we have a vaccine against? It makes no sense. If Al Qaeda has it, I don't believe they'd use it either. They want victory for a people, a culture, a religion. Smallpox is the ultimate boomerang. If released at Chicago-O'Hare, it's only a matter of days before it hits Mecca and Medina. It's not a weapon for war unless one seeks the destruction of both civilizations.[113]

Prof. David Rosner of Columbia gives a second equally cogent argument for the same conclusion:

> Smallpox is the only disease to have been eradicated through human intervention. Yet we saw in it the chance to create a new and better weapon of mass destruction. Both the U. S. and Russia kept the virus in storage awaiting the opportunity to terrorize the world. Both made it immune to the vaccine that had eradicated it by genetically altering the virus. Even if smallpox could be used as a weapon, the fear of it is being used to make fundamental changes in public health. Mundane but indispensable activities like making sure our water is safe to drink, our air isn't too polluted to breathe, and our food isn't too spoiled to eat are being sacrificed for fear of smallpox, which plays into Bush's strategy of militarizing public health.[114]

5. Implications for Health Policy.

In conclusion, I want to apply the broader, more comprehensive viewpoint I have sketched out to try to identify some underlying themes of our present vaccine policy, to correct some of its inadequacies, and to resolve some of the contradictions that follow from them.

The More, the Merrier.

The sequence whereby vaccines originally intended for a limited purpose or target population are awarded a larger and larger market share logically culminates in the prized government mandate enforcing them on everyone. As we saw, such universalization presupposes a deep and abiding faith that vaccines are inherently beneficial and in no sense a major public health risk, which makes it look acceptable to promote all vaccines to the fullest extent possible, and to achieve maximum compliance with each new mandate.

Writing in medical journals and news magazines, prominent advocates routinely exhort physicians to improve their vaccination rates, offer practical tips for overcoming patient resistance, and downplay the risks and contraindications that parents continually worry about, and that still crop up in the literature. Part pep talk and part sales pitch, such motivational efforts have long since reached out beyond any narrowly defined pediatric constituency to target other age groups as well.

In "Adult Immunizations: How Are We Doing," a typical example of the genre, a leading infectious disease specialist calculated the number of lives that could be saved by vaccinating adults with the same zeal and thoroughness that we bestow on our children:

> 30,000 lives could be saved yearly if adult immunization recommendations were implemented. Between 50,000 and 70,000 adults die each year from influenza, pneumococcal infection, and hepatitis B. This exceeds the number of automobile deaths, and far outweighs mortality from these diseases in children. Those for whom vaccines are contraindicated are fewer than those who fail to be immunized because of the following, which are not contra-indications but often thought to be:
>
> 1) local reactions to past vaccines, with fever less than 104°;
>
> 2) mild acute illness, with or without fever;

155

3) antibiotic treatment or convalescence from recent illness;

4) household contact with a pregnant woman;

5) recent exposure to infectious disease;

6) breast-feeding;

7) history of allergies, including to penicillin or most other antibiotics; and

8) family history of allergies, adverse reactions, or seizures[115]

In other articles, similar concerns are expressed for adolescents and young adults, who have been equally neglected by our narrow preference for infants and small children:

> Vaccination programs focusing on infants and children have decreased the occurrence of many vaccine-preventable diseases. But many adolescents and young adults are still being attacked by hep B, chickenpox, measles, and rubella, because our vaccination programs have not focused on these age groups. All not previously or adequately vaccinated should be updated with Hep B, MMR, DT, varicella, and pneumococcus. Influenza and Hep A should be offered to all at high risk.[116]

The most convincing proof for the universality of the concept is its extension to pregnant women, who have always been considered exempt and inviolate, out of concern for the safety of their unborn that the new imperative threatens to render obsolete:

> Adult immunization rates have fallen short of goals because of misconceptions about the safety and benefits of vaccines. This danger is magnified during pregnancy, when physicians are hesitant to give vaccines and patients to accept them. Routine vaccines that are safe to give during pregnancy include DT, flu, and Hep B. Meningococcus and rabies may be considered. Contra-indicated are MMR, varicella, and BCG. Others have not been adequately studied and must be weighed individually. But inadvertent use of any of these is not grounds for termination[117]

Ironically, it is widely agreed that mandated childhood vaccination programs have not only achieved but often outstripped their stated goals. According to the CDC's National Immunization Survey, all recommended vaccine targets were met or exceeded by 1995:

95% of children aged 19 to 35 months received at least 3 doses of DPT;
92% received at least 3 doses of HiB;
90% received the MMR;
88% received polio; and
68% the Hep B.
In fact, the 1996 goals were reached in 1995.[118]

Even in California, where alternative medicine is widely popular, and a thriving subculture openly questions traditional medical practices, vaccination rates have reached extremely high levels, as shown in this 2001 study by the state Health Department:

> The California Department of Health examined school immunization records for all children in the state. In the fall of 2000, personal belief exemptions were listed for 0.77%, or 4000 of the 526,000 attending kindergarten. Seventh-graders have higher exemption rates, probably because of the Hep B requirement. Of 500,000 seventh-grade students, 1.3% recorded personal belief exemptions.[119]

In fact these levels are far in excess of what is necessary to prevent sustained outbreaks of even the most highly contagious diseases, like chickenpox and measles, both of which attack nearly 100% of the people exposed to them for the first time. A study of 1000 Milwaukee-area children found that

> Modest improvements in low levels of immunization among 2-year-olds confer substantial protection against measles outbreaks. Coverage of 80% or less may be sufficient to prevent sustained outbreaks in an urban community.[120]

Whereas all of these campaigns tacitly assume that it is permissible and actually desirable to add on as many different vaccines in as many doses as we think fit, the preponderance of evidence points to exactly the opposite conclusion. If all vaccines have the power to promote, intensify, activate, or reactivate whatever chronic disease tendencies already exist, then the risk of adverse reactions is not rare or incidental, but inseparable from the process, and indeed, I fear, in direct proportion to the total number of vaccinations given. Whether unaware of or simply untroubled by this possibility, in January 2004 the ACIP updated its Recommended Childhood and Adolescent Immunization Schedule as follows:

3 Hep B shots in the first 24 months, beginning at birth;
3 DPT at 2,4, and 6 months, and a 4th at 5-24 months;
3 HiB at 2,4, and 6 months, and a 4th at 12-18 months;
2 injectable polio at 2 and 4 months, and a 3rd at 6-24 months;
One MMR at 12-18 months;
One chickenpox at 12-24 months;
3 pneumococcus at 2,4, and 6 months, and a 4th at 12-18 months; and
One influenza yearly, beginning at 6 months.[121]

This adds up to 22 vaccinations for each child in the first 2 years, many of them with two or more components, and that's only the beginning. For ages two through 18,

One influenza vaccine annually [another 16 from 2-18 years of age];
3-4 Hep A shots recommended, from 2-18 years;
DPT booster at 4-6 years, followed by DT at 11-12 years;
One injectable polio booster at 4-6 years;
One MMR booster at 4-6 years; and
One chickenpox booster at 4-6 years.[122]

This makes 25 more mandatory or recommended vaccinations between 2 and 18, a total of close to 50 by the time they enter college, not to mention whatever new vaccines lie in store for them in the future, while as young adults they will become eligible for yet another series of boosters to carry them into old age. Thus slowly, incrementally, and inexorably, purely as a matter of policy and without any real public health emergency, vaccination has become the normal, acceptable means for reducing the incidence of any identifiable acute infectious disease whatsoever, often simply to save money or time lost from productive work, a strategy which now involves every individual in every age group and necessitates repeated doses throughout life.

To roll back this juggernaut, the top priority must be to reduce the total vaccine burden borne by our population, especially infants and young children. In my view, this should be done, first of all, by postponing vaccination as long as possible, at least until two or ideally three years of age, to give young immune systems ample opportunity to develop in a wholesome and natural way, by learning how to mount fevers and other vigorous, acute responses to infection, before reprogramming them in a more chronic fashion.

Second, we should preserve a clear distinction between diseases that represent a major risk of death and disability, like diphtheria, tetanus, and polio, and others that originate from organisms in our normal flora, like HiB and pneumococcus, or are nuisances that we have elected to vaccinate against for economic or other policy reasons, such as influenza, MMR, and chickenpox, or problem diseases that we feel helpless to influence in any other way, like hepatitis B and undoubtedly AIDS on the horizon.

With no urgent medical need for it, the MMR was brilliantly successful as a public relations stunt, proving that vaccination could work as a general strategy by nearly erasing three ubiquitous acute diseases as a simple demonstration of its validity. Yet it has been wholly counterproductive to impose the MMR on populations like ours, which through centuries of adaptation had already tamed these viruses into routine diseases of childhood that most kids in reasonably good health would benefit substantially from coming down with and recovering from.

In industrialized countries like the United States, a reasonable argument could be made for recommending DT and polio, and making the other vaccines available to those who request them. As for pertussis, I cannot support large-scale use unless a vaccine is developed with a much better safety record than any we have now. Since the pressure to vaccinate early derives mainly from the risk of pertussis in young infants, dispensing with that vaccine will also encourage waiting longer before giving DT and polio. In my opinion, the MMR, chickenpox, and Hep B vaccines have no legitimate use on a mass scale and should not be recommended. Vaccinating the whole population in advance of bioterrorist threats like anthrax and smallpox is useless, since weaponization renders these organisms impervious to vaccines, and also unnecessary, since the likelihood of their use remains vanishingly small.

A Sacrament of Modern Medicine.

In any case, since vaccinating everybody against everything at every opportunity obviously represents an enormously profitable venture for manufacturers, it should not be a surprise to anyone that their aggressive marketing strategies are essentially comparable to what other major industries regularly do to maximize their bottom line if they are able. As we saw, their sweetheart deals with state health departments, foreign governments, and both federal and international agencies, often involving millions of doses guaranteed at their chosen price, along with the famous "hard sell" of doctors and patients that accompanies them, entail nothing more mysterious or unfamiliar than good old crony capitalism getting a free ride.

As we saw, the rotavirus debâcle was largely about greed. With its $30 unit price far beyond their reach, the vaccine was never made available to the poor countries that stood to benefit most from it, while the U. S. government never tried to persuade the manufacturers to lower it, and gladly provided easy access into the domestic market instead. In like manner, the anthrax vaccine controversy ended in scandal because the government's policy of requiring it of all military personnel resulted in too many high-profile casualties and defections for the company's shoddy practices and the Pentagon's condoning of them to be kept hidden any longer.

Thus unrestrained even by market forces, abetted by corporate welfare at the taxpayers' expense, and rubber-stamped by their allies in government, the thriving biotech industry has amplified these problems exponentially by creating new vaccines against any desired viruses or bacteria as fast as they can identify, isolate, and propagate them, often for no better reason than their technical capacity to do so. In the absence of any serious regulatory effort, we can confidently expect a rich harvest of new vaccines in the future, some on the drawing board, others in the pipeline or already in stock and awaiting only a convenient opportunity and marketing strategy to launch them:

> While its incidence has declined in the past decade, hepatitis A is still responsible for nearly 60% of acute viral hepatitis in the United States. It seems unfortunate that outbreaks continue to occur in one of the most affluent countries in the world, given that a highly immunogenic, safe, and effective

vaccine is available. Routine vaccination in early childhood would lead to a dramatic reduction in the infection within a decade. The failure to begin such a program is a missed opportunity.[123]

But corporate greed and ambition are only the most familiar and obvious side of the story. Above all other drugs and industrial products, vaccines alone are uniquely blessed and indeed sanctified by their extraordinary triumph at the unconscious or mythic level, as a veritable panacæa for a health care system that seems embattled and in deep trouble almost everywhere else. No purely financial or commercial motive can account for the sincere and nearly universal veneration accorded to the idea of vaccination by doctors and patients alike, which not only exempts vaccines from the customary ordeal of criticism that every new scientific discovery must rightly endure, but also makes the mere hint of disapproval seem disloyal or sacrilegious, and even inspires the physicians who administer them to volunteer their own children for the latest experiments.

Quasi-religious sentiments of this kind are evident in the writings of Dr. Paul Offit, the aforementioned Merck consultant who recently boasted that young infants can generate protective humoral and cellular responses to multiple vaccines simul-taneously, perhaps as many as 10,000 at a time, by what he calls a "conservative estimate."[124] At a deeper level, the vaccination project must also be understood in mythic and spiritual terms, as a kind of baptismal initiation into the religion of modern medicine.[125]

In any case, regardless of which motives seems uppermost in any given case, the result is the same: compulsory vaccination has promoted a kind of self-righteous fanaticism that is often invoked to justify various abuses and infringements of the rights of parents, children, and the public at large. From the 1940's through the Reagan years, compliance with vaccination laws was achieved mainly by intense social pressure to conform that doctors, school boards, friends, neighbors, and relatives still bring to bear against deviant parents, whose unvaccinated kids were regarded as the chief reservoir of the few diseases at issue and therefore a substantial threat to the vaccinated kids and everyone else as well. In the mid-1980's, as we saw, this simplistic rationale was demolished by the large measles outbreaks in highly vaccinated populations, where most of the cases had been vaccinated, and parents began to wonder how, if the vaccine were as effective as it was claimed to be, unvaccinated kids could threaten anybody but themselves.[126]

During the Clinton years, as both the number of required vaccinations and the public resistance to them began to multiply, the government and public health authorities began implementing a tracking system for identification and surveillance of noncompliant parents, based on computerized government data banks that raised widespread alarm and spread fears of "Big Brother" overriding personal privacy, notwithstanding official denials and reassurances to the contrary:

> Community- and state-based immunization registries are computerized systems that contain data about children's vaccines, a tool to maintain high vaccination coverage. Such registries consolidate records from different providers, generate reminder notices, and produce an official record. Remaining challenges include balancing the need to protect privacy with gathering and sharing information to benefit the public and individuals. $178 million in Federal funds have so far been awarded to state and local health departments to develop such registries.[127]

With the added impetus of President Bush's "War on Terrorism," the Patriot Act, and the huge Homeland Security bureaucracy created in their name, the threat to civil rights began to frighten eminent legal experts and health activists all over the country, as in the following "News Release" that was sent to me over the Internet and gave only a phone number as its source:

> Attorneys for the CDC have advanced legislation that suspends civil rights in case of a declared biological emergency. The Emergency Health Powers Act gives governors and public health officials the power to arrest, transport, quarantine, drug, and vaccinate anyone suspected of carrying a potentially infectious disease. An article by Prof. Lawrence Gostin of Georgetown that tried to balance the need to control disease with protecting individual rights was removed from the *Boston Globe* website. The law gives state public health authorities dictatorial powers with scant legal recourse for internees. Its definition of a public health emergency is highly subjective.

Once it is declared, most civil liberties are suspended, with states declaring ownership of private property. Persons refusing to submit to medical exams and tests are subject to misdemeanor charges and forced isolation. If the authorities suspect that they have been exposed to infectious diseases or pose a risk to public health, detention may be ordered for them. If an attack is carried out or even suspected, thousands could be held in camps, and physicians assisted by police be required to perform medical tests and exams. Individuals may be forcibly vaccinated or medicated, and those refusing would be guilty of a crime and subject to arrest, isolation, or quarantine, while the state and public health authorities are exempt from liability associated with the death or injury of detainees or damage to their property.[128]

In a sizeable number of divorce and/or child custody hearings and lawsuits that have come to my attention, the plaintiff, almost always the husband or ex-husband, seeks to win or regain physical custody of his children on grounds that his wife or ex-wife was negligent or unfit as a parent by failing to comply with vaccination laws, even if he had acquiesced in her position and failed to challenge it for all the time they were together.[129]

In Canada, where vaccinations remain optional but are held in comparable esteem by the medical establishment, the Quebec College of Physicians revoked the medical license of Dr. Guylaine Lanctôt, a physician who strongly opposed routine vaccination, simply for espousing ideas that they found "derogatory to the honor and dignity of the medical profession," and for disseminating information to the public that they proclaimed to be "inaccurate, deceptive, inappropriate, and contrary to accepted medical science."[130]

Vaccination has also lurked behind the scenes in the criminal prosecution of some parents for "shaken-baby syndrome," a form of encephalopathy secondary to traumatic brain injury. In an infamous case from Florida, the father served 8 years of a life term for murder in the state penitentiary, and recently won his release only when the Medical Examiner's testimony that convicted him proved to have been falsified in several key respects,[131] while a review of the baby's medical records by myself and several other physicians found them consistent with the possibility of an encephalopathic reaction to the DPT vaccine, which he had received only a few days before.

But my favorite illustration of the sacramental power of the vaccination concept lies in the voluntary and largely instinctive self-censorship practiced in its favor by the news media, which almost never make statements or issue opinions of their own that vaccines actually hurt anybody, apart from those attributed to interested parties such as parents or medical experts. The only exception to that rule that I know of was this article from the *Boston Globe* that let the cat out of the bag just this once:

> **INOCULATIONS PUT ASPIN IN D. C. HOSPITAL.** Defense Secretary Les Aspin was in "clearly improved" condition but remained in the Intensive Care Unit of Georgetown University Hospital yesterday after suffering breathing difficulties triggered by routine inoculations. "He's definitely on the road to recovery," the spokesman said, but would remain in the ICU to be monitored, because he has a history of heart problems, and fluid collected in his lungs. He entered the hospital because of shortness of breath aggravated by "a mild, pre-existing heart condition," the Pentagon said. He became ill the day before, soon after receiving a number of immunization shots in preparation for overseas travel.[132]

Although Aspin's hospitalization remained newsworthy for several days, there was no further mention of his vaccinations, and readers who had missed the original story were given the impression that he merely suffered a flare-up of his pre-existing heart condition, which was true enough, thus superbly illustrating the theme of invisibility that furnished the basic subtext and starting point of this essay.

To dispel the aura of sanctity that blesses the vaccination concept and protects it from closer scrutiny, it is enough to show that vaccines are no panacæa for the health care system, to see them for what they are, instruments of medical science with ample power to do harm as well as good, like any other drug or procedure, and to hold them accountable to the same standards of safety and efficacy, by obliging them to run the usual gauntlet of lively criticism and open debate.

Who Decides?

I have often wondered who gets to decide that a particular disease represents such a grave or urgent threat to the public health that everyone has to be vaccinated against it, whether they want to be or not. Yet simply asking the question is enough to remind us of what on some level we already know, that such deliberations take place behind closed doors without any public input or oversight. The fantasy scenario that comes to mind cannot be far from the truth: a government conference room where officials of the CDC, the FDA, and the American Academy of Pediatrics meet with the vaccine manufacturers themselves, to decide which vaccine to recommend or mandate next, and to devise a suitable marketing strategy for promoting it. Whatever the outcome, this "good ol' boy network" rarely seems to meet a vaccine that it doesn't like.

I can easily imagine a real emergency where swift actions need to be taken for the public good that some people of conscience might disagree with. But that is not the issue here. Whether because or in spite of the vaccinations that have been mandated in the past, or perhaps for other totally unrelated reasons, no vaccine-preventable disease now poses any urgent threat to the health of the nation, and most of the vaccines now in use are marketed largely from motives of policy, as we saw, whether to save lost wages, to gain access to a group that would otherwise be elusive, to eradicate a disease that has been a problem in the past, or simply to make a lot of money for the manufacturer.

Like many other physicians, I believe it is unwise and illegitimate to privatize our health system to the extent of surrendering decisions in the public domain that clearly affect the health and welfare of everyone to private corporations that are devoted mainly to turning a profit. In conformity with the laws of all other civilized countries, I consider health to be a basic human right of everyone, not merely a privilege of the few who can afford to pay whatever the providers feel entitled to charge for it. The issue of vaccination is too important to be decided in backroom deals behind closed doors, and must be opened to public discussion and debate at every level and at every stage.

I do not believe and have never taught that all vaccines are wholly bad or evil and to be avoided under all circumstances. In all my writings, I have simply tried to show that there is a major downside to their use on such a scale that needs to be acknowledged frankly, studied carefully, and factored into all future deliberations about them. To that end I advocate a simple pro-choice position, that under most circumstances, and in the absence of any genuine public health emergency, it should be left to the free and

165

informed decision of the parents about which vaccines, if any, are given to their children, as is generally the case in all other industrialized countries.

Wanted: a Better Model for Biomedical Research.

Devising adequate vaccine policies will also require more comprehensive studies of their adverse effects and actual mechanisms of action than any previously undertaken; and to succeed they will have to be designed in a new and radically different way. In the first place, they will need to look well beyond the narrow focus of our present studies on the reduced incidence of the typical acute disease and the titers of specific antibodies, our only available standards of vaccine "efficacy," both of which correlate very imperfectly with true immunity, as we have seen. Secondly, estimating the safety of vaccines and identifying adverse reactions to them must include learning to recognize such non-specific effects, as I have described.

To render these phenomena more visible, three major changes will be required. First, it will be necessary to investigate the full range of adverse effects of each vaccine and vaccine combination, involving every organ and tissue of the body, as well as more global measures of health and functioning, such as neurological development, school performance, sensory-motor integration, mental and emotional maturity, and suffering and disability from other diseases. Secondly, these investigations will have to be carried out for enough time to reveal significant chronic patterns, i. e., for years or decades at least. Finally, the overall health status of the children receiving vaccines must be compared with that of those who do not receive them, an obvious requirement which assigns special priority to finding the unvaccinated children. Far from being "spoilers," as they are often regarded, this control group, along with their parents who choose not to vaccinate them, must be sought out and protected as our last, best hope for enabling such studies to be carried out, to whom society as a whole and even the parents who choose to vaccinate clearly owe a major debt of gratitude.

Owing to the profusion of different vaccines and combinations that are currently available and in use, it is impractical to study each individual vaccine separately at the present time. Therefore, I propose the simplest kind of survey to begin with, to compare the overall health picture of those vaccinated according to the official schedule with those minimally vaccinated at age three with tetanus and polio alone, and with those not vaccinated at all. If what I've said so far proves correct, as I fear it will, then the unvaccinated and lightly-vaccinated children should be substantially and measurably healthier, freer from chronic disease, more alert mentally, and more stable emotionally than those who are fully vaccinated, and should also outperform them in school, with fewer absences, higher test scores, and the like. That is my prediction and my deepest concern. If any can prove me wrong, let them come forward, and I will thank them from the bottom of my heart.

Vaccine Laws and Exemptions.

Achieving even these modest reforms also involves rethinking our present vaccine laws and the allowable exemptions from them. Under the U. S. Constitution, which leaves to the states all residual powers not explicitly assigned to the central government, vaccination and the practice of medicine generally fall within the authority of each state, with some important local and regional differences. Regarding mandatory vaccination, all states recognize a medical exemption, based on recommendations from Board-certified pediatricians or other licensed physicians; but these are valid for only one vaccine at a time, for only one of the very few adverse effects it has been unequivocally shown to cause, and must be renewed every year.

Because of these limitations, medical exemptions rarely correspond to what parents feel they need, and are too difficult for most people to qualify for to be of much use. Almost half of the states also recognize a "religious" or "philosophical" exemption, based on membership in some Church or denomination which is on record as being opposed to vaccination, such as Christian Scientists or Jehovah's Witnesses, or in the most liberal interpretation, simply a deeply-held "philosophical" conviction that opposes the practice. In Massachusetts, where I practice, the law as written includes the narrower word "religious," but the courts have interpreted it very liberally to extend into the purely personal realm of the individual conscience.

Much closer to the actual beliefs, attitudes, and special circumstances of most of the parents I talk with, the religious or philosophical exemption has generally been honored whenever they have claimed it; but serious difficulties remain that it does not address. Even in its most liberal interpretation, the religious or philosophical exemption is an absolute, across-the-board rejection of the concept of vaccination per se, designed to accommodate a dogmatic belief system in the "abolitionist" or "conscientious objector" mold.

In other words, the law protects the right of parents to be a kook, to dissent or deviate from the standard practice, but not to make intelligent medical decisions for their children, such as choosing some vaccines but not others. While this "pro-choice" position is respected by some open-minded physicians, nurses, and school boards in certain areas, such wording has yet to be written into the laws of any state, and draft laws proposing such changes have so far been rejected by every state legislature which has considered them, although by smaller and smaller margins each year.

As the biotech industry continues to crank out new vaccines without limit or restraint, and new and ever-broader applications are being found for the old ones, the widespread belief that the total number of vaccinations does indeed matter provides the best indication that the optional or pro-choice position will eventually prevail. As their ultimate strategy for circumventing even this modest ceiling on their profits, the vaccine manufacturers are busily developing a single vaccine containing a dozen or more individual components and administered in a single dose, whether injected, ingested, or perhaps even inhaled, to be repeated at rare intervals, and thus presumably arousing less public outcry.

Cost-Benefit Analysis and the "Bottom Line."

With that in mind, I want to consider the ultimate claim of the advocates of compulsory vaccination, its alleged effect of reducing the bottom-line *costs* of health care. As we saw, this viewpoint attained its peak of inflence during the Clinton era. Borrowing the newly popular "cost-benefit analysis" from the economists who used it to analyze the Federal budget into a list of allegedly discrete "line items," vaccination advocates

1) estimated the number of additional cases of any acute disease to be expected in an unvaccinated population;

2) multiplied it by the cost of caring for each case, including doctor and hospital fees and time lost from work, to obtain the total cost saved by the healthcare system; and then

3) divided it by the cost of vaccinating, i.e., the unit cost per vaccination times the number of doses given, to compute the "benefit-cost ratio."

In 1992, before President Clinton took office, Dr. Georges Peter of Brown University Medical School made the economic case for mandatory vaccination, based on its high benefit-cost ratio:

One of the most important medical developments in the 20th century has been the control of common childhood infectious diseases by the administration of highly effective vaccines. With the exception of safe water, no other modality, not even antibiotics, has had such a major effect on mortality reduction and population growth. Of particular importance in the current era of escalating health care costs is the fact that effective childhood vaccines are highly economical and thus represent an efficient use of society's resources. A highly favorable benefit-cost ratio — the ratio of the reduction in the cost of disease to the cost of the vaccination program — has been substantiated by many studies in the United States. For example, the MMR program led to savings of nearly $1.4 billion in disease costs in 1983, with a benefit-cost ratio of 14.4:1. By a similar analysis, for each dollar spent on pertussis vaccine, $2.10 is saved in health care costs.[133]

While the benefit-cost ratio soon became the favored calculus for promoting childhood vaccinations and silencing effective opposition to them, it systematically overlooks the rampant but still largely unseen epidemic of nonspecific effects that I've been describing, including ear infections, asthma, eczema, allergies, ADD, autism, auto-immune diseases, and the whole spectrum of common pediatric diseases, each of which contributes its own enormous chunk to those same exorbitant costs that vaccinations are supposed to be keeping down.

To give just one familiar example, this study of childhood ear infections was published in 1982, fully ten years earlier:

Otitis media is the most frequent diagnosis made by physicians who care for children. It has been estimated that approximately $2 billion is spent annually on medical and surgical treatment of this disease in the United States. This figure includes expenses for the estimated 1 million children who receive tympanostomy tubes and over 600,000 who yearly undergo tonsillectomies and adenoidectomies, which are mainly for the prevention of such infections.[134]

These figures would of course have been much higher had they been calculated at the time of Professor Peter's study, not to mention comparable figures for asthma, autism, allergies, and the other ailments we have been discussing, all of which have attained truly epidemic proportions in the twelve years since 1992. I do not claim that vaccines are solely responsible for creating these diseases, and cannot estimate with any degree of accuracy the percentage of their total medical and social costs that are attributable to the adverse reactions I have described. But merely recognizing that such reactions occur with the kind of frequency that I see in my practice, and that vaccines are required of every child, is sufficient to establish that this hidden factor is enormous in size, and that the benefit-cost ratio will look shockingly different once we factor it in.

I therefore propose the appointment of a bipartisan government Commission to investigate the medical and social costs of the leading childhood diseases, with the help of a panel of medical economists whom they would select, and the understanding that its deliberations would be conducted in a public forum, and that its final report would include a wide range of testimony from the medical and public health community and all sectors of the general public.

In particular, the Commission should be directed 1) to calculate the total medical and social costs of the common problems that all pediatricians commonly deal with, such as asthma, autism, allergies, eczema, ear infections, pneumonia, sinusitis, ADD, learning disabilities, behavior problems, and the like; 2) to try to measure the fraction of them that should be ascribed to vaccine-related causes; and 3) to multiply the first by the second to obtain the real cost of giving children all recommended vaccines on the approved list. If we estimate that the vaccines contribute even 20% of the total cost for each of these diseases, which I fear is much smaller than the true amount, it is evident that these hidden factors exceed by several orders of magnitude any conceivable savings that even the most rabid vaccine advocates have ever claimed for them.

Far from being a bargain, then, I submit that vaccines are in fact exorbitantly expensive on every level, and must bear an important share of responsibility for the skyrocketing costs of the present health care crisis as a whole, over which representatives of the government, the insurance industry, and the medical profession merely shake their heads in confusion and disbelief. In short, they provide a splendid example of what CFO's often refer to as a "hidden cost center."

Finally, even if vaccination programs could be shown to be effective in achieving their stated goals, the goals themselves may be of dubious value. As René Dubos once aptly warned, in words sounding even more prophetic today,

> The faith in the magical power of drugs often blunts the critical senses, and comes close at times to a mass hysteria involving scientists and laymen alike. Men want miracles as much today as in the past. If they do not join one of the newer cults, they satisfy this need by worshipping at the altar of modern science. This faith in the magical power of drugs is not new. It helped to give medicine the authority of a priesthood, and to recreate the glamour of ancient mysteries.[135]

The idea of eradicating measles, polio, and the rest has come to seem attractive to us because the power of medical science makes it seem technically possible: we worship each victory of biotechnology over Nature in the same way as a bullfight celebrates the triumph of human intelligence over the brute beast. Yet even if we manage to eliminate measles, polio, and all other acute diseases of mankind, nobody of sound mind can seriously maintain that we would be any the healthier for it, or that other at least equally serious ailments would not quickly rise up to take their place. Both medically and economically, I would argue that exchanging the few remaining epidemics of the past for the ubiquitous chronic diseases of today is the opposite of a good bargain, especially in the industrialized world, where the major infectious diseases were already in rapid decline owing to major improvements in basic hygiene, sanitation, air and water quality, and so forth.

In that sense, the quasi-religious fervor of the vaccine establishment offers an appropriate metaphor for the privatization and commercialism of the American medical enterprise as a whole, with its uncritical, idolatrous worship of biomedical science and technology, and its identification, expropriation, and commodification of every available life function for the sacrosanct twin purposes of profit and mastery. The deeply irreligious and infinitely hazardous myth that technical solutions can be found for illness and all other authentic human problems seems seductively attractive because it bypasses the problem of *healing,* which is a genuine miracle in the sense that it requires art and caring and individualized attention and therefore can always fail to occur.

NOTES.

1. Letter to the author.
2. Horton, R., "Vaccine Myths," in *Health Wars,* New York Review Books, 2003, pp. 207-208.
3. Ibid., p. 206.
4. *Morbidity and Mortality Weekly Report* in *Journal of the AMA* 260:198, April 8, 1988.
5. Letter to the author.
6. Letter to the author.
7. Coulter, H., and Fisher, B., *DPT: a Shot in the Dark,* Harcourt Brace Jovanovich, 1985.
8. Mortimer, E., *et al.,* "The Risk of Seizures and Encephalopathy after Immunization with the DTP Vaccine," *JAMA* 263:1641, March 23, 1990.
9. Cherry, J., "Pertussis Vaccine Encephalopathy: It's Time to Recognize It as the Myth That It Is," *JAMA* 263:1679, March 23, 1990.
10. "Vaccine Side Effects, Adverse Reactions, Contraindications, and Precautions," Advisory Committee on Immunization Practices, *MMWR* 45:22, September 1996.
11. Letter to the author.
12. Letter to the author.
13. Scheibner, V., *Vaccination: a Medical Assault on the Immune System,* New Atlantean Press, 1993, pp. xiv-xv, *passim.*
14. Ibid.
15. Bernier, R., et al., "DTP Vaccination and Sudden Infant Deaths in Tennessee," *Journal of Pediatrics* 101:419, 1982.
16. Torch, W., "DPT Immunization: a Potential Cause of SIDS," *Neurology* 32:169, 1982.
17. Ibid.
18. Noble, G., et al., "Acellular and Whole-Cell Pertussis Vaccines in Japan," *JAMA* 257:1351, 1987.
19. Cherry, J., et al., "Report of Task Force on Pertussis ands Pertussis Immunization," *Pediatrics* 81:939, Supplement, 1988.

20. Noble, G., op. cit.
21. Wakefield, A., et al., "Measles Vaccine: a Risk Factor for Inflammatory Bowel Disease?" *Lancet 345:1071,* 1995.
22. Wakefield, et al., "Ileal-Lymphoid Nodular Hyperplasia, Nonspecific Colitis, and Pervasive Developmental Disorder in Children," *Lancet* 351:637, 1998.
23. Ibid.
24. Wakefield, "MMR, Enterocolitis, and Autism," Lecture, *NVIC International Conference on Vaccination,* November 2002.
25. Ibid.
26. Ibid.
27. Megson, M., "Genetics, Vaccine Injury, and Getting Well," and Cave, S., "Vaccine Injury Therapy," *NVIC Conference Presentations,* November 2002.
28. *Family Practice News,* May 15, 2000, p. 49.
29. Ibid.
30. Ibid.
31. ACIP Update, "Vaccine Side-Effects, etc.," *MMWR* 1996, *op. cit.,* pp.7-8, *passim.*
32. Unpublished case.
33. *L. K. vs. Secretary of HHS,* No. 99-624V.
34. *T. O. vs. Secretary of HHS,* No. 99-635V.
35. Mathieu, E., et al., "Cryoglobulinemia after Hep B Vaccination," Letter, *New England Journal of Medicine* 335:356, August 1, 1996.
36. "Hepatitis B Vaccine," *The Vaccine Reaction,* NVIC Special Report, September 1998, p. 7.
37. Ibid.
38. Ibid.
39. Ibid.
40. Ibid.
41. Ibid.
42. Ibid., p. 9.
43. Moskowitz, R., "The Case Against Immunizations," *Journal of the American Institute of Homeopathy* 76:7, March 1983, p. 13.
44. Unpublished case.
45. Moskowitz, *Resonance: the Homeopathic Point of View,* Xlibris, 2001, pp. 177-178.
46. Moskowitz, "Childhood Ear Infections," *JAIH* 87:137, 1994.
47. Moskowitz, *Resonance,* op. cit., pp. 209-210.
48. Ibid., pp. 215-216.
49. Unpublished case.
50. Davis, B., et al., *Microbiology,* 2nd Ed., Harper, 1973, p. 1346.
51. Ibid.
52. Ibid., p. 1418.
53. Neustaedter, R., *The Vaccine Guide,* Revised Ed., North Atlantic, 2002, pp. 69-74.

54. Ibid.,pp.70-71.
55. Ibid., pp. 71-72.
56. Ibid., pp. 76-77.
57. Ibid.
58. Ibid., pp. 74-76.
59. Cherry, J., "The New Epidemiology of Measles and Rubella," *Hospital Practice,* July 1980, p. 49.
60. Gustafson, T., et al., "Measles Outbreak in a Fully-Immunized Secondary School Population," *NEJM* 316:771, March 26, 1987.
61. Chen, R., et al., *American Journal of Epidemiology* 129:173, 1989.
62. Cherry, "Measles," op. cit., 1980, p. 52.
63. National Vaccine Advisory Committee, "The Measles Epidemic," *JAMA* 266:1547, September 18, 1991.
64. Edmondson, M. et al., "Mild Measles and Secondary Vaccine Failure During a Sustained Outbreak in a Highly Vaccinated Population," *JAMA* 263:2467, May 9,1990.
65. Ibid.
66. Ibid.
67. Ibid.
68. Moskowitz, "Immunizations," op. cit., 1983.
69. Moskowitz,"Vaccination: a Sacrament of Modern Medicine," *The Homœopath* (UK) 12:137, 1992.
70. Adams, W., "Decline of Childhood *Hæmophilus Influenzæ* B Disease in the HiB Vaccine Era," *JAMA* 269:221, January 13, 1993.
71. *Family Practice News,* October 1, 1997, p. 9.
72. "Adverse Events Associated with HiB Vaccine," *WHO Printout,* www.who.int/ vaccines diseases/safety/infobank/hib.
73. Ibid.
74. Daum, R., et al., "Decline in Serum Antibody to *H. influenzæ* B Capsule in the Immediate Post-Immunization Period," *Journal of Pediatrics* 114:742, 1989.
75. *Boston Globe,* June 11,1991, p.9.
76. *FP News,* August 1, 1992, p. 23.
77. Pevsner, J., Letter, *American Family Physician,* January 1994, p. 47.
78. Tucker, A., et al., "Cost-Effectiveness Analysis of a Rotavirus Immunization Program for the United States," *JAMA* 279:1371, May 6, 1998.
79. Ibid.
80. Keusch, G., and Cash, R., "A Vaccine Against Rotavirus: When Is Too Much Too Much?" Editorial, *NEJM* 337:1228, October 23, 1997.
81. Murphy, T., et al., "Intussusception Among Infants Given an Oral Rotavirus Vaccine," *NEJM* 344:564, February 22, 2001.
82. Ibid.

83. *AMA Encyclopedia of Medicine,* 1989, quoted in "Chickenpox: the Disease and the Vaccine," Massachusetts Citizens for Vaccination Choice handout, East Arlington, MA.
84. American Academy of Pediatrics brochure, 1996, quoted in MCVC handout,op. cit.
85. "The Vaccine for Chickenpox," *American Family Physician* 53:652, February 1, 1996, Patient Information handout.
86. Spingarn, R., and Benjamin, J., Letter, *NEJM* 338:683, March 5, 1998.
87. Shapiro, E., and LaRussa, P., "Vaccination for Varicella: Just Do It!" Editorial, *JAMA* 228:1529, November 12, 1997.
88. Simberkoff, M., et al., "Efficacy of Pneumococcal Vaccine in High-Risk Patients," *NEJM* 315:1318, November 20, 1986.
89. Eskola, J., "Efficacy of a Pneumococcal Conjugate Vaccine Against Acute Otitis Media," *NEJM* 344:403, February 8, 2001.
90. *FP News,* April 15, 2000, p. 1..
91. Cantekin, E., Letter, *NEJM* 344:1719, May 31, 2001.
92. Damoiseaux, R., Letter, Ibid.
93. *Medical World News,* April 14, 1986.
94. Hurwitz, E., et al., "Guillain-Barre Syndrome and the 1978-1979 Influenza Vaccine," *NEJM* 304:1557, June 25, 1981.
95. *FP News,* June 1, 1999, p. 1.
96. Ibid.
97. Ibid.
98. *FP News,* August 15, 2002, p. 30.
99. Nichol, K., et al., "The Effectiveness of Vaccination Against Influenza in Healthy Working Adults," *NEJM* 333:889, October 5, 1995.
100. *FP News,* August 15, 2002, p. 30.
101. *Boston Globe,* August 25, 1992, p. 57.
102. Heemstra, T., *Anthrax: a Deadly Shot in the Dark,* Crystal Communications, 2002, p. 46.
103. *Boston Globe,* August3, 1999, p. 1.
104. *New York Times,* March 11, 1999, via Internet.
105. Heemstra, op. cit., 2002, pp. 31-35.
106. Ibid., p. 64.
107. Bates, S., "Anthrax Vaccination in the Military: One Pilot's Story," *NVIC Conference Presentation,* November 2002.
108. Matsumoto, G., "The Pentagon's Toxic Secret," *Vanity Fair,* May 1999, pp. 82-98.
109. Heemstra, op. cit., 2002, p. 107.
110. Ibid.
111. *FP News,* July 15, 2002, p. 10.
112. *FP News,* May 1, 2004, p. 41.
113. Quoted in Moskowitz, ed., "Smallpox," *AIH Bioterrorism Report, JAIH* 96:121, Summer 2003.

114. Ibid.
115. Eickhoff, T., "Adult Immunizations: How Are We Doing?" *Hospital Practice,* November 15, 1996, p. 107.
116. Averhoff, F., *et al.,* "Immunization of Adolescents," *American Family Physician* 55:159,January 1, 1997.
117. Sur, D., et al., "Vaccinations in Pregnancy," *American Family Physician* 68:299, July 15,2003.
118. *FP News,* April 1, 1997, p. 2.
119. *FP News,* September 1, 2001, p. 2.
120. Schlenker, T., et al., "Measles Herd Immunity," *JAMA* 267:823, 1992.
121. "ACIP Childhood and Adolescent Immunization Schedule," *FP News,* January 1, 2004, p. 9.
122. Ibid.
123. Koff, R., 'The Case for Routine Childhood Vaccination Against Hepatitis A," Editorial, *NEJM* 340:644, February 25, 1999.
124. Offit, P., et al., *Pediatrics* 109, January 2002, abstract by Sherry Tenpenny, D.O., "Expert Believes Infants Can Tolerate 10,000 Vaccines," March 27, 2002, www. mercola.com.
125. Moskowitz, "Vaccination: a Sacrament," op. cit., 1992.
126. Moskowitz, "Unvaccinated Children," *Mothering,* Winter 1987, p. 34.
127. *MMWR,* reported in *JAMA* 283:2381, May 10, 2000.
128. www.publichealthlaw.net, quoted in "News Release," No. 71_DITA, November 26, 2001,
129. Letter to the author.
130. 'The Vaccine Reaction," op. cit., January 1996, pp. 3-5.
131. *Orlando Sentinel,* August 28,2004, p..l.
132. *Boston Globe,* February 23, 1993, p. 1.
133. Peter, G., "Childhood Immunizations," *NEJM* 327:1794, December 19, 1992.
134. Bluestone, C., "Otitis Media in Children: to Treat or Not to Treat?" *NEJM* 306:1399, June 10,1982.
135. Dubos, R., *Mirage of Health,* Harper, 1959, p. 157.

IV. Writings on Homeopathic Philosophy and Method:

"Childhood Ear Infections"

"Hahnemann's Achievement and Legacy"

Resonance: The Homeopathic Point of View, Excerpts

"The Fundamentalist Controversy"

"For Homeopathy"

Childhood Ear Infections*

Otitis media has become the commonest pediatric diagnosis made by physicians caring for children in the United States,[1] its annual budget reaching $2 billion in 1982,[2] and growing ever since, with no relief in sight. After decades of punishing warfare against the resident nasopharyngeal bacteria, several medical journal articles have recently begun to admit defeat, and have questioned not only the safety and effectiveness of antibiotics and tympanostomy, but also the wisdom of prolonging the essentially military strategy based on them.[3,4,5**]

For those pursuing more holistic approaches, the present stalemate confers the opportunity and indeed the obligation to come forward and present our experience to the medical community and the public at large. Nobody need take my word for it that homeopathic remedies are inexpensive, non-toxic, and can help even the most advanced cases, or that parents, children, and their pediatricians alike will come to appreciate the non-invasive philosophy governing their use. I will feel amply rewarded if more professionals and lay people will simply try them and see for themselves.

Cases.

The following examples are intended to show how the homeopathic viewpoint can assist in diagnosis, treatment, and research for these extremely common ailments. The cases I have chosen are noteworthy not for any particular skill in choosing the correct medicine, but in precisely the opposite sense, that excellent results are regularly attainable with the common remedies and case-taking methods already well-known to every serious student. Indeed, our exemplary success in using homeopathic medicines to treat these children may itself be a clue to solving the mystery of pediatric otitis media and its disturbing pre-eminence in recent times.

---

* "Childhood Ear Infections," *Journal of the American Institute of Homeopathy* 87:137, Autumn 1994.

Case 1. C. Z., a girl of 3, had had recurrent ear infections since the age of 5 or 6 months, typically associated with colds and the production of thick, green mucus in the nose, throat, and sinuses, and treated with antibiotics each time, often for months without interruption. With no fever and perhaps a slight earache, she often became irritable and cranky as the cold ended, when her physician would make the diagnosis by otoscope. Apart from mild eczema, the child was seldom ill otherwise, and rarely had the fevers or acute illnesses to be expected at her age. A strapping 8 lb. at birth, she weighed only 16 lb. at one year, and had remained small for her age ever since. Teething was late and difficult. She had had all the usual vaccines, with no obvious reaction.

I chose *Calcarea sulphurica* 200, one dose, and 2 months later her mother reported "the best winter ever," with no ear infections and two mild colds that soon cleared up with the help of *Calcarea sulph.* 12C. I next saw her a year later, several weeks after an episode of wheezing in the middle of a cold, for which 2 doses of *Pulsatilla* 30X prescribed over the phone had worked splendidly. Despite no more ear infections in all that time, she had had a fever or two, and was still plagued by quantities of thick, greenish-yellow phlegm in her nose and throat. After one dose of *Sulphur* 200, she never came back. When I called recently, some 5 years later, her mother told me that she had never had another ear infection and that there was no need to bring her back, since her general health had remained very good, and the usual remedies had proved quite effective for the typical colds, fevers, and URI's that had developed along the way.

I want to add a few other comments about this by no means unusual case. First, as I reread it now, I doubt that either *Calcarea sulph.* or *Sulphur* was the true *simillimum* for this patient, since she was actually on the chilly side, and even after the treatment she she continued to produce large quantities of thick green phlegm and be subject to frequent colds. Indeed, I can't really defend or explain either prescription at this remove. Yet her mother was more than satisfied: the ear infections disappeared and never came back, the main constitutional issues stayed quietly in the background, and the remedies that she herself came up with continued to help without needing further assistance.

Notwithstanding all the small remedies and "cured" cases that we like to parade at our conferences, I suspect that by far the larger share of our practices and reputations are built upon stories as generic and unspectacular as this one, and can hardly fail to be deeply grateful for a method that adds feathers to my cap even when I bumble or fall short.

My own experience amply confirms numerous reports in the European literature that most kids eventually outgrow their ear infections anyway, if simply allowed to do so without too much allopathic interference.[6]

Case 2. K. G.-S., a boy of 16 months, had already had 5 ear infections and 5 rounds of antibiotics when I first saw him. The first episode at 6 months of age was the only one associated with fever (T. 102.8°) and acute earache, both of which subsided soon after the eardrum burst and discharged the pus that had accumulated behind it. Although he weighed 7 lb. at birth and appeared normal, he was slow to nurse, fell behind in his gross motor development, had had considerable pain and discomfort with teething, and still weighed only 20 lb. His only other complaint was a persistent diarrhea that had begun under antibiotic treatment and had since become chronic. In spite of prolonged and intense crying after his first two DPT s, the 3rd one and the MMR provoked no obvious reaction at all.

I gave him *Sulphur* 10M, one dose, and one month later his mother reported that the diarrhea had worsened, becoming particularly acute the first week, but that, despite a fever of 103° on the third day, the highest in his life, he had had no symptoms of a cold or ear infection since. Because of the diarrhea, I gave him *Calcarea carbonica* 10M, one dose, and by the next visit, two months hence, he was well and had made good progress developmentally, with no sign of an ear infection, one brief cold, for which *Calcarea sulph.* 12C worked well, and no more diarrhea.

After that I didn't see him again for more than a year, about 4 months after another acute otitis episode, with fever but no earache, that was diagnosed by otoscope, and continued for a full week on antibiotics. Previously, apart from a few colds and the reappearance of diarrhea at such times, he had had no more ear infections and was continuing to develop normally. Repeating the *Sulphur* 10M, I never had any further news of him until I had my receptionist call recently, more than 5 years later, and learned that he had been in good health the whole time, with no ear infections and no antibiotics. After buying a kit and studying on her own, the mother had herself found *Belladonna* to be highly effective in the early stages of his colds and acute illnesses, and no longer needed my help.

Again not for any elegant prescribing on my part, much less from any notion that the child was "cured," I treasure cases like this, because our work together helped his mother to take charge of his health and to perform competently in that role. When my own learned prescriptions fail, as they not infrequently do, I feel if anything even prouder when

180

the parents themselves find the remedies that work best for their child. Among the most precious gifts that homeopaths can offer the medical community is our relationships with our patients, which can continue to grow and flourish even when the *simillimum* proves elusive.

Case 3. J. L., a girl of 6, had had ear infections repeatedly since the age of 5 months, particularly when exposed to other kids in crowded day care or classroom settings. With little fever and no earache, the individual episodes were quite mild, with red cheeks, loss of appetite, and grumpy, cross, or irritable behavior. While vulnerable to staying up late and sudden changes of weather, she seldom ran fevers of any kind, the highest around 102° with a "Strep throat," yet had already taken antibiotics over two dozen times. Although vaccinated at the usual times without any obvious reaction, she developed an ear infection after her 5-year DPT booster that persisted for 4 months despite long-term maintenance on antibiotics, and subsided only with chiropractic treatment.

Two days after a single dose of *Sulphur* 10M, she developed a generalized rash that lasted 3 or 4 days, followed by a more bouncy mood and livelier energy than she had displayed in a very long time. At the time of her first follow-up, she had a mild cold, with the usual red cheeks, runny eye, temporary hearing loss, and the dreaded positive Strep culture. It required a considerable leap of faith for her mother to allow even this minor illness to run its course without antibiotics, using only *Pulsatilla* 30X as needed, but soon after she bought a kit of remedies and a book to learn how to use them. Two months later, her pediatrician was happy to report and even take credit for the fact that her ears were uninfected for the first time that anyone could recall.

The following winter, she was back with her usual symptoms, a low fever, and a weakly-positive Strep culture. As it subsided, I repeated the *Sulphur* 10M, and at her next visit the picture had changed to one of recurrent sore throats, foul breath, enlarged tonsils, dark circles under the eyes, and a loose, productive cough. This time I chose *Mercurius vivus* 1M, followed by the 10M one month later, with good results until yet another cold several months later, accompanied by the same swollen tonsils and loose cough as before. This time I repeated *Sulphur* 10M, and I never saw her again, but her mother reported a few years later that she had remained very well the whole time, with no major colds, no ear infections since the first visit, and for the first time a perfect attendance record for the school year just completed. Calling her back recently, we learned she was doing very well in high school, with no ear infections at all in the nine years since she had begun using remedies.

Once again leaving aside my rather crude prescribing in this case, I want to point out a few of the methodological issues it exemplifies, issues so basic as to be readily overlooked. First, the official policy of equating fluid behind the drum with a full-blown "ear infection" calling for antibiotic treatment ignores what every family doctor or pediatrician knows, that most colds or URI's, especially with swelling of the tonsils and adenoids, can be expected to produce secondary congestion of the middle ear and some degree of temporary hearing loss as a result. The girl in this case was subject primarily to tonsillitis, and could be said to have ear infections only to the extent that the pneumatic otoscope can detect even minute amounts of fluid, and that years of war against the resident ear bacteria have culminated in this failed Vietnam-like strategy of killing everything in the vicinity.

Secondly, her longest period of ear involvement followed soon after a DPT booster, a connection that I have verified countless times in my practice for a number of different vaccines, but that is rarely suspected by doctors and parents alike, because vaccines are widely regarded as almost risk-free and indeed sacrosanct, except for a few comparatively rare life-threatening events developing within the first hours or days.[7] Finally, like most of my patients with chronic otitis media, this child seldom ran fevers throughout the time she had received conventional treatment, and began to do so only when her general condition improved. Useful prognostically for reassuring the family, this simple fact also carries major implications for the natural history of the disease and its evolution in recent times.

Case 4. L. P., a girl of 10 months, had already had 4 acute ear infections and received antibiotics for each one. They began at 2 months of age, when her mother was forced to wean her to go back to work, and the baby developed a rash and unusually cranky behavior on a milk-based formula. These early symptoms were all greatly intensified for a full week after her first DPT shot, promptly followed by an acute ear infection with high fever and a violent earache, much like all of the others.

With the help of *Calcarea carbonica* 1M at the outset and *Chamomilla* 30X as needed acutely, she did quite well, with fewer colds and none of her typical acute episodes, but mild symptoms persisted and were aggravated by teething, when the remedies had to be repeated. The following spring, 6 months later, she started all over again, with 3 typical ear infections and as many rounds of antibiotics in the 3 months since her father had insisted on her long-overdue MMR vaccination. At this point I gave her *Lycopodium* 10M, followed by *Sulphur* 10M a month later, and was about to change the remedy yet again, until I learned that the parents had recently separated and were angrily vying over the child. From then on, she continued to do very well on infrequent doses of *Sulphur*, despite a violent bout of gastroenteritis after a DT and polio booster, and a tendency to relapse when she stayed with her father, who let her eat her fill of dairy products and took her to the pediatrician for her regular quota of antibiotics and vaccines.

I have continued to follow this child at irregular intervals for more than nine years, and although she has long since outgrown her ear infections, her underlying health issues have not changed all that much. Already evident in the acute, vigorous responses of her infancy, her basically strong constitution and immune system have matured over the years, enabling her to bounce back more quickly than ever when she does fall ill. While both allergic and mildly addicted to milk and cheese, she has continued to grow and develop relatively normally in the face of a conflicted heritage that she can not as yet understand or change.

In short, this is a child of strong vitality who exemplifies the opposite side of the same issues already discussed:

1) the innate tendency to respond acutely and vigorously to infection, and to recover quickly from it;

2) the tendency to relapse following any vaccination, and to milk allergy which is often associated with it; and

3) the tendency to develop the classic signs and symptoms of acute otitis media that were the rule in the pre-vaccine and pre-antibiotic era, but have since become the exception.

Overview.

With these few representative cases in mind, I will try to summarize my experience with the general phenomenon of otitis media in children, giving special emphasis to the practical issues of diagnosis, treatment, prognosis, and long-term case management.

First, as with my allopathic colleagues, middle-ear infection is one of the commonest presenting complaints of children in my practice, although I do mostly chronic work and provide well-baby and well-child visits only when the parents explicitly ask for them. In an average week, I may triage four or five acute cases over the phone, and see one new and two or three established patients with chronic or recurrent otitis that have been diagnosed and treated repeatedly or on a long-term basis with antibiotics or tympanostomy, or both.

What most of these patients have in common is the absence or relative paucity of strong symptoms like high fever or violent earache, such as would indicate an acute, vigorous response to the illness. With a few exceptions, like the previous case, their symptoms when they do flare up are more likely to be vague and nondescript in character, such as "fussy" or "cranky" behavior, whining or picking at the ear, mild hearing loss, poor appetite, and the like. In quite a few instances, there are no symptoms whatsoever, and the child behaves and functions perfectly normally, but the pediatrician detects some fluid behind the drum at a well-baby visit, signs it off as an "ear infection," and begins the cycle of antibiotic treatment that may prove quite difficult to break.

Similarly, although the symptoms often recede to some extent during conventional treatment, relapse is common afterwards, and even when the child appears clinically well, the presence of fluid is generally interpreted as a persistence of the infection, or in any case as a mandate for continuation of antimicrobial therapy. In this way, a child who may never have been that sick never gets entirely well, and continues to relapse until the pediatrician recommends maintenance doses of antibiotics for months at a time, or indefinitely, as well as surgical insertion of tubes for artificial drainage if the condition persists despite these measures, as indeed it often does. In short, the most striking and disturbing feature of these cases is simply their *chronicity,* their tendency to develop smoldering or persistent responses to illness, to relapse more and more easily, and to fail to heal or resolve themselves in a clearcut or timely fashion.

In treating such a case, the physician need only break this cycle, which may be accomplished quite easily if the parents are willing to co-operate. But here too lies the major obstacle, our own cultural belief and professional indoctrination that reduces the art of diagnosis to the specialized detection of abnormalities and the goal of treatment to the killing or decimation of our resident bacteria. Even more than finding the correct remedy, the most difficult and important requirement for success in treating these kids lies in re-educating the parents and developing an alternative model that works and makes sense for them.

First, I try to redefine the nature of the illness and the best way to detect and diagnose it, beginning with some basic anatomy of the ear, nose, and throat, and the typical clinical and pathological features of a URI with ear involvement (congestion, earache, etc.), contrasting it with that of a full-blown acute otitis media. Always my emphasis is focused on the signs and symptoms that they are already well aware of, that is, how the child feels and functions, or what we homeopaths like to call "the totality of symptoms."

If we've made a good connection and feel pretty much "in synch" so far, I may go a step further and propose that we *not* look in the ear just yet, unless the clinical picture is especially intense, or hasn't resolved after giving remedies, or either of us is so panicked that we just have to know. Since almost any URI can produce detectable fluid congestion behind the drum, and it is not necessary or even desirable to treat the illness all the way to the end, the totality of symptoms is what best defines the illness, and what we can see through the otoscope adds really useful information only in the rarest and most difficult cases.

If there is significant ear involvement, I like to reassure parents that giving antibiotics is no more effective than placebo,[8,9,10] and that in fact it produces more frequent relapses than giving analgesics and simply allowing the children to recover on their own.[11] Only at that point will I add the punch line, that homeopathic remedies are wonderfully effective, both for the acute episodes and "constitutionally," to prevent them or minimize their number and severity.

Finally, I will take a careful vaccine history and look for any other underlying chronic or constitutional influences that may contribute to the problem, such as a difficult pregnancy, traumatic birth, or other established illness, food allergy, emotional upset, and the like. Quite often, the first episode can be traced to shortly after a DPT, MMR, or some other vaccination, even when no acute or obvious reaction was noted at the time,[12] or the old pattern of chronic or recurrent otitis is reactivated by a booster after a long period of remission.[13] Many times, a relapse following this or that booster after a long period of good health is what first convinces the parent of the connection, which has also been

183

independently corroborated by the curative effect of homeopathic nosodes prepared from the vaccine or natural disease in such cases.[14] Citing these experiences, I will ask the parents not to vaccinate the child at least until the condition has been resolved, and refer them to my various writings on the subject for further study.

While they are by no means the only important factor in the background of such cases, and I have seen my share of chronic otitis even in unvaccinated kids, vaccines stand alone in being legally mandated for every child, and in being regarded as so uniformly safe and beneficial that the mere possibility of chronic, long-term sequelæ is seldom if ever taken seriously.[15]

With this important preparatory work done, I'm ready to proceed with homeopathic remedies. The guidelines I follow and the remedies I use are no different from the ones that we use in general pediatric practice, and I see no need to elaborate on them here. If the child is not acutely ill at the time of the first visit, I usually begin with a single dose of the indicated preventive or "constitutional" remedy in perhaps a 200 potency, often a typical polychrest, such as one of the *Calcareas* or *Kali* salts, or *Sulphur,* or sometimes with a so-called "acute" remedy like *Aconite, Belladonna,* or *Chamomilla* if it is indicated for the acute episode but clearly discernible in the chronic pattern as well.

I also find it very helpful to suggest the 12C or 30X of a remedy to have on hand for acute flare-ups, often the same one as the 200, or perhaps another complementary to it, and to see the child or at least coach the parents through the episode with words of encouragement, changing the remedy if necessary. Once remedies have helped them through an acute episode without antibiotics, the remainder of the treatment is apt to proceed quite smoothly. If the child has never had a fever or responded acutely or intensely before, it is prudent and even reassuring to prepare the family for such an eventuality beforehand.

By no means grounds for discouragement, relapses many months or even years later are even simpler to treat, since the precipitating factors will be much more obvious after a period of good health, and the remedies that worked well before will most likely perform even better the next time, as the children often know by asking for it themselves. This uncanny ordering and clarification of the case over time is the predictable legacy of effective treatment, and the awe and wonder that they inspire in doctors, patients, and family members are among the most treasured and lasting rewards of every homeopathic practice.

Chronicity.

Thus what is most mysterious and problematic about ear infections in children does not lie in the manner of their treatment, which is not especially difficult, and typically involves the same remedies as are indicated for many other chronic ailments, but rather, as we have seen, in the nature, causes, and effects of that chronicity itself.

When I was a medical student in New York City in the early 1960's, otitis media was pre-eminently an acute disease, often presenting in the Emergency Room with a high fever and piercing shrieks of pain, both of which ended abruptly as soon as the eardrum burst and discharged its purulent contents. While certainly not a pleasant experience for doctor or patient, it seldom lasted very long, indeed had often taken care of itself before we had the chance to interfere with it, and was unlikely to come back for a long time to come. In short, it closely resembles the type of acute flare-up which, when I see it in one of my patients today, I have learned to interpret as a favorable prognostic sign.

When I moved to Boston in 1982, stopped doing births and primary care, and limited my practice to classical homeopathy, I started to see large numbers of chronic otitis patients such as I have just described. Why the occasional acute ear infection I knew in medical school had mushroomed into a chronic disease of epic proportions was also precisely the question with which I began this article. Both my clinical experience and the research I have conducted to support it have amply confirmed my intuitive sense that the modern pandemic of chronic otitis media can be attributed largely to two cruel, fanatical, and ultimately self-defeating wars that embody the same militaristic philosophy:

1) a decades-long war on the nasopharyngeal bacteria, fought with antibiotics, tympanostomy tubes, and the cultivation of fear of communicable disease; and

2) the vaccination of entire populations against a growing list of acute diseases, essentially on principle, with no end in sight, and no inclination to consider the possible long-term consequences of doing so.

Based on Koch's postulates and their considerable predictive value, the war on our own resident bacterial flora is both undesirable and unwinnable, even in thought. Unwinnable, because as among this planet's most basic life forms, bacteria can reproduce themselves in an average of six hours, and through natural selection rapidly become resistant to even the most lethal antibiotics. In clinical medicine, some important examples include nosocomial or hospital-borne outbreaks of resistant *Staphylococci* and *E. coli,* and the emergence of infections with new, mutant organisms such as *Mycoplasma,* and PPLO, which lack cell walls, obvious adaptations to penicillin-rich environments. In a recent *Newsweek* article, the propagation of resistant strains made hospitals into veritable centers of germ warfare, from which virulent organisms are widely disseminated out into a general population more or less powerless to stop them.[16]

In the case of childhood ear infections, resistant strains have similarly been implicated in the weakened primary immune responses and high relapse rates associated with antibiotic treatment.[17] Other common sequelæ include superinfection with yeasts and other common fungi, as well as the food and environmental allergies that often accompany them.

Studies of the fluid isolated from kids' infected ears have shown that the predominant organisms are simply the common pathogens of the tonsils and nasopharynx, such as the "pneumococcus," or *Streptococcus pneumoniæ,* Group A ß-hemolytic *Streptococcus*, the main culprit of "Strep throats," *Hemophilus influenzæ* type B (HiB), and *Staphylococcus aureus,* all of which are commonly found in healthy throats as well.[18] Indeed, in 20% of the children with acute otitis media, and 80% of those with the chronic serous variety that is now most prevalent, the effusions are sterile and no longer contain any organisms whatsoever.[19,20] Once the resident bacterial flora are destroyed, the common result is "glue ear," an important cause of chronic and sometimes permanent deafness. Thus even more injurious than the drugs themselves is the fanatical strategy of attacking and killing everything in sight that makes such imagery seem attractive.

A further application of the same military approach is the pneumatic otoscope, the tight seal of which permits the detection of even minute amounts of fluid and thus facilitates both early diagnosis and ongoing surveillance. Yet diagnosing more infection has only unleashed still more firepower, with the same ruinous results as described above. With tympanostomy, the war against otitis media attains its final dead end, looking like an obvious practical solution to the mechanical problem, yet itself recently found to be a major cause of otosclerosis and *permanent* hearing loss, ironically the same spectre used to browbeat reluctant parents into accepting it in the first place.[21] Even more ironic is the fact that such ear tubes merely substitute a fixed, artificial conduit for the natural process of perforation and drainage that the acutely infected ear heals so well by itself and with so few complications.

In any case, it makes no sense to search out and destroy the mostly friendly bacteria that have already established residence in our bodies and police them so effectively for our benefit, or to suppose that making war on them could ever produce anything but more war, more devastation, and the emergence of still other and for the most part even more hostile types of bacteria capable of surviving it.

As for vaccine-related illness, comparatively little of my experience is of the kind that Harris Coulter and Barbara Fisher described in their book, *Shot in the Dark,*[22] which like most of the anti-vaccination literature is limited to what appear to be specific effects of specific vaccines, in their case, different types of encephalopathy or brain damage from the DPT. While such reactions are likely to be the most dramatic and severe, as well as those for which the corresponding homeopathic nosodes would probably be most useful, most of my own clinical experience has to do with subtler, more generic reactions of what I would describe as a *non-specific* type. By that I mean that they appear to represent exacerbations of a pre-existing chronic state, as is evident from the fact that they appear more or less the same in a given individual, regardless of which vaccine is given, and are benefited by the same group of remedies that we already use for the general population, whether vaccinated or not. While such reactions are rather more difficult to recognize and verify, they are also much more common and in the overall scheme of things, I suspect, considerably more important.

In particular, two of the four cases I presented exhibited prolonged, severe relapses of their chronic state after a vaccination; one patient suffered almost identical relapses after two different vaccines; and all four first developed their chief complaint soon after their first dose of the DPT series. In no case were their responses acute or obvious enough to be identified as a repeatable symptom of that particular vaccine. Indeed, as I've said, all that was repeatable in all of the cases, and with all of the vaccines, was simply the chronicity of the responses, the fact that they occurred more frequently, persisted for longer periods of time, and showed less of a tendency to resolve themselves spontaneously.

It is precisely this congruence between vaccine-related responses and the original illnesses that they make worse, that suggests how vaccines act nonspecifically on the immune system as a whole, and so implicated vaccines in the still more basic riddle of chronicity itself. As biotech firms are busily cranking out new genetically-engineered vaccines almost as fast as they can identify possible organisms to attack, the all-out war against identifiable acute diseases has already added to the pre-existing chronic disease burden a full complement of new DNA- and RNA-like fragments looking for chromosomes to recombine with, and thus inadvertently to engender new diseases of which as yet we know nothing. In short, I'm afraid that doctors, like politicians, are here to stay.

NOTES.

1. Koch, H., *Office Visits to Pediatricians,* National Center for Health Statistics, Washington, 1974.
2. Bluestone, C., "Otitis Media in Children," *New England Journal of Medicine* 306:1399, 10 June 1982.
3. Cantekin, E., et al., "Antimicrobial Therapy for Otitis Media with Effusion," *Journal of the AMA* 266:3309, 18 December 1991.
4. Frenkel, M., "Acute Otitis Media: Does Therapy Alter Its Course?" *Postgraduate Medicine* 82:83, October 1987.
5. *Family Practice News,* 15 December 1990.
6. Van Buchem, F., et al., "Therapy of Acute Otitis Media," *Lancet* 2:883, 1981.
7. Moskowitz, R., "The Case Against Immunizations," *Journal of the American Institute of Homeopathy* 76:7, March 1983.
8. Cantekin, op. cit.

9. Van Buchem, op. cit.

10. Townsend, E., "Otitis Media in Pediatric Practice," *New York State Journal of Medicine* 64:1591, June 1964.

11. Cantekin, op. cit.

12. Moskowitz, R., "Vaccination: A Sacrament of Modern Medicine," *Journal of the AIH* 84:96, December 1991.

13. Ibid.

14. Ibid.

15. Ibid.

16. "The End of Antibiotics," *Newsweek,* 28 March 1994.

17. Cantekin, op. cit.

18. Bluestone, op. cit.

19. Ibid.

20. Cantekin, op. cit.

21. *Family Practice News,* op. cit.

22. Coulter, H., and Fisher, B. L., *DPT: A Shot in the Dark,* Avery, Garden City, NY, 1991.

Hahnemann's Achievement and Legacy*

I am grateful for this opportunity to reflect on and pay tribute to the life and achievements of this extraordinary man, which are almost without precedent in the history of science. For as far as I know, homeopathy is the only extant methodology for medicine or any other learned profession that was conceived and brought forth fully-formed from a single human brain, and has continued to grow and develop while remaining essentially intact for a period of two hundred years.

Similarly, there is no other profession that I know of in which those who carry on its work are content and even proud to acknowledge their greatest achievements as basically footnotes to the books he wrote and the principles he enunciated so long ago. Nor is there a more precise or suitable measurement of the gulf which still separates the homeopathic viewpoint from that of conventional medicine. While the latter rightly prides itself on its readiness for change, its astonishing capacity to remake itself on short notice, not only the Law of Similars, but the "Vital Force," the Totality of Symptoms, the Single Remedy, the Minimum Dose, and other basic principles remain as fresh and timeless today as when the Master first proclaimed them.

In part the uniqueness of Hahnemann's achievement lies in the fact that what we have come to know as "homeopathy" actually comprises two radically different projects in a single package, each closely bound up with the other, and both rightly bearing his name. To the public, it is best known as a set of techniques for healing the sick, a *methodology* that includes detailed instructions for interviewing patients and for preparing, investigating, selecting, and administering medicinal agents. Indeed it is at this technical level that Hahnemann continued to experiment throughout his career, and where homeopathy has always seemed utterly strange and even improbable to most people, and thus controversial and vulnerable to its many detractors as well. And it is here, too, that its practitioners are most grateful to him at that moment of truth when we

---

* "Hahnemann's Achievement and Legacy," *American Homeopath* 6:65, 2000.

place a bit of fairy dust on the patient's tongue and get to to savor the look of incredulity that heralds the miracle to come.

But to those of us who practice it, homeopathy is also a *philosophy,* not only in the ordinary sense of a set of ideas and opinions about health and disease, but also technically, as a coherent system of principles that all follow logically from a few axiomatic premises that cannot themselves be proved, quite in the spirit of Bertrand Russell's whimsical definition:

> . . . the point of philosophy is to start with something so obvious as not to seem worth stating, and to end up with something so paradoxical that no one will believe it.[1]

Not only the Law of Similars, but also the *Materia medica,* the single remedy, the minimum dose, the "Laws of Cure," and the other cardinal principles of homeopathy all seem to follow inevitably from the concept of the "vital force," without which they make very little sense, and the "totality of symptoms," its applied or clinical aspect, upon which the methodology itself depends.

Homeopathy owes its peculiar longevity to this happy conjunction of both elements, of philosophy and method. Gifted thinkers have always left behind enduring philosophies that still speak to us across the centuries, but without a practical method of applying them in the world they survive only as ideal possibilities as yet unrealized. Conversely, modern physicians and scientists have contributed a wealth of technical innovations that by transforming medical knowledge and practice have also engendered new operating principles to keep pace with them.

Only homeopathy, Hahnemann's brainchild, has managed to sustain itself without fundamental change, because it is *both* philosophy and method, such that even its practical applications, while reflecting and keeping abreast of technical progress, remain firmly grounded in principles that still generate relevant and valid conclusions, and are therefore still operative to that extent. While it does not qualify as "hard science" like physics and chemistry for precisely that reason, because the "Law of Similars," the "Vital Force," and the "Totality of Symptoms" are not subject to experimental proof or disproof like ordinary hypotheses, homeopathy remains thoroughly scientific in its attitude and its subject matter, and is entirely amenable to objective, scientific, and even experimental corroboration as to the consistency, accuracy, relevance, and predictive value of the system as a whole.

Perhaps its closest analogue in modern history is Freudian psychoanalysis, which was likewise conceived and developed by a single great mind, and which not only combined a rigorous analytic philosophy of experience with a detailed methodology for professional practice, but also gave rise to a disciplined and committed *movement* that still plays an important part on the world stage.

The similarity becomes even closer and more fruitful when we consider the practical difficulties that have beset homeopathy from the very beginning and are still very much in evidence today. For Hahnemann as for Freud, his tireless quest for immutable Laws of Nature, his overriding ambition to see his discoveries made good in the world, and the sheer force of his intellect all conspired to found a sectarian movement, based on strict adherence to his principles, that demanded the absolute loyalty and obedience of its adherents, and increasingly isolated itself from and fortified itself against dissenting cultural influences from outside.

In spite of his distinguished reputation as an expert chemist and authority on the preparation of medicinal substances, Hahnemann's unorthodox discoveries and often strident claims were greeted with silence from many of his colleagues, and actively opposed by the local apothecaries, whose livelihood seemed threatened by his insistence on the single remedy, and on physicians preparing it themselves.[2]

Even after his success in treating epidemic diseases earned him a lectureship and made him famous throughout Europe, Hahnemann continued to be ridiculed and persecuted for his heresies until 1822, when a wealthy patron gave him shelter and a regular stipend to publish his writings.[3] In addition to the *Organon of Medicine,* his original text, which ran to six editions, and the *Materia Medica Pura* and *Chronic Diseases,* his other major works, he wrote dozens of technical articles and monographs, as well as maintaining a voluminous correspondence, and continuing to teach, practice, and conduct experimental research until the very end of his long life.

In his old age he remarried and moved to Paris, where at last he enjoyed wealth and celebrity, and died secure in the knowledge that his students and followers were practicing quality homeopathy throughout Europe and in America. Over fifty years after his death, his remains were finally laid to rest in the Père Lachaise, fitly crowned by his own epitaph, *Non inutilis vixi,* which means "I have not lived in vain." Gifted by intellect and driven by ambition, he left us an elegant philosophy of health and illness and a practical methodology of healing the sick that have stood the test of time.

At the same time, his autocratic style and imperious temper not only alienated many promising students, but also inadvertently encouraged a profusion of opposing factions and interpretations, each claiming legitimate inspiration and descent from some aspect or phase of his thought. The unending flood of invective against faint-hearted prescribers who still cling to allopathic philosophy, use several remedies at a time, or treat the disease category rather than the patient all originated with diatribes emanating from the pen of the Master himself.

Defending the principles of homeopathy as sacred, quasi-religious truth, Hahnemann and his disciples were, as indeed many still remain, harshly intolerant of all who appear to deviate from his vision, creating an absolutist dogma that still expects and indeed attracts persecution, as well as a tradition of internecine ideological warfare that has continued to divide the movement through periods of success as well as decline. A tragic example was the abortive career of the Leipzig Homeopathic Hospital, a project which Hahnemann had long cherished, and which would undoubtedly have succeeded had he not turned the Law of Similars into a kind of loyalty oath by insisting that anyone claiming the title of homeopath be made to swear allegiance to it.

In 1832, physicians of the Leipzig Homeopathic Union put up the money to establish a hospital and medical school, and selected Dr. Moritz Müller, a prominent, reputable clinician and enthusiastic supporter of homeopathy, as acting Medical Director. It was understood that Dr. Benjamin Schweikert, an experienced classical prescriber, would eventually relocate to the area to take over the post, but the latter refused to serve without pay, and then backed out entirely when the original sponsors voted to admit all interested physicians, even if they were not yet ready to practice homeopathy exclusively.[4]

This seemingly well-meaning compromise infuriated Hahnemann, who turned on Müller and the "half-homeopaths" of Leipzig in a scathing letter to the local newspaper that not only ruined the former's long and illustrious career, but also effectively insured the failure of the hospital itself. I quote a few choice passages:

> I have heard that some in Leipzig who pretend to be Homeopathists allow their patients to choose whether they shall be treated homeopathically or allopathically. Whether they are not as yet thoroughly grounded in the true spirit of the new doctrine, or lack due benevolence to their species, or do not scruple to dishonor their profession for the sake of sordid gain, at least let them not expect me to recognize them as true disciples!

> Bloodletting, the application of leeches and Spanish flies, the use of setons and mustard plasters, salves and aromatics, emetics and purgatives, destructive doses of mercury and quinine: these and other quackeries, combined with the use of homeopathic remedies, identify these crypto-Homeopaths as surely as a lion is known by his claws. Let such be avoided, for they regard neither the welfare of the patient nor the honor of the profession. Practice honorably as an Allopath, as yet ignorant of anything better, or a pure Homeopath for the welfare of mankind. But as long as you wear this double mask, you will be a contemptible hybrid of a physician, of all the most pernicious.

> From now on, he who hesitates to prove himself a Homeopath in word and deed should never come to me expecting a friendly reception. We are considering an institution for demonstrating the efficacy of pure Homeopathy on the sick before the eyes of the whole world. Therefore I solemnly protest against the employment of such a bastard Homeopath either as teacher or attendant. Should any false doctrine be taught in the name of Homeopathy, or patients be treated with any imitation of Allopathic practice, I will raise my voice and warn the world against such treachery.[5]

But Hahnemann's all-too-human character flaws cannot detract from the greatness of his achievement. It does us as little credit to blame him for the intransigeance and fanaticism of our debates today as to abdicate responsibility for how we behave by writing it off to abusive parents or a difficult childhood. Indeed if Hahnemann or his disciples had been any less zealous about preserving his principles, it is quite possible, if not likely, that neither the method nor the philosophy that we find so elegant and beautiful today would have survived in the face of both the persecution and the seductiveness of conventional medicine, which tried for so long and so powerfully to destroy it and very nearly succeeded not so long ago.

To understand our *own* sectarian mentality, we shall have to re-examine that part of Hahnemann's legacy that we still reaffirm today for reasons of our own. What has always divided us amongst ourselves and from the medical profession as a whole is simply a logical consequence of the absolute moral force we do in fact accord to the basic principles of homeopathy, first as an objective law of health and disease, and above all as a prescriptive guide to our conduct as health professionals, which does indeed imply the right and even the duty to set standards for ourselves over and above those of our various licenses.

It should therefore occasion no surprise or excessive disappointment if Hahnemann turns out to have been a flesh-and-blood human being not unlike ourselves, with his full quota of human failings and unattractive qualities. We can still be thankful for his mastery of the healing art, and for his having used his splendid gifts so long and so well for the improvement of our understanding, the development of our practice, and the benefit of mankind. He left us an art that is still beloved throughout the world, and a philosophy of health and illness that will endure long after the homeopathic method as we now know it becomes obsolete. For these great blessings we remain deeply grateful.

NOTES.

1. Russell, B., "The Philosophy of Logical Atomism," in *Logic and Knowledge: Essays, 1901- 1950,* Allen and Unwin, London, 1968, p. 193.
2. Bradford, T. L., *Life and Letters of Hahnemann,* Boericke & Tafel, Philadelphia, 1895, pp. 113-116.
3. Ibid., pp. 120-134.
4. Ibid., pp. 292-313.
5. Ibid., pp. 300-302, *passim.*

Resonance: the Homeopathic Point of View*

When I began studying homeopathy in 1974, the sleepy little town where the course was held and the advanced age and semi-retired status of the instructors didn't augur well for the future of the movement. By the time I moved to Boston eight years later, no homeopathic physician had prescribed in the area for twenty-five years, as if a whole generation of active, full-time practitioners had never materialized. With no year-round schools, clinics, and teaching hospitals to its name, American homeopathy seemed obsolete and unlikely to survive much longer.[1]

Today, against all odds, reputable schools and training programs for physicians and allied health professionals are thriving as never before, while homeopathic ideas and products enjoy growing popularity and visibility at the retail level and in the media. After generations of aging and decline, this renewed interest in a method nearly two centuries old is so improbable that it is worth asking why Americans are rediscovering it now, as if for the first time.

To that little conundrum should be added the deeper mystery of homeopathy itself. Its basic claim that medicines have healing power over the same array of symptoms that they can elicit in healthy people is far from self-evident, to say the least, and has never been proved or disproved in the same way that ordinary scientific hypotheses are expected to be. Still less has anyone ever satisfactorily explained how a dose too minute to be detected chemically could possibly have *any* effect on a patient, let alone a beneficial one.[2] Confronted at every turn with riddles like these, I can't help feeling a little uneasy when patients seem prepared to swallow them whole without question or demur.

Finally, homeopathic theory and practice have changed remarkably little in two centuries, an era when technical achievements like surgical anesthesia, blood transfusion, the germ theory of disease, molecular biology, and the detailed anatomy and physiology of the human body

---

* *Resonance: the Homeopathic Point of View,* 372 pp., with Epilogue and Historical Appendix, Xlibris, Philadelphia, 2001

196

have transformed how we live and think almost beyond recognition. If homeopathy cannot match or even keep up with these developments, why should we bother to resurrect it today, when the same forces that superseded it long ago now control the entire health care system? Before attempting to explain it, then, it seems fitting to ask a more basic question: Who *needs* homeopathy?

Why Patients Seek Homeopathic Treatment.

The short answer is to be found among the reasons our patients give for coming to see us. The first is simple curiosity about other philosophies and approaches, coupled with the natural instinct to try a gentler approach before more drastic methods are called for. The second is that many who are seriously or chronically ill come for homeopathic treatment as a last resort, after conventional methods have failed, or created even worse problems of their own.

Common to both groups is the assumption that homeopathy will at least be less harsh and dangerous than drugs or surgery, albeit tempered with a healthy skepticism as to its effectiveness. Much the same mix of feelings are expressed by patients wanting evaluation and treatment of strange ailments as yet undiagnosed, and by some with no pressing complaints at all, who seek mainly a caring, accessible physician and a style more congenial than the prevailing one. In short, the growing interest in homeopathy is no ignorant repudiation of science as such, but simply a faithful indicator of dissatisfaction with the limitations and shortcomings of the current medical system.[3]

Why I Became a Homeopath.

A more detailed answer is provided by the life histories and autobiographical statements of homeopaths and other like-minded physicians, many of whom have chosen to give up more prominent, lucrative, or respectable careers for the sake of alternative methods and philosophies still regarded as unscientific if not heretical by the bulk of the profession. *Why do they do it?*

My own core beliefs and attitudes about doctoring grew out of my experiences as a medical student in the 1960's, long before there was such a thing as "alternative medicine."[4] Practical dilemmas encountered daily on the wards of a large city hospital impelled me to study philosophy before going into practice and have continued to influence my career ever since.

One is the often glaring discrepancy between how patients actually feel and function and how we expect them to behave as specimens of their disease, which has taught me to trust our subjective feelings and intuitive hunches at least as much as objective measurement of the abnormalities we were trained to substitute for them.

Another is that drugs powerful enough to control life functions as we expect them to do automatically pose a significant threat of destructive force, one that is multiplied exponentially when the treatment must be continued over extended periods of time.

As a result, my first priority as a physician became simply to avoid invasive diagnostic procedures, elective surgery, and pharmaceutical drugs for long-term maintenance as much as possible. I began investigating older, more traditional methods, like acupuncture, herbal medicine, and home birth, all of which are effective only to the extent that they are congruent with the individuality of the patient and thus much less likely to harm.

From that point of view, chemical drugs and surgery are best held in reserve as extreme measures for special situations, exemplifying a type of causal thinking far too rigid to accommodate the richness and complexity of actual illnesses, in which all aspects of experience are represented, a wide variety of influences are discernible, and patients tend to respond uniquely and more or less unpredictably to them.

Even before I'd seen it work in a patient, homeopathy offered the kind of systematic philosophy of health, illness, and the art of medicine that I'd been seeking all along. Ideally gentle and non-invasive, it uses minute doses of natural remedies artfully chosen to match the individuality of the patient and assist the natural self-healing capacity. Conducive to building non-adversarial relationships based on consensus and respect, it also suggests holistic models of medical research that could be of great benefit to the medical profession as a whole. Quite apart from its practical value in diagnosing and treating the sick, it merits a respectful hearing and careful study as a patient-centered approach and a humanistic style of doctoring.

Does It Work?

On top of that, my career itself bears witness to the effectiveness of the method, which has helped me practice family medicine for several decades without needing to write prescriptions, or refer patients for surgery except as a last resort. Having used remedies effectively in every phase of pregnancy and childbirth,[5] and in many other acute and threatening situations, I have seen them save life, ease the pain of death, and give dramatic, long-lasting relief where conventional methods had failed or seemed totally inapplicable. Two examples from long ago come to mind.

The first was an eight-pound baby girl, born covered with thick, green meconium, who took one gasp and then breathed no more. After brisk suctioning produced nothing but more of the same, the child lay limp, white, and motionless, with a heartbeat of 40 per minute, responding feebly to mouth-to-mouth resuscitation but unable to breathe on her own. I put a few tiny granules of *Arsenicum album* 200 on her tongue, and she awoke with a jolt, crying and flailing, her heart pounding at 140 per minute, her skin glowing pink with the flame of new life. The whole evolution took no more than a few seconds. After a night in the hospital to be on the safe side, mother and baby went home in the morning with no outward sign that anything untoward had happened.

Experiences like these are imprinted for life in every practitioner's mind.

The second was a 34-year-old R. N. with a history of severe endometriosis since her teens. After four surgeries to remove large, blood-filled cysts from her bladder and pelvic organs, and several courses of male hormones to suppress the condition, she came seeking only to restore her menstrual cycle, having long since abandoned any hopes of childbearing. While quite painful at first, her periods had become scanty, "dead," and dark-brown as a result of so many operations and years of hormones and oral contraceptives in the past. In the course of treatment, her menstrual flow became fuller and richer, and within six months she was pregnant. By the time I next saw her for a different ailment eight years later, she had had two healthy children after uncomplicated pregnancies and normal vaginal births, and had remained in good health ever since.

While no one can attribute such an outcome to a homeopathic remedy or indeed to any other agency in precise, linear fashion, my patient has never stopped thanking me for it, which is reason enough to honor and be grateful for a process by its very nature catalytic and persuasive rather than forcible or compulsory.

It would be a great mistake to impute these happy endings to any unusual skill of mine, since they are wholly compatible with what every experienced prescriber has seen or could easily duplicate; and I could just as well cite other patients whose conditions were far from hopeless, who believed in the remedies and in me, but whom I was unable to help.

Finally, I am deeply grateful that most homeopathic remedies are available without prescription, and that the knowledge of how to use them is readily accessible to everyone, with or without professional training, a state of affairs I take as further proof that self-healing and self-care are fundamental elements of our experience, and even a political and human right, which no government or medical bureaucracy can rightfully abridge or take away.

Remedies as Placebos.

I do not believe and have never taught that homeopathy is the only way to heal people, or the best way for everyone. But the standard argument that remedies are merely placebos cuts both ways. To begin with, it's just *wrong,* since the method has an impressive track record in the treatment of animals, newborn babies, and comatose patients, for whom the influence of suggestion is generally thought to be negligible.

Second, if giving placebo or natural remedies or doing nothing at all can accomplish the same result as suppressive drugs or crippling surgery, then it is surely worth asking which method really works better, and who of sound mind would not prefer the cheaper and safer alternative, at least to begin with.

And third, while it is certainly true that when homeopathic remedies succeed, our patients quite rightly feel that they have healed themselves, and may even wonder if they might have done so on their own, without our help, this delicious quandary is hardly cause for complaint. Indeed I can imagine no higher compliment to pay to a medicine than that its action cannot be readily distinguished from a gentle, spontaneous, long-lasting cure requiring no further treatment. Rather, it strikes me that the irony lies entirely in the opposite direction, that this optimal response is relegated to the placebo side of the ledger, while drugs are considered effective only to the extent that they can overpower the physiology of as many patients for as long as possible. It is absurd if not contemptible to boast of standards that prize brute force over elegance of fit, and subordinate the difficult task of healing the sick to the prideful thrill of manipulating their biological functions artificially and more or less at will.

The Homeopathic Phenomenon as a Legitimate Object of Study.

However admirable and useful it may be in certain extreme circumstances, the ideal of technical mastery tends to work like a strait-jacket in restraining not only alternative methods but also medicine and surgery themselves, by insisting on standards too rigid to accept any but the most punishing treatments, and too old-fashioned to make use of the most promising trends in contemporary science. What J. Robert Oppenheimer once told a group of psychologists is even more relevant for the medical community as a whole:

> We inherited at the beginning of the century a notion of the physicaworld as a causal one, in which every event cold be accounted for if we were ingenious, a world characterized by *number,* where everything interesting could be measured, [and] anything that went on could be broken down and analyzed. This extremely rigid picture left out a great deal of common sense which we can now understand with a complete lack of ambiguity and phenomenal technical success. The first is that the world is not completely determinate. There are predictions that you can make about it, but they are purely statistical. Every event has in it the nature of a surprise, a *miracle,* or something you could not figure out. Every pair of observations taking the form "we know this and can predict that" is global and cannot be broken down. Every atomic event is individual: it is not in essence reproducible.[6]

Historically, the basic argument against homeopathic remedies has always been not that they *don't* work, which would require careful and unbiased study, but merely that they *can't* work, that their use flatly contradicts the atomic theory of matter and is therefore unworthy of serious consideration. That homeopathy does challenge some cherished scientific beliefs I freely admit. But two hundred years of experience with it furnishes ample reason for a serious, dispassionate investigation of the method on its own merits, free of the ideological biases that are themselves at the heart of the dispute.

From Copernicus and Galileo to Darwin and Freud, the history of culture has repeatedly been enriched by scientific discoveries that were considered impossible or repugnant by leading thinkers of the time, because they presupposed major "paradigm shifts" in our way of thinking about the natural world, and in how our knowledge of it can be acquired and verified.[7]

In future generations, even if the homeopathic method as currently practiced becomes obsolete, the easily verifiable phenomena on which it is based and the more comprehensive ways of looking at health and illness that have resulted from it will continue to stretch the envelope of what we can perceive, and to promote a more integrated and wholesome medicine for humanity. In that spirit I have tried to write this book, and will feel amply rewarded if I can interest my readers enough simply to consider this extraordinary idea and try it for themselves.

NOTES.

1. Cf. Kaufman, M., *Homeopathy in America: the Rise and Fall of a Medical Heresy,* Johns Hopkins, Baltimore, 1971.
2. Cf. Holmes, O. W., "Homeopathy and Its Kindred Delusions," in *Medical Essays,* Houghton Mifflin, Boston, 1895, pp. 1-102.
3. Cf. Eisenberg, D., *et al.,* "Unconventional Medicine in the United States," *New England Journal of Medicine* 328:246, 1993.
4. Cf. Moskowitz, R., "Why I Became a Homeopath," *Journal of the American Institute of Homeopathy* 89:74, 1996.
5. Cf. Moskowitz, *Homeopathic Medicines for Pregnancy and Childbirth,* North Atlantic, Berkeley, 1992.
6. Oppenheimer, J. R., "Analogy in Science," *The American Psychologist* 2:134, 1956.
7. Cf. Kuhn, T., *The Structure of Scientific Revolutions,* 2nd Ed., University of Chicago, 1970, Chapters 1 and 2.

From Chapter One: *Principles.*

Homeopathy is both a philosophy of health and illness and a method of healing the sick, employing minute doses of medicinal substances. In its use of remedies to assist and enhance the natural self-healing capacity, homeopathy exemplifies the "vitalist" tradition in medicine, whose teachings are beautifully summarized in the aphorisms of Paracelsus, the great Renaissance physician and alchemist:

> The art of healing comes from Nature, not the physician . . .
> Every illness has its own remedy within itself . . .
> A man could not be born alive and healthy were there not already a Physician hidden in him.[1]

Evoking a venerable philosophy of ancient lineage, these sayings may be interpreted roughly as follows:

1) *Healing implies wholeness.* Derived from the same root as "whole," the English verb "to heal" literally means to make whole [again], represents a definitive property of all living systems, and implies a concerted effort of the entire organism that cannot be achieved by any part in isolation.

2) *All healing is self-healing.* As an intrinsic function of all living creatures, healing continues automatically throughout life, and tends to complete itself spontaneously, with or without outside help. In other words, all healing is self-healing; and the proper rôle of drugs, surgery, and of professional or designated "healers" of every kind is simply to facilitate and enhance the natural process that is already under way, rather than to interfere with or substitute for it.

3) *Healing pertains solely to individuals.* Healing is always *possible,* but also inherently problematic, even risky, and can always *fail* to occur or at least complete itself. That is because it pertains only to individuals, in concrete, here-and-now situations, rather than to abstract diseases or abnormalities. To put it another way, healing is inescapably an *art,* which can never and should never be reduced to any technique or formula, however scientific its foundation.

The Law of Similars and Its Implications.

The homeopathic notion of using medicines or physical agencies to imitate or reproduce and thus *resonate with* the symptom-picture of the illness is actually an ancient one, appearing frequently in the Hippocratic writings;[2] and even the testing of medicines on the healthy had already been proposed by a number of physicians in the Eighteenth Century.[3] But the elaboration of these ideas into a systematic philosophy and method of healing was the singular achievement of Samuel Hahnemann, M. D. (1755-1843), a noted physician, chemist, and pharmacologist, and the author of a standard textbook for the preparation and use of the medicinal substances of his time.

In 1790, while experimenting with Peruvian cinchona, the source of quinine, Hahnemann decided to take a therapeutic dose of the bark himself, and soon felt cold, numb, and drowsy, with thirst, prostration, and aching in the bones, a syndrome he immediately recognized as "the ague," or intermittent fever, which it was then being used to treat. Allowing the dose to wear off, he took a second and a third to make sure, with exactly the same result.[4] Awed by this unlooked-for correspondence, he began to investigate other medicines in the same way, testing them on himself, his colleagues, and his students, and recording their detailed responses to each. In his painfully methodical fashion, he discovered

1) that every medicinal substance produces a distinctive combination of signs and symptoms in healthy volunteers; and

2) that those whose symptom-pictures most closely match the illness to be treated are the ones most likely to initiate a curative response, by virtue of that correspondence.[5]

Coining the term "homeopathy" for his method of choosing remedies with the power to reproduce the illness as a whole instead of simply opposing this or that symptom with superior force, he proclaimed it as a universal law of healing with medicinal substances, *Similia similibus curentur,* or "Let likes be cured by likes."[6]

Sounding improbable to most people, and profoundly mysterious even to homeopaths who use it every day, the "Law of Similars" makes sense once we reflect that the outward manifestations of illness represent the automatic self-healing mechanism at work, so that the similar remedy need only assist and strengthen such efforts to lead them to their proper conclusion. In clinical medicine, familiar examples include

1) fever and cough, now generally recognized as immune-system responses to infection, promoting the expulsion of foreign organisms from the blood; and

2) other common pathological processes (inflammation, tumor formation, hypertension, allergy, etc.), now generally understood as exaggerated versions of normal homeostasis.

In other words, homeopathy differs from established medicine not so much in its interpretation of these phenomena as in its subtler and more elegant method of correcting them. Unlike pharmaceutical drugs, designed to control biochemical abnormalities by the application of superior force, homeopathy utilizes the gentler influence of the similar remedy to help the natural healing process complete its work as promptly and efficiently as possible. Thus wholly compatible with our lived experience of illness, the Law of Similars feels out of step primarily with our impatience to replace subjective feelings with objective disease categories to be fought and measurable abnormalities to be corrected.

As a disciplined way of thinking about health and illness, homeopathy also qualifies as a philosophy in a more technical sense, that its basic principles all follow deductively from a simple, self-evident axiom like the "vital force," the unitary life principle, and the counter-intuitive Law of Similars, neither of which can be *proved* in the usual sense, much in the spirit of Bertrand Russell's whimsical definition:

. . . the point of philosophy is to start with something so obvious as not to seem worth stating, and to end up with something so paradoxical that nobody will believe it.[7]

As the defining principle of a logical system, the Law of Similars is not amenable to conclusive proof or disproof by itself, independently of the others, like ordinary scientific hypotheses, but only by continual re-evaluation of the consistency, relevance, accuracy, and predictive value of the system as a whole. As a basic rule or guideline of medical science, on the other hand, it stands or falls by the same test of clinical experience as any other empirical generalization, namely, by how well it *works* in the treatment of the sick.[8]

Provings.

In Hahnemann's classic formulation, the Law of Similars postulates a direct correspondence between the signs and symptoms that medicinal substances can provoke or elicit in healthy people and those that they can help to cure in the sick. By thus defining what it *means* to be a medicine, this basic duality provides a method for investigating the therapeutic powers of each substance on healthy volunteers that is wholly experimental and almost ideally safe and gentle as well.

Using minute doses sufficient to produce symptoms but far below the threshold of organic toxicity, and keeping a detailed record of the physical, mental, and emotional responses of each individual ingesting it, provings yield a composite symptom-picture of each medicinal substance that is uniquely characteristic of it and recognizably different from that of every other substance.[9] When homeopaths describe the characteristics of a particular remedy, they mean essentially the sum of observable responses of all the people who have ever taken it, a *Gestalt* or ensemble that must be studied as a whole and for its own sake, and not merely as a weapon against a particular disease or abnormality.

Moreover, what qualifies as a medicine is defined equally broadly to include *any* substance with the power to alter human health in either direction, to provoke illness or cure it, to elicit symptoms or to relieve them, so that the distinction between medicines and poisons becomes one of degree only, of the dosage and the individual sensitivity of the patient.

In his typically painstaking fashion, Hahnemann completed and published detailed provings of more than ninety medicines in his own lifetime, a truly heroic achievement.[10] With more than two thousand remedies in use by homeopaths today, provings remain the lifeblood of the method and its most distinctive contribution to medical science, with important applications in pharmacology, ethnobotany, toxicology, and industrial medicine.[11]

The Homeopathic *Materia Medica.*

By far the most numerous in the Homeopathic Pharmacopoeia are the *remedies of plant or vegetable origin,* including seeds, roots, leaves, flowers, barks, fruits, resins, and their various alkaloids and extracts, which may be roughly subdivided as follows:

1) *poisons* that can kill or intoxicate (aconite, cockle, hellebore, hemlock, henbane, ignatia, jimson weed, *Nux vomica,* poison ivy, tobacco, water hemlock, yellow jasmine, etc.), including many used in allopathic medicine as well: belladonna (atropine, scopolamine), coca (cocaine), curare, digitalis (digoxin, digitoxin), ergot (ergonovine, ergotamine), ipecac, opium (morphine, codeine, papaverine), pilocarpine, physostigmine, etc.;

2) *medicinal herbs:* aloe, chamomile, comfrey, echinacea, eyebright, ginseng, golden seal, hawthorn berries, mistletoe, mullein, peyote, poke root, skullcap, tansy, witch hazel, yarrow, yellow dock, etc.;

3) *foods, beverages, and spices:* cayenne, chickpeas, chocolate, coffee, garlic, mustard, oats, onions, nutmeg, pepper, radish, rhubarb, rosemary, sage, tea, thyme, wild hops, wild yam, etc.;

4) *fragrances, resins, oils, and residues:* amber, charcoal, gasoline, kerosene, kreosote, paraffin, petroleum, phenol, turpentine, etc.;

5) *flowers, trees, and shrubs,* both wild and domesticated: aspen, bittersweet, buttercup, cimicifuga, daisy, delphinium, juniper, marigold, meadow anemone, meadow saffron, peony, rue, tiger lily, etc.; and

6) *mosses, lichens, molds, mushrooms, fungi,* and derivatives: club moss, *Amanita muscaria,* penicillin, streptomycin, tetracycline, etc.

The second-largest group comprises the *mineral remedies,* which may be classified more or less as follows:

1) *metals:* copper, iron, gold, lead, mercury, nickel, osmium, palladium, platinum, silver, tin, titanium, uranium, zinc, etc.;

2) *metalloids:* antimony, arsenic, bismuth, germanium, etc.;

3) *salts:* bromides, carbonates, chlorides, fluorides, iodides, nitrates, oxides, phosphates, silicates, sulfates, etc., with barium, calcium, lithium, magnesium, potassium, sodium, and various metals;

4) *acids:* boric, fluoric, hydrobromic, hydrochloric, nitric, phosphoric, sulfuric, etc.;

5) *elements:* bromine, chlorine, fluorine, hydrogen, iodine, phosphorus, selenium, sulphur, tellurium, etc.; and

6) *constituents of the earth's crust:* aluminum oxide, silica, ores, rocks, lavas, mineral waters, etc..

As yet the smallest group are the *remedies taken from the animal kingdom,* including

1) *venoms:* jellyfish, honeybee, wasp, Spanish fly, mosquito, black widow, brown recluse, and other spiders and tarantulas, scorpion, eel toxin, frogs and toads, cobra, rattlesnakes, coral snake, vipers, bushmaster, and other snakes, lizards, etc.;

2) *secretions and extracts:* ambergris, beaver, coral, cockroach, cuttlefish ink (sepia), milks of various mammalian species (cat, cow, dog, dolphin, goat, horse, human, lion, tiger, etc.), musk, ox bile, skunk, etc.;

3) *hormones, metabolites, glandular and tissue extracts* ("sarcodes"): thyroid, parathyroid, pituitary, adrenal, estrogen, testosterone, cortisone, insulin, adrenaline, cholesterol, spleen, blood, saliva, urine, placenta, dog and cat hair, etc.; and

4) *disease products,* or "nosodes;" cancer tissue, tuberculous abscess, syphilis, gonorrheal discharge, yeast, pus, measles, toxins of diphtheria, botulism, tetanus, rabies, polio, and other pathogenic viruses, bacteria, fungi, parasites, extracts, and vaccines.

In fact, the technique of proving can be used to investigate the medicinal action of any substance whatsoever, including traditional and folk remedies as yet unproven (several thousand in the Indian and Chinese pharmacopoeias alone); major pharmaceuticals (Prozac, Valium, etc.); and toxic chemicals, commercial and industrial products, and their wastes (dyes, paints, solvents, insecticides, car exhaust, acid rain, cigarette smoke, etc.). Ultimately the homeopathic *materia medica* is as vast and limitless as the creation of the earth and its transformation and breakdown by planetary and cosmic forces, including human action.

The "Vital Force."

As we have seen, the Law of Similars becomes intelligible only when the signs and symptoms of the illness are identified with the defense mechanism of the patient, so that the similar remedy is chosen to facilitate the natural self-healing process, to calm its excesses and strengthen its deficiencies.

In words sounding almost prophetic today, Hahnemann recognized a unified energy field in the complex array of activities and functions that distinguish the living organism from a dead body. Calling it the "vital force" to emphasize its purely energetic character, he included within it the full range of sensations, movements, and internal processes of self-healing and self-preservation.[12] Homeopaths similarly redefine illness as an energetic disturbance of the organism as a whole, and study the aggregate of signs and symptoms as its true outward reflection or mirror-image, the internal state being hidden and unknowable apart from it.[13] In parallel fashion, the action of medicines is fully and directly observable in the ensemble of clinical manifestations they can elicit in provings on the healthy.[14]

Whatever terminology we use to designate it, the vital force or something like it forms the conceptual basis of the entire system, from the Law of Similars, which makes no sense without it, to the totality of symptoms, its applied or clinical aspect, on which everything else depends. Four interrelated properties make it indispensable for clinical work:

1) It is *unitary,* affecting all parts of the organism simultaneously, such that all responses are concerted and felt everywhere, and no disturbance is purely local;[15]

2) It is *energetic,* rather than material in character, thus not confined to particular structures (cells, organs, tissues), and is capable of responding to stimuli without delay;[16]

3) It is *individual,* showing itself uniquely and idiosyncratically for each person and at every moment;[17] and

4) It is *perceptible to the senses,* in the form of signs and symptoms, and thus amenable to detailed examination by the physician.[18]

Although modern medicine has long been critical of vitalistic concepts as too vague to define and too crude to measure,[19] doing without them entirely has proved to be a costly blunder, on the order of throwing out the baby with the bath water. Whatever we choose to call it, the unified, self-organizing aspect of living beings remains indispensable not only for homeopathy, but at least as much for the medical system as a whole.

First, the overall effect of treatment in general, whether improvement or worsening, and of drugs, vaccines, chemicals, or vaccines in particular, cannot be evaluated unambiguously apart from how patients feel and function as a whole and according to their own individual standards.[20]

Second, some global sense of the individual as a whole is implicitly or explicitly used by every physician to assess each patient's general vitality, to offer a prognosis of curability or incurability, and to make wise decisions regarding complex issues of case management, such as setting appropriate and realistic goals for the treatment. Precisely because they were driven to it by calculations of profit and loss, the fact that many HMO's now routinely include the quasi-homeopathic "quality of life" assessment in their outcome research has transformed these ungainly bureaucracies into unlikely agents of genuine reform in the health care system.

The Totality of Symptoms.

Just as provings define each remedy as the unique ensemble of signs and symptoms that it can elicit in healthy subjects, homeopaths define illness as the totality of observable responses that is equally characteristic of the patient. As the true reflection of the inner state, the overall symptom-picture becomes the chief goal of the clinical examination of the patient and the search for the remedy that best matches it.

Admirably rich and lifelike if enough time and attention are given to it, to a trained homeopath this composite portrait represents the illness and condition of a patient much more faithfully than any diagnostic category or printout of laboratory abnormalities. On the other hand, it is simply a working description, which need not and cannot include every single manifestation. As in a proving, it is effectively complete when a reasonable facsimile, including the peculiar flavor of the condition as a whole, is clearly discernible, such that further questioning merely elicits more of the same material.

To illustrate, I will present the case of an elderly patient with many pathological diagnoses, allopathic drugs, and signs and symptoms all mixed up together, just as we typically find them. Whether or not the outcome was attributable to the remedy, I tell a bit of her story merely to show that examining an illness with sufficient care to find an effective remedy for it requires an intimate acquaintance with the lived experience of the patient, including the full range of human thoughts and feelings:

> Diagnosed with inoperable lung cancer and lately undergoing radiation treatments for it, a spry, energetic woman of 78 felt constriction and oppression in her chest when she walked, and a dry cough that made her gag, choke, and gasp for air. Although quite healthy for most of her life, she came bearing diagnoses of aneurysm of the abdominal aorta, diverticulitis, asthma, high blood pressure, and hypothyroidism, for which she took a formidable array of diuretics, thyroid hormones, beta-blockers, broncho- dilators, and antihypertensives daily.

> Further questioning revealed that the soles of her feet were sore with walking, and that her legs were wobbly and easily fatigued, causing her to stagger as if drunk and hold onto things to steady herself. All of these miseries were catalogued in a stoical, matter-of-fact tone, devoid of fear or anguish. as if much to be expected and taken in stride. Others included neck pain and stiffness, associated with osteoarthritis of the cervical spine, carpal tunnel syndrome in both hands, and stitching pain in the area of her kidneys, mainly in the right in the morning, and the left at bedtime; but these too she mostly ignored. Recently, she had been plagued by a severe headache that radiated up the back of her neck, accompanied by a loss of appetite, and had lost 10 pounds in a matter of a few weeks.

> At this point she admitted that her cancer would undoubtedly kill her, and that she was tired and ready to give up, but went on living mainly for the sake of her daughters. Based on this and other information, I gave her one dose of *Calcarea carbonica* 200 every 2 to 6 months, and despite inoperable cancer and her roster of diseases and medications, she lived another three years of generally happy and productive life.

As a global energy disturbance that is not restricted to any particular organs, the totality of symptoms always includes mental and emotional states as well as physical complaints, just as the provings do. While the interview elicits symptoms of all kinds, and there is no need for prior assumptions about mental states "causing" the physical, or *vice versa*, psychological states often weigh heavily in the choice of the remedy, for two reasons.

First, while physical symptoms tend to be localized to a specific part of the body, as indicated by the adjective "my" (*my* back, arm, head, nose, stomach, or whatever), mental and emotional states refer to how patients feel *as a whole,* so that they use the pronoun "I" to describe them (*I* am sad, happy, angry, afraid, etc.). Because the basic energy disturbance is always global and systemic, the totality of symptoms accords special priority to symptoms which reveal the condition of the patient as a whole.

Second, an incomplete, poorly-taken case is an assortment of heterogeneous, seemingly unrelated items, while the common threads uniting them are striking, peculiar, or uncommon characteristics that set each patient apart from others with the same diagnosis. Distinctive features of this kind are often found in the personality and character of the patient and displayed in important areas of the biography, such as career, interests, and relationships.

The Single Remedy.

As old as homeopathy itself, this cardinal rule follows directly from the totality of symptoms. From the beginning, *homeopaths are trained to choose one remedy at a time for the whole patient,* comparing the totality of the symptoms of the illness with those of various remedies until the best possible match is found.[22] Instead of giving part of a drug to part of the patient and dismissing the rest of its actions as "side effects," the single remedy matches the whole of its effects to the whole of the patient, its "power" consisting solely in the ability of the patient to *respond* to it as a whole, by virtue of that correspondence.

More than any other, the principle of the single remedy has divided the minority of homeopaths committed to the "pure' or classical method from the larger body of sympathizers who are attracted to the philosophy in a loose way, but balk at various aspects of the discipline. Right from the beginning, "pluralists" using the lower dilutions have advocated using two or more remedies simultaneously,[23] and most manufacturers likewise market combinations of ingredients to pharmacies and health-food stores for first aid and the relief of common domestic ailments,[24] most of them safe and reasonably effective if properly used.

While such combinations have undoubtedly given symptomatic relief to many people, only a single remedy in its totality can approximate the richness and individuality of a living patient, help a serious student to accumulate a detailed experience of the remedies, and thus generate the pleasure and excitement of learning how to use them. Since giving parts of remedies to parts of the patient makes it difficult to know which one has acted, practitioners are then reduced to choosing them according to the generic indications of folk medicine or the technical language of abnormalities, which is not all that different from allopathic drug treatment.

Under these circumstances, what little of value can be learned will not yield an experience that can build on itself, or a method that can or need be taught. To an extent undreamed of in the past, the improbable revival of American homeopathy in recent years has been achieved primarily on the strength of the classical or single-remedy method, because only the totality of symptoms can do justice to remedies and patients as unique individualities supremely worthy of study for their own sake.

The Minimum Dose.

As he began choosing medicines homeopathically, Hahnemann found that many of his patients would only get better after a definite and sometimes prolonged period of aggravation from the standard therapeutic dose.[25] At times these reactions were so severe that he felt obliged to experiment with diluting the substance, and in his methodical fashion was able to demonstrate

1) that remedies continue to be effective at concentrations too minute to be detected chemically,[26] and

2) that brief, vigorous shaking or "succussion" of the remedy before each dilution actually enhances its healing effect in a subtle way that has never been fully understood.[27]

The seeming impossibility that such highly dilute remedies could still act at all helped to convince Hahnemann that their effect must be chiefly dynamic or energetic rather than chemical in nature.[28] Assuming that the process of dilution greatly multiplies the amount of surface area available for reacting with the solvent, he theorized that succussion acted to liberate the medicinal energy of substances from chemical "bondage" and release it into the solution,[29 thus] in a sense foreshadowing the discovery of subatomic forces in the Twentieth Century.

From Oliver Wendell Holmes to the professional "quackbusters" of today, the use of such "infinitesimal" doses has always aroused controversy and ridicule,[30] so much so that quite a few professing allegiance to Hahnemann's Law of Similars have never ventured to follow him into this realm.[31]

While the action of highly dilute remedies has never been satisfactorily explained, their apparent defiance of the laws of physics and chemistry makes much better sense in the light of the diametrically opposite purposes for which prescription drugs and homeopathic remedies are given. Whereas the former are designed to correct measurable abnormalities by the application of superior force, are administered in doses as large as the patient can tolerate, and must be repeated as soon as their effect wears off, homeopathic remedies are intended simply to catalyze, facilitate, and enhance whatever self-healing processes are already under way, such that only minute doses are required, and too many or too frequent repetitions of even the correct remedy can actually spoil the effect.

Using only the smallest possible doses, and repeating them only when their action is exhausted, homeopaths are trained to allow ample time for the cure to complete itself spontaneously and without further interference. In most situations, the term "minimum dose" refers not to its size or degree of dilution, but only to the number and frequency of its repetitions.

Finally, homeopathic remedies usually have little or no effect unless they are correctly chosen, unless their total symptom-picture matches that of the illness closely enough to render the patient highly susceptible to their action. Otherwise, in the event of a poorly-chosen remedy, one which does not adequately fit the totality of the illness or the individuality of the patient, the minuteness of the dose makes it extremely unlikely that anything untoward or dangerous will occur, a crucial safety feature.

By its own choice, allopathic medicine aspires to be rigorously quantitative, by titrating the usual therapeutic dose against the risk of toxicity, and walking the narrow margin of safety like a tightrope stretched between them. Homeopathy, on the other hand, is essentially *qualitative,* in that its remedies can act only to the extent of their fit or congruence with the unique energy pattern of each patient, a phenomenon of resonance that still awaits a science capable of explaining it.

As we smell the lilacs in bloom, the concentration of lilac molecules in the olfactory bulb remains vanishingly small,[32] and what delights us is the unique quality of the fragrance, so unmistakably different from a rose or an iris, while our organ of smell, as if hard-wired to respond to such minute amounts, would suffer infernal torments if forcibly exposed to a vat of lilac essence in a perfume factory.

In analogous fashion, the physics of ultradilute solutions generates a series of riddles that our customary notions of quantity are simply unable to solve. In the case of an ordinary 200C dilution, for example, which already lies well beyond the molecular threshold of Avogadro's number,[33] it generally makes no difference whether a patient ingests 10 granules or 10,000, so that if an inquisitive child swallows the contents of an entire vial, it is still only one dose, and not at all dangerous. Similarly, in clinical practice, the size of the dose, the actual number of granules or tablets ingested, is ordinarily of no importance, a fact which suggests that what the patient receives is not a *quantity* of something, but rather *a specific kind of information,* like an energy blueprint, one hopefully clearer and more efficient than the one they are currently operating with.

On the other hand, provers failing to react to the first few doses are instructed to take larger ones, while some patients who overreact to the usual tiny amounts seem to do better with less, or even by carrying the remedy in a vial on their person and not ingesting it at all, suggesting that dose size does indeed matter at times.[34] Like the atom of quantum physics, the higher dilutions seem to behave like a particle with mass under some conditions, and purely energetically like a wave in others, but not both at the same time.

Equally ambiguous and misleading is the common tendency to equate potency with the degree of dilution. It is true that colicky babies soothed by chamomile tea, for example, are likely to need it again the next day, while others given a high dilution of the same remedy, with no molecules to break down or excrete, are presumably better able to initiate a more sustained response if the remedy fits them. To that extent, the higher dilutions are indeed capable of a deeper, subtler action, and are thus more "potent" in that sense.

On the other hand, some patients respond more profoundly to the lower dilutions, and which dilution will be the most potent for a given patient cannot be known with certainty in advance of his or her actual response to it, any more than how many times or how often it is best to repeat it, or indeed which remedy will work optimally. At every turn, the physics of highly dilute solutions traps us in riddles that negate or render meaningless the standard assumptions of quantitative chemistry and the atomic theory of matter, . .

With remedies now detectable by laser spectroscopy and bioassay,[35] hormones, enzymes, and vaccines available in microgram and nanogram amounts, and ultradilute phenomena regularly making headlines in the media, homeopathy has at last come full circle, from fossilized relic of a bygone age to futuristic paradigm for a new integrative medicine still unborn.

The "Laws of Cure."

In addition to helping clinicians define the illness and select the remedy, the totality of symptoms provides the basic criteria for improvement and worsening at the follow-up visits, and thus for assessing the effect of the remedy and tracing the evolution of health and illness as a whole and through time. With the aid of detailed case-taking and careful record-keeping, homeopaths learn to judge improvement and worsening simply by comparing the observed totality of symptoms from one visit to the next and over extended periods of time.

A woman of 46 was brought in by her daughter-in-law for "memory problems," which had become increasingly severe over the past three years. On returning from a trip to her native country, she had had trouble walking and keeping her balance, and had twice fallen in the street and been taken to the hospital. There the diagnosis of hydrocephalus was made; and as if on cue, she began to hallucinate and drop things. Although she improved a lot after a shunt was put in place, it soon plugged up and had to be removed, and her mental state continued to deteriorate. By the time I saw her, a second one had also been inserted and removed without significant change.

As her daughter-in-law hastened to add, she had been depressed for many years, even in her homeland, to the point that her current psychotic state seemed almost easier for her and everyone else to bear. Severely constipated and lately incontinent as well, she sat on the floor of my office and barely spoke above a whisper. Her meds included Navane, Ativan, and Desipramine, without which she grew restless and agitated, with hallucinations of visitors from abroad, plus Dilantin and Cogentin for seizures and spasticity.

After the first remedy had no effect, *Plumbum* 200 was given; and within a month her family reported that she was able to speak coherently, walk without falling, read a newspaper, cut vegetables, and enjoy watching TV, all of which made her feel and seem much more like her old self. When symptoms of tardive dyskinesia appeared (smacking and pursing her lips, grinding her teeth, biting her tongue), her psychiatrist stopped the Navane. Although she still hallucinated at times, the images were pleasant and no longer distressed her, and her bowels had improved greatly. Three months later, I repeated the remedy; and she has since returned to her native country, much improved overall and in her mental state, albeit still with some dyskinesias and occasional mood swings.

However complicated and difficult to make, evaluations of improvement and worsening are of paramount importance to patients and loved ones alike. The follow-up interview is designed to ascertain changes in the global energy state after treatment, a capability almost entirely obscured by reliance on the theory of disease processes, each of which must be diagnosed and treated separately.

Thus in the previous case, the evolution of her condition before and after treatment shows meaningful patterns and raises complex issues that cannot even be formulated intelligently apart from some version of the totality of symptoms. These include

1) the pathogenetic rôle of disappointment;

2) the daughter-in-law's observation that the psychosis was less painful than the depression and seemed to have arisen from it as a deeper or more profound state; and

3) the increase in spasticity and dyskinesia, and thus heightened efficacy of her allopathic drugs, as her mental and general condition improved.

Although Hahnemann clearly understood the importance of these issues, the guidelines most widely used in practice today were formulated by his student, Constantine Hering, M. D. (1800-1880). In his so-called "Laws of Cure," Hering proposed four directions in which the totality of symptoms tends to redistribute itself in the process of recovery and cure, those for falling ill and worsening being precisely the opposite:

1) *from above downwards,* from the head end of the body to the feet or bottom end;

2) *from inside outwards,* from the more central or interior parts or regions to others more external, peripheral, or superficial;

3) *from more vital to less vital organs,* from deeper, more important, or visceral structures to others less essential to life; and

4) *in the reverse order of their appearance* in the life history of the patient, from the most recent symptoms to the oldest.[36]

The first three are anatomical, representing successive generalizations or refinements of the same basic idea, that as healing proceeds the force of the illness tends to be displaced away from the vital centers and toward the more peripheral or less critical areas. Thus, for example, a marked improvement in the psychiatric or emotional sphere could be tempered by the appearance of neurological symptoms, as if the "center of gravity" or main force of the illness had descended from the higher brain centers to the lower, e.g., from the cerebral cortex to the basal ganglia.[37] Other examples might include the reappearance of eczema or a skin rash following improvement of a deeper condition, such as asthma, or the development of a nasal or vaginal discharge after the cure of an internal complaint in the same anatomical region, like sinusitis or endometriosis.

Like many homeopathic principles, these first three "Laws of Cure" can be rather difficult to interpret, since which structures and functions are more or less "vital" or important are subject to interpretation, may differ widely from one patient to another, and require Solomonic judgments as tricky and ambiguous as any the Laws were devised to simplify.

The most reliable and important of Hering's Laws, the fourth is chronological and biographical, tracing in reverse order the deposition of successive "layers" of illness at important junctures or milestones in the life history of the patient, and thus offering valuable clues and insights into how our illnesses are made. Because older symptoms can be more deeply embedded, and more recent ones somewhat less so, the follow-up interview can often recapitulate the sequence in which different groups of symptoms were acquired and established at various phases of life, like the annular rings of a tree.

A related application is the "never well since" phenomenon, in which certain features of the present condition are traceable to a specific physical or emotional trauma in the past, or to an acute illness that never healed completely, as if the patient's energy field became fixated or "stuck" at that point, creating a chronic focus for new symptom-patterns to crystallize around it.

> Disabled with chronic ovarian pain, a woman of 40 unhesitatingly traced her problems to a tubal ligation six months earlier, complicated by a major pelvic infection requiring IV antibiotics and an extended hospital stay. Ever since these events, she had had severe burning pains in her right ovary with each period, and numerous attacks of cystitis in between. However restrained and dignified in the telling, she could not conceal her anger and resentment against the gynecologist who had performed the surgery and seemingly ruined her health. Radiating down her right leg, the pain was somewhat better from heat and pressure, but had recently spread to the left side and to odd times between the periods as well.

> After a single dose of *Staphysagria* 200, her next period was the worst ever, but the pain lasted only a few hours and was much more localized. From then on, her periods became less and less painful, her cystitis cleared up and did not return, and she had no further problems.

The Place of Allopathic Diagnosis and Treatment.

Although orthodox methods appear at times to be incompatible with the homeopathic philosophy, in practice they actually complement each other quite nicely in a number of ways, and fit together a lot better than might be expected. In both, the technique of making an anatomical or pathological diagnosis is the same, although in allopathic medicine the diagnosis is the endpoint of the investigation and dictates the treatment, whereas for the homeopath it is only the beginning, only one factor in the choice of the remedy, and rarely the most important one. In any event, it bears repeating that homeopathy should not be thought of as a substitute for trained and experienced medical or surgical help when necessary.

An attractive first option for patients with functional ailments and minimal organic pathology, like PMS, attention deficit disorder, or chronic fatigue syndrome, to whom standard treatments offer only palliative relief in any case, homeopathy also performs very well in intractable, incurable, or terminal cases, where chemical drugs have failed or reached the end of their usefulness.

Conversely, in emergencies and other conditions evolving rapidly and threatening death or irreversible tissue damage, drugs and surgery are typically the methods of first choice, and are equally indispensable as a backup or last resort when gentler approaches prove inadequate. In many instances, both methods complement each other quite effectively, and potential conflicts can almost always be avoided if caregivers of differing traditions and beliefs are willing to work together and learn from each other, respecting the wishes and best interests of the patient.

NOTES.

1. Paracelsus (P. A. T. B. Von Hohenheim), *Selected Writings,* ed. J. Jacobi., trans. N. Guterman, Bollingen XXVIII, Pantheon, New York, 1958, pp. 50, 76, *passim.*
2. Hahnemann, S., *Organon of Medicine,* 6th Ed., ed. W. B. O'Reilly, transl. S. Decker, Redmond WA, 1996, Introduction, p. 57.
3. Ibid.
4. Bradford, T. L., *Life and Letters of Hahnemann,* Boericke & Tafel, Philadelphia, 1895, pp. 36-37.
5. Hahnemann, "Essay on a New Principle for Ascertaining the Curative Powers of Drugs," *Lesser Writings,* transl. R. E. Dudgeon, Wm. Radde, New York, 1852, p. 265.
6. The term "homeopathy" is derived from 2 Greek roots, *omoios,* meaning "similar," as in "homeostasis," and *pathos,* meaning "suffering," or simply "feeling," as in "sympathy," "pathology," or "pathos" itself. "Allopathy," another Hahnemannian coinage, comes from the root *alloios,* meaning "other," and refers to the two non-homeopathic modes of treatment, namely the "antipathic" or palliative method of *opposing* the symptoms by contraries, *contraria contrariis,* and the "heteropathic" method of drawing off diseased humors through some different and as yet unaffected channel, as by purging, bleeding, salivating, etc. Both methods are savaged and disposed of in the *Organon.*
7. Russell, B., "The Philosophy of Logical Atomism," in *Logic and Knowledge: Essays 1901-1950,* Allen and Unwin, 1968, p. 193.
8. Hahnemann, *Organon,* ¶ 25-28.
9. Ibid., ¶118-120.
10. Cf. Hahnemann, *Materia Medica Pura,* transl. R. E. Dudgeon, B & T, New York, 1880-81, and *Chronic Diseases,* transl. L. H. Tafel, B & T, Philadelphia, 1896.

11. Cf. Moskowitz, "Homeopathic Reasoning," *Homeotherapy* 6:135, 1980.

12. Hahnemann, *Organon,* ¶ 9, 10.

13. Ibid., ¶ 11-13.

14. Ibid., ¶ 11n, 106-108.

15. Ibid., ¶ 9, 189.

16. Ibid., ¶ 11, 11n.

17. Ibid., ¶ 108-120.

18. Ibid., ¶ 12, 14, 18.

19. Cf. Moskowitz, "Some Thoughts on the Malpractice Crisis," *British Homœopathic Journal* 77:17, 1988.

20. Ibid.

21. Hahnemann, *Organon,* ¶ 18.

22. Ibid., ¶ 272-274.

23. Demarque, D., "The Several-Drug Way or Plural Prescription," in *How to Study Homeopathy,* Centre d'Études et de Documentation Homéopathiques, Boiron, Lyon, 1992, English Ed., pp. 166-181.

24. Moskowitz, "Options in Homeopathic Self-Care," *East/West Journal,* January 1990.

25. Hahnemann, "The Medicine of Experience," *Lesser Writings,* pp. 461-469.

26. Hahnemann, "On the Power of Small Doses," ibid., pp. 385-389.

27. Hahnemann, "How Can Small Doses of Such Highly Attenuated Medicine Still Possess Great Power?" ibid., pp. 728-734.

28. Hahnemann, "The Medicine of Experience," op. cit., p. 466.

29. Hahnemann, "How Can Small Doses . . . ," op. cit., p. 734.

30. Holmes, O. W., op.cit.

31. Hughes, R., "Homeopathic Posology," in *Manual of Pharmacodynamics,* 4th Ed., Heath & Ross, London, 1880, pp.93-106.

32. Best and Taylor, *The Physiological Basis of Medical Practice,* 6th Ed., Williams & Wilkins, Baltimore, 1955, pp. 1219-1220.

33. See Chapter 2, "Pharmacy."

34. Hahnemann, *Organon,* ¶ 129.

35. See Epilogue, "Homeopathic Research."

36. Hering, C., "Hahnemann's Three Rules Concerning the Rank of Symptoms," *Hahnemannian Monthly* 1:5, 1865, and *Analytical Therapeutics,* B & T, 1875, p. 24.

37. Vithoulkas, G., *The Science of Homeopathy: a Modern Textbook,* Ed. W. Gray, Grove Press, New York, 1980, pp. 25, 47-48.

From Chapter Three: *Patients.*

The art of caring for the sick transcends simply taking down information and doling out remedies, which may not work or even be chosen properly until an appropriate setting and a healing relationship are created for them. Most people afflicted with pain, suffering, and disability need relationships with others,

1) to help them make sense out of what is happening to them;

2) to help them construct a working mythology of their illness;

3) to help them find and navigate a safe passage through it; and

4) to help them envision a way beyond it insofar as possible.

Largely because of its emphasis on the totality of symptoms, the individuality of the patient, and the ordinary language of daily life, the homeopathic interview is a powerful healing experience in its own right, which prepares the way for remedies to continue the work of making whole again when the patient goes home.

A girl of ten was brought in for treatment of enuresis, which began when she was three, when her parents separated for a year, and had continued ever since, but only at home in her own bed, never while visiting relatives or sleeping over at a friend's house. In addition, she was prone to developing acute cystitis, with stinging pains in her urethra that often woke her in the night and made her scream.

After her father returned, she became frightened of him and his booming voice, especially after he refused to believe her story that a neighbor boy had sexually molested her. Ever since then, she had become hypersensitive to any teasing or criticism from her father or older brother, or whenever her friends told secrets or did anything to exclude her, often to the point that she would leave the scene in tears and vent her anger and sense of humiliation to her mother.

Four weeks after a single dose of *Staphysagria* 10M, her mother wrote that the wetting was worse than before, and that the girl felt quite discouraged at times, and impatient for the remedy to work, but also "talked a lot about our visit and the way you listened, and seemed relieved to have been able to share the sexual stuff with you." That was the last I saw or heard of her for two years, at which point the mother brought her back for a different complaint and told me that the bedwetting had stopped a few weeks after sending the letter and never came back.

The Homeopathic Interview.

Above all else, the chief purpose of the case-taking is to provide the opportunity for patients to tell their story in their own way, and in its entirety, using their own words as well as the observations of friends and loved ones, and continuing without interruption until they have nothing else to say. Always on the alert for any hint of predisposing causes or factors influencing the present condition, the interviewer then inquires about stressful events, life crises, and previous illnesses, which are usually well known or suspected by the patient, and which attentive listening and careful questioning van usually uncover. Provided our own biases don't frighten it away, the actual experience of sick people can detect pertinent factors that a strictly pathological orientation would never suspect or countenance, like ailments provoked by a chemical exposure that would barely affect most people, or by a vaccination not consistently associated with such symptoms.

Listing them one after the other down the page, homeopaths record the symptoms *verbatim* as much as possible, leaving ample space for further clarification. While greatly expanded in content, the interview adheres in every particular to the form of the standard medical history, including whatever physical and laboratory examinations are necessary to establish a pathological diagnosis.

In acute conditions, much of the past history, family history, and review of systems may be omitted, since the illness is pretty much limited to what is immediately manifest or differs from the usual pattern, and the symptoms themselves are fewer, more intense, and more often volunteered by the patient or evident in the body language without having to be asked about.

When the patient is finished speaking and has nothing further to say, direct questioning is needed to characterize the main symptoms in further detail, and to inquire about other aspects of the history that have not yet been mentioned. Questions should be open-ended and framed to require thought, avoiding simple yes-or-no answers or signaling a preferred response.[1]

When described well enough to help choose a remedy, symptoms should include at least some if not all of the following elements:

1) *Subjective sensations,* like pain, dizziness, fatigue, anger, etc., which can only be described imaginatively, e. g., in the case of pain, as an instrument capable of inflicting it, or of emotional states, by using typical vignettes or clues such as a close friend or loved one might observe, and so forth.

Even without overt manifestations to corroborate them, sensations provide direct access to the patient's inner state and thus often point to the central disturbance and the remedy that best matches it. Notable examples are the so-called "strange, rare, and peculiar" symptoms, which describe idiosyncratic elaborations so striking, improbable, or unusual as to overshadow and at times even explain the others. Thus when one chilly patient with severe bronchitis told me that on bad days the inspired air felt cold all the way down into her lungs, I was prompted to seek and happily found a nearly identical symptom in the provings of *Cistus canadensis,* the rock rose, a correspondence which gave me every confidence that the remedy would help her, as in fact it did.

2) *Localization,* e. g., symptoms in a particular place, on the same side, or alternating sides; pains that wander or radiate (like menstrual cramps extending down the thighs), are diffuse or circumscribed, or always occur in the same spot, details which most patients are well aware of and will usually describe by using body language when asked to point to them.

Helpful for conventional diagnosis, localizing can be equally important as an individualizing factor, as when several different symptoms occur consistently on the same side, indicating an asymmetrical energy pattern that is characteristic of that organism, rather than of any known pathology. Without detailed provings of the snake venoms, for example, it might never have occurred to anyone to recognize lateralization as a *bona fide* phenomenon warranting serious study. In the same way, provings of remedies with symptoms that alternate from side to side, or wander or fly about from place to place, have helped to identify and validate these and other localizing phenomena, on the way to finding suitable treatment for them.

> 3) *Modalities,* agencies by which or circumstances in which symptoms are relieved or intensified, such as times of the day or night, changes in the weather or climate, emotional states, foods, or just about anything that the patient has noticed.

Generally less unusual or outlandish than the "strange, rare, and peculiar" symptoms, modalities identify natural cycles and subtle influences that operate powerfully but inconsistently in many people, like diurnal and sleep rhythms, seasonal or annual periodicity, and atmospheric conditions, each of them unique in degree and combination, none affecting everyone or even a given individual the same at all times.

Especially useful when applicable to several symptoms at once, in such cases modalities reflect then energy state of the patient as a whole, and when consistent and well-marked can help narrow the choice of possible remedies to a much smaller group. Equally valuable for teaching purposes, they document subtle forces, influences, and causal factors at work in many patients that our customary double-blind standard is designed to exclude or override.

> 4) *Concomitants,* symptoms that accompany other symptoms, or precede or follow them in a definite sequence, like nausea with headache or vertigo, fever and thirst, followed by chills or sweating, and so forth. Concomitant symptoms are related synchronistically rather than causally, are peculiar solely in their connectedness, and may be so unexpected and strange as to illuminate a whole case or remedy picture.

Ever on the lookout for anything striking, odd, or unusual about an illness or a patient, the skilled homeopath becomes a kind of connoisseur, not only of the symptoms themselves, but also of the feeling-tone of the interview, an engaged yet neutral stance that encourages people to unburden their darkest secrets, many of which don't fit any preformed diagnostic category and thus easily fall through the cracks of our disease-oriented system. . .

Homeopathy: For and Against.

With no absolute contra-indications to trying them, homeopathic remedies may at least be considered before resorting to more drastic methods, or after they have failed. Almost ideally safe and gentle, as well as economical and easy to use, the remedies are not harmful and rarely produce serious or enduring ill effects. While often subtle at first, responses to treatment are typically prompt, thorough, and long-lasting, requiring infrequent repetition of the dose, and posing minimal risk of chronic drug dependence. In many cases, patients, friends, and loved ones alike notice a renewed vitality and emotional well-being that seem genuine, spontaneous, and attributable at least in part to the patient's own efforts.

Although the encyclopedic scope and richness of the homeopathic *materia medica* demands years of study to practice the method with skill, its basic principles are easy enough to understand that even a novice can obtain creditable results with only a small number of remedies. As long as a few simple rules are observed, it is perfectly safe for untrained people of average intelligence to learn and use at their own pace.

On the other hand, it is far from a panacea for all ills. However admirable for first aid and the self-care of wounds, injuries, and simple domestic ailments, it is no substitute for the repair of structural and mechanical problems, such as lacerations needing to be sutured, fractures demanding open or closed reduction, emergency surgery, and the like, or for well-trained and experienced professional help when necessary. Naturally, patients with severe or disabling illnesses and established dependence on corticosteroids, antipsychotics, anticonvulsants, and other potent drugs are much more difficult to treat successfully. In addition, the remedies themselves are somewhat delicate and easily inactivated, so that certain precautions in administration, handling, and storage must be observed.

Finally, homeopathy is a difficult and exacting art. Even in comparatively easy or uncomplicated cases, a well-trained and competent prescriber may have to try several remedies before any benefit is obtained, while in other cases, despite the most conscientious efforts, there is little or no improvement at all. Perhaps most important of all, nobody understands how the dilute remedies really act, or can reliably predict how different patients will respond to the remedies chosen for them, or which symptoms will come, go, or change in what order. However sound its principles or scientific its methodology, and no less than acupuncture, midwifery, or even medicine and surgery for that matter, homeopathy remains essentially an art, having to do with the unique life energy of individual human beings.

NOTE.

1. Hahnemann, *Organon,* ¶ 87.

From Part Two, Introduction: *The Study of Remedies.*

The core of homeopathy lies in its peculiar conception of medicinal substances and its elaborate methodology for studying and using them. With the vital force, the totality of symptoms, and other basic principles at least tacitly acknowledged by healers of every stripe, the homeopathic philosophy has always exerted a considerable influence far beyond the relatively small circle of its adherents. But its peculiar yoga of preparing, selecting, and administering remedies remains uniquely its own, speaking a private language both elegant and beautiful, but accessible only to those who take the trouble to learn it.

While the ultimate goal of studying remedies is to recognize them in the life of the patient, the actual procedure consists of learning how to distinguish each one from all the others, and especially from those most closely resembling it. Quite laborious and exacting under any circumstances, the discipline is also intensely gratifying and pays handsome rewards as long as certain peculiarities of homeopathic thinking are kept clearly in mind.

Medicines Produce Symptoms as Well as "Curing" Them.

First, the Law of Similars is dualistic in its teaching that remedies can cause symptoms or cure them, can act as medicines or poisons, depending on dosage and the individuality of the patient. Thus remedies known for a particular keynote symptom, like *Bryonia,* with its profound aggravation from movement, may also be useful at times for patient with the opposite modality. Just as opposite emotional states regularly co-exist in dreams and the unconscious, remedies stand for basic themes or issues more than a fixed resolution of them, so that fixed "essences" that exclude or require a specific characteristic, or rest smugly on what is already known, are likely to mislead or fall short.

Reasoning by Similarity.

Second, our knowledge of remedies is built up by *analogy* or multi-level similarity between older, more limited formulations of a symptom, and its subsequent application to other areas of functioning, which results in broadening and eventual redefinition of the symptom itself.

"Worse from movement," the classic *Bryonia* modality, is again a perfect example, being ordinarily associated with physical symptoms like headache or pleuritic pain, but equally applicable to the mental state, typically a mild delirium that shuns intellectual activity or sensory stimulation of any kind. When generalized in this manner, the original modality comes to represent the *Bryonia* energy pattern as a whole, no matter what the illness, on both sides of the psycho-somatic frontier, and thus prior to the mind-body distinction itself. Similarly, the homeopathic *materia medica* grows and develops in unforeseeable ways defying pat or rigid formulation, and a lot of the art and fascination of using remedies lies in this recognition of the old themes in newer and ever more inclusive variations.

Patients Can Get "Stuck" at Any Point.

Third, the "never well since" phenomenon means that chronic ailments often date from finite, memorable acute illnesses that have never resolved, leaving behind a residue of "stuckness" to which new symptoms and layers of illness may adhere. Frequently healed by the same remedies that would have been indicated for the original acute episode, this process of fixation is well illustrated by

1) *Arnica,* the classic first-aid remedy for blunt trauma to the soft tissues, and also indicated for chronic ailments appearing in the wake of such injuries.

Star pitcher of his high-school baseball team, a boy of 16 was hit in the face by a line drive, knocked unconscious for about 30 minutes, and subsequently developed fainting spells that kept him on the bench for the rest of that season and well into the next. A neurological exam and EEG were negative, and most of the episodes occurred when he tried to pitch a game or in batting practice. These complaints quickly disappeared after one dose of *Arnica* 1M.

2) *Ignatia,* unrivalled for first-aid treatment of acute grief and bereavement, and also beneficial in the treatment of various chronic complaints appearing later as a result.

A girl of ten was brought in for a nasty sore throat that had been interfering with her sleep for weeks. Complaining of a lump there in the morning, and especially before lunch, she said that the pain was actually better after eating, and hurt most when *not* swallowing. This odd pattern led me to the further discovery that her best friend's mother was receiving chemotherapy for breast cancer, of which a close family member had recently died, and that the girl had recently been troubled with nighttime thoughts of illness and death and sometimes awoke in a panic if her mother wasn't there to comfort her. After a round of *Ignatia* 200, she bounced back from this embryonic illness in a few days. When it returned in a milder form about a year later, she asked for the remedy herself, and this time it acted at once and didn't have to be repeated.

3) *Gelsemium,* a superb remedy for influenza, and equally beneficial to some patients with chronic fatigue syndrome (CFS) and other illnesses dating from a flu-like illness or flu vaccine in the past.

4) *Staphysagria,* the standard remedy for healing surgical or other cleanly-incised knife wounds, also without equal for patients who have never been well or fully recovered from a traumatic surgical procedure in the past.

With almost any remedy potentially useful in this way, the perpetuation and elaboration of acute ailments into an ongoing state illustrates the importance of "stuckness" in the pathogenesis of chronic disease. By defining what is out there to be healed, remedies can also help teach us how our illnesses are made.

The Fundamentalist Controversy: An Issue That Won't Go Away*

I am honored by your invitation to speak, and delighted to participate in your 25th Anniversary celebration by talking about what we all know and love, yet never quite seem to get to the bottom of. But I warn you that my subject is one of those doctrinal and almost theological matters about which there is right and wrong in every position, yet everyone feels the pressure to declare unequivocally for one or the other. In America, where the dispute became so contentious that old friendships were broken on account of it, individuals on both sides are reaching out to compose their differences, such that fellowship and civility may yet prevail over abstract ideologies, however deeply felt.

I must also point out that the terms "innovation" and "fundamentalism" were both coined by me after the fact to characterize the two main opponents, and not chosen or used by the major players themselves.[1] In fact the whole controversy began with a series of attacks on the teachings of Rajan Sankaran, Jan Scholten, Jeremy Sherr, Nancy Herrick, and others, largely based on the accusation that they are speculative in nature. So I need to begin by examining the arguments of these critics in some detail.

The Fundamentalist Critique.

In North America the first broadside came from Julian Winston, Editor-in-Chief of *Homeopathy Today,* which enjoys the largest circulation of any homeopathic journal in the United States and represents the official views of the National Center for Homeopathy. In his lead editorial, Julian lampooned several of the new teachings asspeculative and therefore contrary to both the spirit and the letter of the generally-accepted classical style:

---

* "The Fundamentalist Controversy," *American Journal of Homeopathic Medicine* 97:28, Spring 2004

The earliest remedy "pictures" were popularized by Kent, whose students used them as shortcuts to find the curative remedy. In 1974 Vithoulkas brought out his "essences," which were misapplied by students to make homeopathy easier to understand, and which Künzli spoke out against. Now we have Sankaran's "core delusions," Scholten on the Periodic Table, Herrick anthropomorphizing animals and dinosaur bones, and remedy "families" and "kingdoms," all leading to prescriptions based on theory and speculation. Some who consider themselves classical homeopaths and eschew combination remedies, radionics, etc., don't see that overpsychologizing, dream provings, and all aren't homeopathy either![2]

In the same issue Julian also reviewed Nancy Herrick's book on animal provings and found it wanting in almost every detail:

Hahnemann cautioned against "weaving empty speculations," and Hering warned, "if our school gives up the strict inductive method, we are lost and deserve to be mentioned only as a caricature in the history of medicine." I'm afraid this book is guilty on both counts. If it had just presented the raw data, the provings could stand by themselves, and a picture of the remedy would emerge, developed through use. But the author has added "themes" that are nothing but empathic thinking and anthropomorphic speculation. Thus the mating of elephants is described as "an all-out party atmosphere," in which "everyone gets in on the act," and young male lions trying to dethrone the leader is read as "problems with authority figures." A piece of fossilized dinosaur bone found in a nest led Herrick to potentize it and to infer nurturing behavior under the theme "helping or no one helping." What about letting the symptoms stand on their own? Can't a cigar just be a cigar?[3]

The same themes are still being sounded today. This summer, German homeopath Dr. med. Klaus Habich and two colleagues wrote a piece in the *American Journal of Homeopathic Medicine* which contrasts some of the new teachings with the methodology of Hahnemann:

What is so special about homeopathy? It is not the prescription of potentized substances according to the Law of Similars, which is also used by spagyric, anthroposophic, and Bach flower treatment. It is its scientific mode of working. Hahnemann despaired of the speculative, arbitrary practices of his day and tried to develop rules for a reliable art of healing. It is no accident that the call for "clearly perceptible reasons" comes at the beginning of the *Organon*, before the word "homeopathy" is ever mentioned. In homeopathy, each step is subject to verifiability. All provings, dynamizations, and remedy selections can be confirmed by impartial observers. Those who deviate from this practice should expect to be asked what is homeopathic about whatever they do.[4]

Also identifying homeopathy with the scientific world-view, Dr. Jennifer Jacobs wrote Julian a letter supporting his position from the radically different perspective of experimental medicine, and promoting the double-blind model and other modern research standards:

> Many of us are concerned about the direction in which we are moving. Provings without a blinded supervisor and symptoms elicited in group discussion are subjective and only preliminary to a formal double-blind process using symptoms of individual provers independently reported. Applying plant or animal characteristics from biology to human subjects is both seductive and speculative without solid evidence of provings and clinical verification.

> It is disturbing when new students know more about new or small remedies than time-tested polychrests. It is suspicious when three cases of a new remedy show up in the office a week after attending a seminar featuring it. Wouldn't they have been helped before the remedy was known or the practitioner learned of it? Those offering new ideas must accept criticism without taking it as a personal attack.[5]

But the most learned, detailed, and impassioned opposition has come from André Saine, the Canadian naturopath, whose long, scholarly diatribe appeared in *Homeopathy Today, Simillimum,* and the *American Journal of Homeopathic Medicine.* In the following excerpt, he equates homeopathy with the method of individualization and the hypothetical generalizations of Sankaran and Scholten with the abstract diagnostic entities of allopathic medicine:

> Making use of hypothetical generalizations contradicts two fundamental principles of homeopathy. First, the *Materia medica* must be kept free from all hypotheses and conjectures. Second, in homeopathy we must individualize at all times, even though our human nature entices us to generalize. Didn't Hahnemann teach us to individualize each case and every remedy, and warn us against generalization? Individualization is the essence of homeopathy, generalization a trademark of conventional medicine. Those who individualize succeed in curing, while those who generalize fail.[6]

In a later editorial, Julian softens his criticism a bit, granting that such methods could be acceptable in the hands of experienced teachers well-versed in the classical method, but admonishing them to be more conscientious in teaching their students the fundamentals:

> For most of our teachers, *Materia medica* study and repertory work are second nature: they look at homeopathy from new perspectives, as if unaware of how much the basics still guide them. But what about their students? Kent's *Lectures on Materia Medica* were for graduates with anatomy, physiology, pathology, and four years of homeopathic education. The problem with most seminars today is that there are no such prerequisites. The material is post- graduate level, where knowledge of the basic principles is assumed. They should be for experienced practitioners, not beginners. Teachers may say, "It's not our fault if the students don't do it right," but I believe it is. There must be accountability in the process.[7]

The remaining criticisms were directed at generalization and speculation in specific areas, such as "essences." The most pertinent argument against essences in particular, and overly-mentalized remedy pictures in general, actually dates from the early 1980's, when the great Swiss homeopath Jost Künzli roasted the non-physician Vithoulkas for using them, despite knowing of his work solely from hearsay:

> In Vithoulkas' courses, too much attention is paid to the mental and emotional symptoms and the psychological approach. Students analyze these aspects as if they were qualified psychologists and come up with a hypothetical answer. Since it is impossible to duplicate such a train of thought, he can easily prove them wrong by taking them into a labyrinth from which he alone can find the way out. It is also wrong in my opinion to judge the success of treatment mainly on the emotional level. The whole patient must be improved. I don't care if my hypertensive feels better or likes me if his blood pressure isn't down. I also dislike assigning each remedy an "essence." If the essence of *Lycopodium* is cowardice, this should be the core of the remedy and explain its entire symptomatology. But *Lycopodium* has many other facets. With this schema we can miss 90% of the cases.[8]

Another pet peeve of the critics is the alleged emphasis on "signatures," i. e., correspondences between the non-homeopathic features of remedies, such as their natural history or chemical properties, and their actual use in

233

treating patients. Once again, the alarm is sounded by Dr. Saine, who can quote Hahnemannian catechism on demand for any fundamentalist cause:

> For Hahnemann the doctrine of signatures meant looking for therapeutic meaning in all external, perceptible properties or characteristic features of a substance: "All our senses applied with utmost care to studying the external properties of medicinal substances furnish no information as to their power to alter human health." In examining patients, "the physician sees, hears, and observes what is altered and peculiar," writing down all that is noticeable, his "behavior, habits, activities, domestic situation, way of life, diet, etc., these signs representing the whole of the sickness, its true and only form." He excludes "preconceived notions, conjectures, classifications, or guesswork," and insists that homeopaths refrain from "prejudice and speculation:" 'This healing art derives no knowledge from impure sources of *Materia medica,* pursues no dreamy, false path, but the way consonant with nature, giving no medicine before testing it experimentally on healthy men."[9]

Even though the teachers in question rarely emphasize the actual use of such signatures in practice, Habich et al. likewise raise a considerable fuss about their willingness even to talk about them:

> The question as to whether signatures should become a component of the *Materia medica* is a decisive one. We believe that only remedy provings and toxicology can be *materia medica* sources. Signatures may be useful didactic models, but statements of fact can only result from direct observations, and the model often becomes confused with the fact. As Hahnemann said, "The inner nature of remedies is not recognizable by the intellect alone, but solely by the experience of perceiving their action in individuals."[10]

On the issue of remedy families, André is even more contemptuous:

> Dr. Morrison generalizes that "common threads run through the *Nitricum* remedies: craving fat, fissures, splinter-like pains, and imminent sense of danger," and that "most *Kali's* wake between 1 and 3 a.m." How can he be taken seriously about the nitrics when only *Nitric. acid.* and *Arg. nit.* have all 4 symptoms, while *Kali nit.* lacks splinter-like pains, none but *Glonoin* has a sense of impending misfortune, and *Amyl nit., Benzin. nit., Natrum nit., Nitr. spir. dulc., Nitrog. oxyd., Nitromur. acid., Stront. nit.,* and *Uranium nit.* have none of the 4? What about waking at 1 to 3 a.m. for the *Kali's,* when only *Kali carb., Kali bich.,* and *Kali nit.* are listed for these hours, while the rest are not?[11]

234

Habich et al. also take issue with remedy families and kingdoms, but their tone is rather more judicious, thoughtful, and not wholly dismissive of the concept *per se:*

> Snake venoms share discomfort from tight clothing around the neck. But can we extrapolate to snakes in general, since some venoms are hemolytic, while others are neurotoxic? Similar plants can also have similar effects, as we know from the *Solanaceae.* But we doubt if such generalizations are applicable to the vegetable or animal kingdom as a whole, such as that all animals are jealous.[12]

Oddly enough, André, Julian, and Habich, et al. have very little to say against Sankaran's ideas on miasms, which are by far the most hypothetical and admittedly speculative of his numerous contributions, a paradox which I will discuss presently.

The Battle Lines Are Drawn.

As the pages of *Homeopathy Today* were increasingly filled with such criticisms, and little space was given for favorable or even neutral reporting about the new teachings, Roger Morrison wrote a letter to Julian complaining that he had misused his editorial position on behalf of a stridently partisan viewpoint that was unrepresentative of the American homeopathic movement as a whole:

> While Mr. Winston clearly has great love for homeopathy, his use of the editorship to advocate his personal beliefs has become divisive. We don't like his ridiculing serious people. He says Scholten's work lacks provings, ignoring the dozen reported in his book. Where Sankaran uses dreams, he's not interpreting or theorizing, only asking how the patient *feels,* about his "state," as Hahnemann puts it. Mangialavori speaks of families, Sankaran of kingdoms, Vithoulkas of essences, Herrick of animal behavior, Scholten of chemical groupings. They don't propose throwing out the Repertory, but only looking at cases in another light when repertorization gives no clear answer.[13]

This letter was co-signed by Sankaran, Scholten, Herrick, the Editors of *Links,* two NCH Directors who removed their names when the Board so ordered them, and about a dozen senior American homeopaths, including myself. In the ensuing months, Julian published a spate of fan mail thanking him for his principled stand and accusing the signers of attempting to censor his words. These letters culminated in the long article by André cited above, "Homeopathy vs. Speculative Medicine: a Call to Action," which congratulated him for defending Hahnemann's work and placed the blame exclusively on the infamous twenty-one:

Twenty-one prominent homeopaths accuse Julian of being intolerant and divisive by advocating his personal beliefs. Such accusations are not new, because Homeopathy is based on fixed principles, despite practitioners taking license to practice contrary to them. Divisions in homeopathy are always initiated by approaches incompatible with Hahnemann's: his disciples must keep denouncing such mis-representations. The present will be remembered for its extravagant deviations: teachers taking chronic cases in 15 minutes and prescribing on clothing worn at the visit, provings given to some attendees but including symptoms of the others, provings of doses kept under the pillow.[14]

What infuriated me at the time was his one-sided definition of heresy as the fact, appearance, or mere possibility of meaningful change in our art. Now what strikes me is his absolutist sense of right and wrong, so eerily reminiscent of fundamentalisms everywhere, which gave me the idea for my title, and is indeed, as he says, so deeply and inextricably rooted in our history.

In any case, the Inquisitorial tone of his words continues to reverberate through the movement, as in the Declaration that followed the article of Habich et al., which seems to have been drafted by them as well, and was co-signed by an equally large and impressive roster of homeopaths from around the world, including several former LIGA Presidents:

With great concern we have observed attempts to introduce speculative and metaphysical elements into homeopathy. Homeopathy was founded as rational medicine, with its guiding dictum of treating the sick on clearly comprehensible principles. Fantasy, free association, signatures, and other such analogies can not be the basis for such an art. Association and speculation are tempting from a didactic viewpoint, but to augment the *Materia medica,* drug provings, toxicology, and clinical verification are the only reliable basis. Knowledge from other sources should be carefully separated from *Materia medica.* Whoever uses different methods should name them differently to avoid misleading patients and public and has no right to call them homeopathy.[15]

Notwithstanding its carefully measured tones and its acceptance of clinical verification as a legitimate *Materia medica* source, the flavor and spirit of this Declaration are likewise essentially those of a loyalty oath, a creed or solemn declaration of faith to be signed and sworn to, and thus a basis for excommunication in the event of future backsliding and as binding as any latter-day Torquemada could possibly wish.

So the battle lines are drawn. Just as the new teachings have arisen more or less independently in many different parts of the world, the opposition to them is also global. Much as we might prefer to forget the whole thing as an aberration or bad dream that we wandered into by mistake, the overblown rhetoric on all sides has come to designate a serious issue at the heart of what we all do, so that no matter which side we favor, we have no choice but to develop acceptable criteria for deciding whether and to what extent the new teachings are speculative, and if, when, and how they deviate from the letter and spirit of our rule, or might even then serve a valid and useful purpose.

Moreover, while the charges of speculation and heresy are as old as homeopathy itself, applying them to the teachers under scrutiny is unprecedented and indeed superbly ironic, given that every one of them would have no difficulty qualifying as a good classical homeopath, according to the strict criteria of the International Hahnemannian Association, the same fundamentalist group that André throws up to us for our edification:

Declaration of Principles.
Hahnemann's *Organon* is the only reliable guide to therapeutics.
Homeopathy consists of the Law of Similars, dynamization, the single remedy, and the minimum dose.

Resolutions.
Homeopathy should free itself from
1) Mixing or alternating two or more medicines;
2) Using topical medications or mechanical appliances in non-surgical cases; and
3) Giving medicine in quantity to suppress symptoms by primary action.
The utmost possible relief from suffering in incurable cases is obtained by the *simillimum*, while antipathic or allopathic palliatives are injurious and unnecessary. Provings on the healthy are the basis of our *Materia medica*, but we may cautiously supplement these by frequently verified clinical experience.[16]

Remedy "Essences" and *Materia Medica* Study.

With that as background, I want to return to *Materia medica* study, the issue we began with, to show you that the concept of a remedy "essence," like everything else in homeopathy, is already central to Hahnemann's thought, e.g., in the opening paragraphs of the *Organon,* where he develops the axiomatic concept of the "vital force:"

> In the healthy condition of man, the spirit-like vital force that animates the material body rules with unbounded sway, and retains all parts of the organism in harmonious co-operation, so that our reason-gifted mind can freely employ this living, healthy instrument for the higher purposes of existence. When a person falls ill, it is only this spirit-like, automatic vital force, everywhere present, that is primarily deranged. Only the vital force can furnish the organism with its disagreeable sensations.
>
> As a power invisible in itself and only cognizable by its effects on the organism, its morbid derangement makes itself known by morbid symptoms, and in no other way. In like manner the disappearance of all morbid phenomena under treatment necessarily implies the restoration of the integrity of the vital force and therefore the health of the organism as a whole.[17]

The same theme is recapitulated when introducing the concept of homeopathic *Materia medica:*

> There is no way to ascertain the peculiar effects of medicines other than to administer them experimentally to healthy persons, and to observe the signs and symptoms that each individually produces on body and mind. As certainly as every species of plant differs in its form and mode of life from every other, and every mineral and salt as well, so they all differ in their pathogenetic and therapeutic effects. Each produces alterations in health in a different, peculiar, and determinate manner so as to preclude the possibility of confounding one with another.[18]

All of these passages stress the dynamic character of the vital force -- and thus of the curative remedy that matches it --as ubiquitous, unbounded, indivisible, and therefore seamlessly unified, but also unknowable apart from the particular signs and symptoms it exhibits. In short, the homeopathic enterprise is thoroughly empirical and scientific in its method; but the totality that it implies, the life energy of both patients and the remedies that cure them, remains a mystery that cannot be analyzed or fully comprehended, but only *approximated,* a task for which science alone is inadequate, and art and imagination are also required.

The implications of this paradox were already entirely evident to the great E. A. Farrington, the first American homeopath who clearly foresaw both the need and the possibility of what we now call remedy "essences:"

> We include all the symptoms that we observe. Then what have we? A mass of symptoms seeming to have no connection at all. When you have the changes *in toto* that this substance makes on the system, you have the pathology of the case. This grand effect of the drug must always be kept in mind, qualifying the individual symptoms, or these latter are worthless. You must know what the whole drug does, or you will not be able to appreciate any part of it. You can find twenty drugs with the same symptoms. How will you decide between them? By study of the drug as a whole.[19]

The critical importance of this passage is drummed into the soul of every well- trained classical homeopath, fundamentalist or otherwise, who before choosing a possible remedy in the case knows to read it in the *Materia medica,* to ascertain how well it fits, not just symptom by symptom but globally, and including such elusive and indefinable properties as "flavor," style, and the *Gestalt* or arrangement of the symptoms as a whole. But this is also the problem with Farrington's instruction, for there is and can be no rule or formula for carrying it out, no royal road or shortcut for comprehending the esoteric and mysterious unity of our living patients and the remedies that can heal them. So Farrington's words live on as a vision or prophecy of what is possible, which neither he nor his successors had the tools to fulfill or bring about in any practical or uniformly reproducible way.

Most early *Materia medicas* were compiled after the fashion of Hahnemann's *Materia Medica Pura,* i.e., as simple lists of symptoms arranged by region or system, beginning with "Mind" and ending with "Generalities," a custom that has been preserved right up to the present. From Lippe, for example, a fine text of this older type, rightly admired by André, I have extracted an abridged version of the mental and general symptoms he offers for *Ignatia:*

Mind and disposition.
Sensitiveness of feeling; delicate conscientiousness.
Fearfulness, timidity.
Irresolution: anxious to do this, now that.
The slightest contradiction irritates.
Intolerance of noise.
Taciturn, with continuous, sad thoughts.
Still, serious melancholy, with moaning.
Anger, followed by quiet grief and sorrow.
Inclination to grief, without saying anything about it.
Great tenderness.
Changeable disposition: jesting, laughing, changing to sadness. (Hysteria.)

Generalities.
Convulsive twitchings, especially after fright or grief.
Convulsions alternating with oppressed breathing.
Hysterical spasms.
Trembling of the limbs.
Pressing pains, as from a hard-pointed object pressing outward.
Sensation as of dislocation in joints.
Lancinating stitches, as from sharp knife.[20]

In trying to characterize the remedy as a *totality* rather than merely an arithmetic sum of items, Hahnemann and Lippe simply added a final list of "general" symptoms that, like those of the "mind" section, referred to the organism as a whole rather than a part only. Notice too that Lippe identifies *Ignatia* with grief, but not yet with "ailments from grief," a far more complex and long-term connection that lies beyond the scope of the provings, emerges only gradually with repeated clinical verification, and even then requires a significant component of logical inference and imaginative synthesis that is a lot of what actual medical practice tends to be about.

A generation later, in his popular *Lectures on Materia Medica,* Kent added illustrative vignettes to highlight the most important themes of the remedies, often including a number of variations, and comprising portraits or "remedy-pictures" that are lifelike, readily accessible to students, and highly evocative even today, with strong and at times uncanny resemblance to people we know:

Ignatia is suited to sensitive, delicate women and children, to gentle, fine-fibered, refined, educated women with nervous complaints similar to hysteria. When overwrought, excited, or emotional, a woman will do things that she regrets or cannot account for. She has undergone controversy, is excited, and goes into cramps, trembles and quivers, goes to bed with a headache.

A sensitive, nervous girl finds she has misplaced her affections: the young man has not been true to his word; she has a weeping spell, headache, trembling, is nervous and sleepless. A delicate, sensitive woman loses her husband or child, suffers from grief, has headaches, trembles, weeps, is excited, can't sleep or control herself, feels ashamed.

Quivering of limbs, nervous excitement, sudden weakness, hysterical fainting, jerking, convulsive twitching. Children convulse in sleep, during dentition, or after punishment. Hysterical paralysis. She does unaccountable things, the opposite of what would be expected[21]

In these synthetic or composite portraits we see again with particular clarity the importance of clinical verification, for filling in the gaps between the individual proving symptoms and providing the interpretation that glues these disparate elements together and gives them meaning within an integrated whole.

In the 1980's George Vithoulkas appeared on the scene as another world-class prescriber who inspired a whole generation of homeopaths by both precept and example. As with Kent's, his *Materia medica* first appeared in the form of lecture notes, and his remedy-portraits or "essences," as they came to be known, had to be "stolen" by his students, i.e., compiled and circulated unofficially and in fact against the master's often-stated wishes. Time and again he repudiated all written formulations of his remedy pictures, which he insisted were continuously evolving and forever elusive and incomplete. Here is one such version of *Ignatia,* very much in the Kentian tradition, but with a more idiosyncratic and contemporary feel, featuring a wider latitude for interpretation and at times a provocative edge:

Frequently indicated today because of women's liberation. She tries to assert herself, to be equal to men. Sensitivity with romanticism, which eventually comes into conflict with reality. Overstrained by grief or vexation, she breaks down with spasms or hysteria, unable to talk or think, or faints, unresponsive and unable to cry. Then she locks her door and cries, sobbing spasmodically. Physical problems after feeling better emotionally: becomes cold, hard, irritable, or insulting, and tries to compose herself. Moods change very frequently. Symptoms begin after a death or the breakup of a love affair, suppressing feeling until it comes out in a hysterical reaction.

Torticollis: emotions go into the physical plane with great force. Chorea and cramping in response to internal or external stimuli. Unexpected reactions: emotionally nasty when you are nice to her; unpredictable mentally and physically.[22]

It was just such alleged overmentalization and oversimplification that led the great Künzli to repudiate the whole project, and motivated Vithoulkas himself to equivocate or disappear whenever his students tried to pin him down to any concrete or definitive formulation. Yet almost all classical prescribers accept the special priority of the mental and emotional symptoms in choosing the remedy, as did Hahnemann himself, not only because they refer to the patient as a whole rather than any part of the body, but also because they offer a glimpse of the "vital force," that which transmutes the particulars into a unity and can thus impart *meaning* to them, can fashion them into a *story*. This simplest kind of "essence" is perfectly illustrated by a short case from the early years of my practice:

A girl of ten was brought in for a nasty sore throat that had interfered with her sleep for weeks. Complaining of a lump there in the morning, especially before lunch, she said that the pain was actually better from eating and hurt most when *not* swallowing. This odd pattern led me to the further discovery that her best friend's mother was receiving chemotherapy for breast cancer, which a close family member had also recently died of, so that the girl herself had been troubled with thoughts of illness and death, and often woke in a panic if her mother was not there to comfort her.

After a round of *Ignatia* 200, she bounced back from this embryonic illness in a few days. When it recurred in somewhat milder form about a year later, she asked for the remedy herself, and this time it acted at once and didn't have to be repeated.[23]

However elusive in practice, the quest for meaning or essence helps us look past the narrowly physical and mental dimensions of cases and remedies, and to peer into Hahnemann's dynamic realm, where remedies

242

and patients are comprehensible as unified energy systems, independent of "mind" or "body" and conceptually prior to both. How *Materia medica* study propels us forward in this way is evident in the historical evolution of a remedy like *Bryonia*. First associated with particular symptoms like headache or pleurisy, its grand modality, "worse from motion," eventually proved applicable to mental and emotional states as well, such that patients needing the remedy were found to be gruff, withdrawn, frequently uncommunicative, and averse to human interaction, sensory stimulation, or mental effort of any kind. When generalized in this global fashion, "worse from motion" has come to preside over the *Bryonia* state or energy pattern as a whole, no matter what the illness, on both sides of the psychosomatic frontier, and thus in a sense prior to the mind-body distinction itself.[24]

Another example is *Staphysagria,* which began its career as a remedy for healing surgical incisions and other linear knife wounds. After a time it was successfully applied to miscellaneous ailments developing in the wake of a surgical procedure in the past, a "never-well-since" pattern in which the energy of the original insult becomes chronically "stuck" or fixed in place and then branches out unpredictably through the organism in the form of both physical and mental symptoms. Others found the remedy equally beneficial for obscure, idiosyncratic complaints arising from suppressed anger, as after humiliation or physical or sexual abuse.

These seemingly unrelated applications led to the further revelation that surgery offers the ideal energetic prototype for ailments from suppressed anger: the continuity and integrity of the vital force are interrupted by the surgeon's knife, while the anesthetized patient remains helpless to express or even fully experience the "anger" that such a violation implies. The mere existence of such illnesses, and the usefulness of the remedy in treating them, cannot be adequately explained in either the medical language of cells, tissues, and organs or the psychological language of ideas and emotions, or both. Such dilemmas indicate the need for an energetic language that is mind-body neutral and thus comfortable in either mode and on both sides of the boundary. By defining what is out there to be healed, remedies can teach us how our illnesses are made.[25]

There is nothing new or even remotely speculative about any of this. All good homeopaths of every persuasion make connections and analogies like this all the time, but they are the fruit of clinical verification, nowhere to be found in provings or the works of Hahnemann, and require considerable art and imagination as well. These are undoubtedly the reasons why our fundamentalist critics have so little to say about them. But they *use* them just the same, or they couldn't be the effective prescribers we know them in fact to be.

In his *Materia medica,* even the great Lippe, whom André considers the finest prescriber of all time, limits himself to "the most characteristic symptoms of the best-proved and most used of our remedies;" in other words, *he makes a selection.* But on what basis? What criteria does he use in deciding that some symptoms are more important, more characteristic, more "essential" than others? When Kent and Vithoulkas try to articulate the essence of a remedy, what they offer is merely their own version of these choices, augmented by clinical verifications for unity and dramatic effect. The only real difference between "illuminists" or essence prescribers like Kent or Vithoulkas and "fundamentalists" like Lippe and Künzli is that the former are brave or rash enough to talk about what they've learned from clinical experience, while the latter are careful to keep their innermost thought-processes to themselves, as if sacred and inviolable.

Sankaran's *Materia medica* is simply a further attempt to locate the dynamic or energetic core of the remedy, such that physical, mental, and emotional symptoms can all be understood and located within the same framework. His "essences" thus include the chemical grouping or biological family, the miasmatic affiliation, and his own selection of the most important rubrics that illustrate his sense of the remedy as a whole, just as Lippe has done:

> *Ignatia: Loganiaceæ,* cancer miasm [the need to keep in control]
> Grief, undemonstrative.
> Mildness: bears suffering, even outrage without complaining.
> Silent grief, cannot cry.
> Ailments from death of a child, of parents, or of friends.
> Ailments from shock, grief, or disappointment.
> Ailments from embarrassment, from shame.
> Dreams of unsuccessful efforts.
> Delusion he has done wrong.
> Conscientious about trifles.

Fixed ideas.
Back pain, lumbar region, extending down legs.
Change of position ameliorates.[26]

As a rough guideline, then, I offer the simple compromise that essences are valid and useful if helping us to organize our study of remedies, but misleading and inaccurate when memorized and used as a *substitute* for that process: to that extent, the fundamentalists are quite correct. Like the Repertory from whence they come, essences are merely another way to suggest possible remedies we might not have thought of without them. They should not and must not be allowed to spare us the final task of reading the remedy as a whole, in search of the best possible fit.

Sankaran's quest for the essence further reminds us to pay attention to the imagery and indeed the exact words of the patient, which sometimes lead straight to the goal without needing the Repertory at all:

A 57-year-old engineer came to see me for muscle cramps in his legs after heavy physical work, and was also bothered by tightness in his muscles that made him feel "all locked up," especially in the cold, from a draft or a fan, or when his throat felt cold. Sciatica also "pulled" and "tugged" at his left hip, making exercise difficult. Some arthritic changes were found on X-ray.

Testing materials for an electronics firm, he drove himself to finish any project he started, no matter how late he had to stay. Born and raised in Germany, he came to America at the age of eleven, with his father dead in the War, his mother traumatized, and the political situation "all locked up" in the tense atmosphere of the Cold War.

Proud of his squeaky-clean habits, and devoted to keeping his house and yard in top shape, he rarely paused to relax and enjoy life, while his defiant teen-age daughter, whom he could neither influence nor even talk to most of the time, presented yet another "locked-up" situation, the oft-repeated phrase thus becoming a central metaphor linking his health problems to the character of his life as a whole.

Six weeks after a single dose of *Causticum* 1M, he was much better. His feet felt warm, the "bounce" was back in his legs, and he felt much less sensitive to cold in general. Infrequent doses of *Causticum* 30 were helpful whenever symptoms returned. He has needed no remedies for over two years.[27]

On the other hand, although this man's choice of words certainly helped me find a good remedy for him, I think I probably could have found it using the Repertory just as well. I tell his story primarily to show that the primary validity and usefulness of essences is as a study aid, while in finding the remedy it is only one strategy among many, and not always the best or most important for everyone.

Non-Proving Data: Families, Chemistry, Natural History, and "Signatures."

As we have seen, this broad, heterogeneous area has drawn almost a greater variety and intensity of criticism than any other. I am still rather mystified by the almost puritanical resistance to this kind of information, doubtless in part because I myself am unashamedly addicted to it, and have found it to enrich and enhance my practice in countless ways, all entirely homeopathic as far as I can tell, and wholly innocent of any heretical imputation.

I begin with the concept of remedy "families," because it is the oldest, and, like that of essences, arises directly out of our earliest homeopathic training, which urges us to study each remedy by learning to differentiate it from all others, but especially from those which most closely resemble it. The old way of doing this was symptom-by-symptom, e.g., by comparing all the remedies listed for a particular keynote; but the enormous number of rubrics and almost infinite diversity of remedies conspire to make this strategy too cumbersome for ordinary daily or practical use.

Once again, it was Farrington who first clearly understood the value of looking for deeper and more systematic levels of similarity by following the trail of biological and chemical groupings that already exist in nature:

> It is my duty to show you the genius of each drug, and the relations which they bear to one another. The first I have called the family relation, derived from their similarity in origin. When drugs belong to the same family, they must have a similar action. The halogens chlorine, iodine, bromine, and fluorine have many similarities because they belong to one family. So too with drugs from the vegetable kingdom. In the family to which *Arum triphyllum* belongs, you also find drugs which resemble one another from their family origin. Among ophidians, you will be perplexed to tell the differences between *Elaps, Lachesis,* and *Crotalus*.[28]

As with essences, his words envisioned a whole new way of studying remedies; but both the smaller number of remedies then available and the limited technical means for studying them kept his splendid prophecy from being fulfilled in his own lifetime and for many generations to come. It was the development of computer hardware and software with enough memory power to access the vast homeopathic literature and scan it at high speed that has allowed Farrington's great project to be carried out in a reproducible way for the first time. It is thus surely no accident that the new teachings under discussion have all arisen within the past few years more or less independently of one another and in widely separated locations, but with remarkable similarities in purpose and direction.

In an early example, the great Italian homeopath Massimo Mangialavori analyzed the symptoms of the snake remedies using *MacRepertory* and *Reference Works,* and found, exactly as Farrington had said, that most familiar keynotes of *Lachesis* were in fact characteristic of the family as a whole:

Bilateral asymmetry: one-sided symptoms.
Intolerance of tight clothing, especially around the neck.
Aggravation during and after sleep.
Affinity for the ENT and neck region, with choking and constriction.
PMS, general aggravation of all symptoms before menses.
General relief of all symptoms during menses, from talking, or discharge.
Passionate, sexual, competitive nature.
Deadly cunning, deviousness.
Psychic, clairvoyant, intuitive predilection and ability.
Thrombotic and hemorrhagic phenomena.[29]

He did not claim that every snake has all of these symptoms, but only that each keynote is found in other remedies in the family, so that those we once thought were peculiar to the most thoroughly proved venom must now be attributed to the whole family and thus eventually to other members which have not yet been shown to have them. Far from being an empty generalization of the kind that André is rightly exercised about, his work offers more precise, accurate criteria for distinguishing the various snake remedies from one another, and also carries such *predictive* force as makes it possible to test the validity of the family model itself.

The concept of remedy families merely provides a schema for clarifying which symptoms are peculiar to the individual remedy, and which are shared by the group. As with essences, such schemas are not yet available in every instance, and would not always be necessary even if they were. As the following case shows, the family dimension often proves useful when the most prominent member of the group appears well-indicated but fails to act well or deeply enough to hold:

> Her face swollen and disfigured by crops of red pustules, a woman of 41 was tormented by hot, stinging, stiletto-like pains that were worse from heat, better from ice, and made her angry at everyone. Afflicted with impetigo as a child, she'd had a bad case of chicken pox at 13, followed by recurrent boils and a persistent *Staph.* infection, for which she had taken antibiotics many times.

> Her skin flared up all over after the death of her father, a convicted felon who had left at her mother's insistence when she was 20, and got even worse when she was carrying her second son, who was 3 when I first saw her. *Apis* 200 worked beautifully at first, but soon wore off, and she didn't come back for a year, by which time her face stung so intensely that it reminded her of being attacked by a swarm of yellow-jackets in her teens.

> This little bit of history led me to study *Vespa crabro,* the hornet; and in hours after a dose of the 200, her whole face was flaming-red and hugely swollen, followed by rapid disappearance of all signs and symptoms of inflammation. By her next visit her skin looked clearer than it had for years, and she has remained well ever since.[30]

Sankaran often uses the pain rubrics to describe the sensations of remedies energetically, confirms them with the fears, dreams, and delusions, i.e., with the mental and emotional state, and then compares individual family members to extract the common features and distinguish each remedy within it. As with essences, there is nothing speculative about this: the rubrics are all there in the literature, well documented and confirmed. One could argue with his *selection* of rubrics, just as with Lippe's or anyone else's, since their relevance and importance will require years of clinical experience to verify and sort out. But that caveat does not invalidate the concept or the *procedure,* which is simply to use the computerized literature to facilitate our study of the rubrics. Just as with essences, his preference for the energetic language of sensations also provides another possible focal point around which other rubrics may group themselves:

> With a history of back injuries, a woman of 45 complained of sciatica and numbness in her buttock and thigh, which made it difficult for her to drive or sit, especially in cold, damp weather. The pain felt "hot, inflamed, and burning," and the sole of her foot felt "cushioned, as if walking on a waterbed."

> With her mother unpredictably violent, her father ineffectual, both of them alcoholic, and her older sister absent, she always felt "lost" as a child, with no one to turn to for help, and prayed for her mother to be taken away so that she could have a life of her own. In one dream she was rowing a boat but not moving ahead, and felt the same confusion she had known as a child. In another she was driving a school bus with no brakes, while her spirit guide "floated in and out" trying to fix them. Again the feeling was confusion and bewilderment as to why they were there and where they were going. She also recalled other dreams in which people "floated in and out" or she found herself in a place with no idea how she had got there.

> Using her themes "confused" and "bewildered," I studied the family *Magnoliæ,* which includes *Asarum, Aristolochia, Camphora, Cinnamon, Myristica,* and *Nux moschata,* which in Sankaran's analysis share the following common themes:

> **Sensations:**
> Confused, bewildered, beclouded [and isolated as a result].

> **Passive reactions:**
> Faint, sleepy [shutting out the bad reality, living in one's own world].
> Floating, divided, withdrawn, unconscious.
> Fear of sleep or anesthesia, agg. on waking.
> [Transition from inner to outer world difficult or threatening]

> **Active reaction:**
> Clarity.

> Under *Nux moschata,* I found rubrics that seemed to fit her very well:

> "Beclouded, delusion that everything has changed."
> "Delusion that the world or surroundings don't exist."
> "Delusion that time and space are confused."

> One month after a dose of *Nux moschata* 200, she reported feeling "much better," sleeping 18 hours that first night; her back and leg pain subsided very quickly, and she resumed yoga and bike riding, even losing five pounds. She came back in 7 months for aching joints and a swollen sensation in her back,

but no sciatica. I gave her another dose, and she has continued to do well ever since.[31]

Much the same is true of Scholten's method of group analysis of related mineral remedies, such as the halogens, or metal elements in the same row of the Periodic Table, or the various salts of calcium or barium; in each instance he identifies the common characteristics of the group and then distinguishes the individual members within it:

> Until now the most important method of studying homeopathic remedies has been to look at each one separately. In group analysis we look at groups of remedies and extract what is in common. These symptoms will then be used in the various remedies which contain that element.

> The method is least successful on the level of local complaints. On the level of general characteristics it can be applied very well. But it is on the level of mind that group analysis offers the greatest benefit. Once the central themes of the components are known, it is possible to deduce the themes of the compound. A great advantage is getting not only the separate themes of the component elements but also those of the combination. An incidental effect is that certain aspects of remedies we already know can become clearer.[32]

While his themes are not always identical to Sankaran's, they overlap to a great extent, and their methodologies are similar. He also uses group analysis to deduce the symptoms of unproven remedies, not instead of proving them, but as an *incentive* to do so, as a test of his thinking, precisely in the spirit of modern science, which judges hypotheses by the accuracy of the predictions they generate. As once suggested by Kent, a common application is to consider the salt when the symptoms of the case are comparatively nondescript and both elements composing it rank high in the repertorization:

> Brought in for treatment of asthma, a boy of five clung tightly to his dad, whispering to him in answer to my questions. For the past year he had wheezed with every cold and from running in cold air, but needed no inhalers in between. Athletic and talented in all sports, he played to win but was never wild, persevering until he mastered the skill, and finishing what he started. Cheerful and even-tempered, he was less affectionate outside the family, shunned loud noises, and kept his life and surroundings as orderly as possible.

After *Carcinosin.* 1M, he developed fever and asthma for a few days, followed by excellent peak flows for months; but by autumn he was wheezing and coughing even at rest and in warm weather, coming down with colds and Strep throats, and burping repeatedly during attacks. Since the repertorization pointed equally to *Natrum mur.* and *Phosphorus,* I gave him *Natrum phos.* 200. He never came back. In the four years since then, he has had few colds, almost no asthma, and has needed no medication of any kind.[33]

Much the same considerations apply to the use of non-proving data of any kind, such as natural history, chemistry, and the infamous "doctrine of signatures," which has provoked intense antipathy and opposition from critics as diverse as fundamentalists like Saine, Habich, and Winston on the one hand, and modern scientists of the double-blind persuasion like Jennifer Jacobs on the other.

Of course, André is entirely correct about Hahnemann's insistence that the *Materia medica* be kept free of such impurities, so that even those of us who like to use them, like Sankaran, Manigialavori, Herrick, and myself, assign them at most a secondary importance. But our understanding of remedies would be very much the poorer without them. Thus even Julian always took his students on plant walks to identify the remedies and teach them some of the folklore associated with them, while Clarke regularly introduced his remedies with chemistry, toxicology, and/or natural history wherever possible. In Whitmont's *Psyche and Substance* and Vermeulen's *Prisma,* the non-proving data transport us straight into the mythic realm and even the unconscious, where essence and meaning are intertwined.

How useful is such information to the prescriber? Consider *Lachesis,* a favorite example of mine. The snake is named for the second of the three Greek Fates, who were said to determine the length of a person's life: namely, Clotho, who spins the thread; Lachesis, who draws it out to its appointed length; and Atropos, who cuts it. Even hard-core fundamentalists can hardly fail to be moved by the coincidence that Hering, who proved the venom on July 28, 1818 and continued to exhibit symptoms of it for the rest of his life, died on July 23, 1880, 52 years later, almost to the day.[34]

This is partly a matter of toxicology, I suppose, which we're told is OK, but it speaks to the imaginative gifts of whoever named the animal, evidently referring to another level of "signature." My book *Resonance* teems with other examples. I connected the classic *Arsenicum* delusion of

251

being poisoned with the biochemical fact that arsenic is toxic to all living cells, and used "auto-intoxication" as a kind of metaphor to derive and even "explain" the other keynotes as well: coldness, restlessness, anxiety, fastidiousness, etc.[35] Is this not precisely the sort of "didactic value" that Habich et al. were talking about? It won't help you repertorize, and can assuredly be treacherous in inexperienced hands, as we all agree. But it does often remind me to think of the remedy, which is why I wrote it down; others will no doubt prefer the metaphors that work best for them.

What of *Pulsatilla,* whose common name, the "windflower," aptly corresponds to its mutable nature, both in the provings and clinically, for patients too easily swayed and influenced by outside forces;[36] or *Natrum mur.,* about which the Biblical tale of Lot's wife and the pillar of salt come aptly and indeed irresistibly to mind;[37] or *Sulphur,* the business end of insulin and Coenzyme A, which govern our basic energy production, as does the remedy itself?[38]

True enough, these are all simply metaphors, or teaching aids. No more nor less so than "essences," they are indeed seductive and unnecessary for good practice. But neither Sankaran nor Herrick nor Mangialavori nor I in our wildest dreams covets more than a didactic role for them, or lies in wait hoping to smuggle them into the Repertory or *Materia medica* without anyone noticing. In this matter at least, the fundamentalists are merely beating a dead horse, conjuring up the spectre of new age psychobabble that only our most credulous groupies are actually guilty of; and I have no doubt that André draws his own fair share of these in his entourage. In any case, it sounds a but like the pot calling the kettle black; if you can swallow classical homeopathy, minor details like ESP, radionics, kinesiology, dowsing, clairvoyance, spiritualism, and all the rest surely pose no insuperable obstacles!

For non-proving data, then, just as for essences and families, the bottom line is mainly to suggest remedies we might not otherwise think of:

Brought in by her grandmother for bronchitis that tended to last all winter, a girl of five had been orphaned as a baby when her drug-abusing parents were both brutally murdered. Although described as "a happy child who gets along with everyone," she sulked whenever she felt left out, blew her nose almost constantly, hawking up thick, green mucus from her throat, and wet the bed almost every night. When she smiled, her upper teeth were rudimentary, brown-stained, and broken off in places. Her eyes turned in, alternating from side to side, and she craved salt and milk primarily and was intensely allergic to cats.

Calcarea sulph. 200 did nothing. In a month she was back, sniffling loudly, and this time sporting a new sweatshirt that featured dogs of every description, which immediately reminded me of her alternating strabismus. In this absurdly logical sequence I was led to study and eventually give her *Lac caninum* 1M. At her next visit her cough was gone, she wet the bed much less often, and was breathing freely through her nose. I repeated it in the fall, and that winter was her best ever, with minimal cough and no bronchitis. I've not seen her for five years, but another patient and family friend assures me that she has continued to thrive[39]

In this instance, the dogs on her shirt merely reminded me of the remedy I'd already thought of for other reasons. In the following case, the details of the history and physiognomy added up to a kind of totemic "signature" that was almost all I had to go on, and may therefore be taken to represent the furthest possible application of this admittedly outlandish type of clue, which I would be the last to recommend for general use:

With a history of benign fibroadenomas that had already resulted in four breast surgeries, a 45-year-old artist came in hurting from a fifth and hoping to prevent them in the future.

A painter of horses especially, she had suffered chronic back pain ever since falling from a horse and crushing three vertebræ in her teens, but never gave up riding, having grown up with horses and still feeling mystically drawn to them. Estranged and enraged by abusive relationships in her family of origin, she was raised by a grandmother, spent her childhood mostly alone in the woods, and thought of herself as an Indian brave riding her pony bareback in the wilderness.

Lean and lanky, with a long, graceful neck, two buck teeth jutting out in front, and a craving for lumps of pure cane sugar, in her physique and constitution as well she conjured up the equine archetype as a kind of personal totem.

With little else to prescribe on, I studied *Lac equinum* and decided to give her the 200C as an experiment. Within 6 weeks, I'm almost ashamed to admit, the walnut-sized tumor was no longer palpable. I haven't seen her for six years, but she phoned recently to say that she was well and the tumors hadn't come back.[40]

Now don't get me wrong: I'm far from advocating this "Hail-Mary pass" as a *strategy*. The truth is, I was out on a limb, and tried the remedy because I couldn't think of anything else to do. I freely admit, it's bad homeopathy, or rather, not really homeopathy at all. But it also shows that uncanny signatures and other non-homeopathic similarities do indeed exist in nature, that they can be highly individualized in just the way we need our patients and their remedies to be, and thus may occasionally even be relevant and useful in our prescribing.

So in the end, whether a Hahnemannian Supreme Court or Inquisition of the highest repute, perhaps even one presided over by André himself, is willing to proclaim such adventures as strictly homeopathic or not is not of very great moment to me. But I do most emphatically believe that the discriminating use of non-proving data can enrich and indeed transfigure us all, and that the imaginative faculty is as indispensable to the science as to the art of good medical practice, homeopathic or otherwise; and it grieves and saddens me beyond measure to hear these truly divine gifts maligned by grown men, let alone old friends and esteemed colleagues who should know better.

The Theory of Miasms.

As I've said, I'm especially curious about the dearth of critical attention that Sankaran's ideas about miasms have received, pro or con, since they are by far the boldest, most brilliant, and most avowedly speculative of his many innovations; and moreover, unlike his work with essences, remedy families, chemical groupings, and signatures, they are uniquely his own, and have not been uniformly accepted even by his own followers, who eagerly devour almost everything else he says.

If I'm right, the reasons are intriguing and instructive, and again take us all the way back to Hahnemann himself. Listen to the master in his later years, grappling with the dark and mighty enigma of the chronic diseases, like Jacob wrestling with the angel:

> After being removed time and again with proven remedies, the non-venereal chronic diseases always returned in varied form and with new or increased symptoms. This gave me the clue that the homeopath must combat not only the disease presented before his eyes, that he meets but a separate fragment

of a more deep-seated original disease. He must therefore ascertain the whole extent of the symptoms belonging to the unknown primitive malady before he can discover medicines to remove it. Once it has advanced to a certain degree, it can never be removed by any robust constitution, be overcome by the most wholesome diet or regimen of life, or die out of itself, but rather increases from year to year until the end of life.

> Then I found that the obstacle to cure often lay in a past eruption of itch that was not noticed or told of, and that all later sufferings dated from this time. *So far as is known, only three chronic miasms are found which manifest through local symptoms, and from which most if not all chronic diseases originate,* namely, psora, sycosis, and syphilis.[41] [Italics mine: R. M.]

From watching the underlying disease worsen even after the remedy had acted beautifully, he realized that the symptom-picture as it appears at a particular moment is only a fragment of the totality that needs to be considered, that our prescription must encompass the whole symptom-picture as it has evolved throughout the patient's lifetime. In a *tour de force* requiring decades of careful scholarship, he claimed to trace these underlying maladies to "psora, the itch disease," and two other chronic styles, the venereal "miasms" of gonorrhea and syphilis. In short, he formulated a speculative *hypothesis,* which he backed up with an enormous mass of documentation; but he remained appropriately tentative about it, using such qualifying phrases as "so far as is known" and "from which most if not all chronic diseases originate," to leave room for us of future generations to confirm, refute, and/or build upon.

Similarly, I suspect that the reason why the fundamentalists have let Sankaran's additional miasms alone is that building on Hahnemann is precisely what he has done, so that to go after Sankaran here is to go after the master as well. From Hahnemann's time right up to the present, the whole concept of miasms has remained so controversial and even embarrassing from the viewpoint of contemporary medicine that many eminent homeopaths have declined to follow him into this realm, which remains even further beyond the pale of what passes for science these days than the Law of Similars, the Vital Force, and the totality of symptoms.

Thus in his splendid text, *The Science of Homeopathy,* even the great Vithoulkas offers only the briefest formulation of the miasm concept, almost as a footnote to the idea of predisposition, accepting Hahnemann's basic principle but refusing to limit its application to his three main pathological styles, or indeed to any fixed number:

> A miasm is a predisposition toward chronic disease which is transmissible from generation to generation and may respond curatively to the corresponding nosode prepared from the pathological tissue, drug, or vaccine. From this definition it is clear that there are a large number of miasms, and that the total number is constantly increasing with the advent of suppressive therapies.[42]

My conjecture is that Vithoulkas favors as broad an interpretation of the concept as possible, and as many examples of it as possible, simply to avoid having to take a position for or against Hahnemann's venerable triad. But he is certainly right about the value of the concept in general. Hahnemann's exegesis of the scabies vesicle, the venereal wart and gonorrheal discharge, and the syphilitic chancre as simply external *stigmata* of the underlying miasms or pathological styles, which are transmissible across the generations and require a lifetime to develop their mature form and global extent, is a masterpiece of pure theory and empirical elaboration combined, and has been repeatedly validated through the successful use of the nosodes corresponding to them.

In any case, Sankaran's work lies entirely within this Hahnemannian tradition. First, through computer-assisted study of the corresponding nosodes, he was able to preserve, redefine, and reinterpret the original three, and eventually to identify a new one, the "acute" miasm, which has no nosode but encompasses a group of remedies like *Aconite, Belladonna, Camphora, Arnica, Veratrum,* and others typical of ailments that appear suddenly and heal completely without residue, making a total of four basic miasms.

Then he found five others that had qualities of two of the four and could thus be conceptualized as lying between them, each imaginatively named for a well-known disease with its own distinctive lesions and other features suggestive of the type. Thus "cancer" and "tuberculosis," which had been proposed long before, and whose corresponding nosodes were already familiar and well-studied, were placed between sycosis and syphilis, as was the new "leprosy" miasm, with its nosode *Leprominium,* which has long been used in India. Three others are the "typhoid" or

256

subacute miasm, lying between the acute and the psoric; the "malaria" or intermittent miasm, between the acute and the sycotic; and the "ringworm" miasm, between the acute and the sycotic.

He freely admits that these names and sitings are tentative, approximate, and will take years to evaluate properly. But in each case, by studying the nosode and the remedies that correspond most closely to it, he has recognized and identified a nexus of sensations and systemic features that has repeatedly proved its worth in practice, as in the following case of my own:

A 70-year-old artist and writer consulted me for arthritic attacks in her hand that she described as "terrible, *so bad,* incredible!" Also nursing her husband for a ruptured disc, she was sure that exhaustion played a major role in her problems. Primarily in her fingers, the pain made it hard to write, weakened her grip, and was better from warmth. But she insisted that her main problem was her sense of family responsibility, such that "if something has to be done, I do it," while "I never needed anything for myself!"

The intermittent character of the pains, with an intensity unmatched by any objective findings, plus the curious blend of self-pity and moral superiority in her complaining, suggested a remedy of the malarial miasm, which Sankaran describes as follows:

Sensations:
"Stuck," limited, unfortunate
Imprisoned, dependent
Intermittent attacks

Attitude:
You have to bear it
Fixed limitation, dependent

Successful Stage:
Accepting limits,
    not fighting them
Intermittent anger
Sentimental, phobic
Pathology (partial list):
Migraine, neuralgia
Colitis, labyrinthitis

Failed Stage:
Miserable, brooding,
    sees no good anywhere
Complaining, lamenting
Paroxysms of rage

Rheumatism, arthritis
Asthma

Remedies (partial list):

Antimonium crud.	*Cactus grand.*	*Capsicum*
Chelidonium	*China*	*Cina*
Colchicum	*Colocynthis*	*Eupatorium perf.*
Natrum mur.	*Ranunculus bulb.*	*Spigelia*

I found what I was looking for under the *Compositæ, a* family of wound remedies like *Arnica, Bellis perennis, Calendula,* and *Eupatorium:*

Sensations:

Injured, hurt	Fear of being hurt, touched, or
Shocked, insulted	approached

Passive Reactions:	**Active Reactions:**
Numbness	Touchy
Anesthesia	Hurting, hurtful
Stupor	Cruel, violent, strikes

Compensation:
Tough guy: "I can take it!"
Protective of others

With the help of this summary, especially the part about the "tough guy" who bears his own pain to protect others from theirs, I studied and eventually gave her a 200 of *Eupatorium perfoliatum,* the malarial remedy of the family. Six months later, she reported, "That remedy really made a difference! No pain, no complaints!" None, that is, until recently, when I repeated it. In the last two years, she has only needed it after her "annual *kvetch"* every spring, each time with excellent results.[43]

This case also illustrates Sankaran's technique of "mapping" plant remedies as points of intersection between the miasm and the family. As with essences, families, and chemical groupings, each miasm is defined using the exact words and imagery of the patient, and is thus capable of more precise individualization than the usual repertorization alone.

Provings.

As we have seen, the provings of Rajan Sankaran, Nancy Herrick, and Jeremy Sherr have also drawn a lot of criticism, both deserved and otherwise, which undoubtedly reflects the iconic status of this uniquely Hahnemannian procedure as well as the current obsession to nail down what is or is not "the real thing." I leave aside for the moment the inconvenient fact that we continue to manage very nicely with those hundreds of remedies that have been proved inadequately or not at all. Homeopathy did begin with a proving, after all, and the procedure does beautifully epitomize the whole of what we do, from how to study remedies to the uncannily fruitful parallelism between them and our patients. So it is only fitting that we should feel inclined to fight for our sometimes differing visions of how to conduct them. I begin with a digest of what Hahnemann has to say on the subject:

> Each medicine is taken in pure, unadulterated form, without any other medicine being taken during the time we wish to observe. The diet must be simple, nutritious, and free of spices and stimulant drinks. The prover must be in good health, avoid all passions, dissipations, and overexertion of mind and body, and have no urgent business. He must devote himself to careful and undisturbed observation and be intelligent enough to describe his sensations accurately. Weak medicines do not exhibit their powers as fully in their crude state as when given in the 30th potency.

> All changes in health during the proving are said to belong to the medicine, even if the prover had experienced them in the past. He must record all the sensations he experiences after taking it, as well as when and for how long they occur. If the physician gives the drug to others, he must examine their report afterward, or daily if the trial lasts for several days, amending it if necessary. From such a *Materia medica,* everything that is conjectural, imaginary, or mere assertion must be strictly excluded. All must be the pure language of nature, carefully and honestly interrogated.[44]

The provings of Sankaran, Herrick, and Sherr do indeed depart slightly from the letter of these instructions in varying degrees, and in overlapping but not identical respects. As we saw, Sankaran has been castigated mainly for importing foreign elements from contemporary psychology, namely, the idea of "group mind," exemplified by his interest in the symptomatology exhibited by the "controls" who attended the seminar but did not actually take the remedy; and the use of "dream provings," a wholly novel procedure in which only the dreams are recorded, making straight for the unconscious material and ignoring the physical symptoms altogether.

I will not say much about dream provings, because they are intended only as a supplement to the usual kind, to bring out and highlight an important dimension of remedies that is likely to be missed amid the welter of physical sensations. As mere addenda to the usual procedure, I can't see how dream provings raise any serious methodological issues. On the related issue of group mind, those who can't resist the impulse to ridicule what they know only by hearsay will do well to read Rajan's own words:

> The provers, students or practitioners at a seminar, were all given a dose of 30C. Another dose was given after four days if there were no symptoms or they had ceased. They were asked to record all symptoms, dreams, and non-ordinary experiences; all physical symptoms with exact modalities; all dreams, with exact feelings; all incidents occurring around them; all observations by others about changes in their state; and all persons, movies, books, etc., that they liked or disliked.

> Some not taking the dose experienced symptoms, which were also recorded. I met each prover alone each week, recorded all their symptoms, and video-taped every session. We met as a group after two weeks and again after three or four weeks. At this stage provers' experiences often elicited memories in others, creating a powerful effect in the room, so the underlying state could be more clearly defined. Only then would I reveal the name of the remedy.

> The only symptoms recorded here are a transcription of the video interviews of each prover. I have tried to gather and report the data with a minimum of error, bias, and subjectivity. Provers were instructed not to discuss their experiences among themselves. I elicited mental and emotional symptoms in the interview without prompting or suggestion, just as in casetaking. No summaries or conclusions are offered, to be faithful to the data and not prejudice the result.[45]

As in all his work, the spirit of Sankaran's provings is Hahnemannian through and through. As the above makes clear, the symptoms of non-provers are only recorded for comparison, i.e., as a built-in control group, and are therefore subtracted and omitted from the final or published result. In short, the motive is essentially one of scientific curiosity, stimulated by his actual experience of the phenomenon, which while unknown to Hahnemann has been well documented by modern psychology.

In our laudable zeal to defend the integrity and scientific rigor of his work, we often forget that Hahnemann the fundamentalist was also our greatest and boldest innovator, and that apart from the redevelopment of homeopathy itself throughout his lifetime, including provings, dynamization, miasms, LM potencies, and all the rest, he maintained a lively curiosity about the science of his time, especially in the "etheric" realms of clairvoyance, spiritualism, mesmerism, mediumship, and the like:

The curative power of animal magnetism or mesmerism streams upon a patient by contact with a well-intentioned person powerfully exerting his will. It can act homeopathically, by producing symptoms similar to those of the state to be cured, or otherwise, by redistributing the vital force uniformly throughout the organism.

For the former purpose, a single pass, made with the palms from head to toe, is useful in uterine hemorrhage in the last stage. For the latter, the restoration of the vital force to the whole organism or some weakened part cannot be attained by any other treatment as certainly and with least interference as by mesmerism. Many rapid cures in all ages belong to this class. It is done by concentrating a very powerful and well-intentioned will and placing the hands on the weakest parts. The effect is most notably shown in the resuscitation of persons who had lain seemingly dead for some time, of which history records many notable examples.[46]

Nancy Herrick's methodology is very close to Rajan's, with a few important exceptions and modifications that I will consider in a moment. Unfortunately her Preface is ambiguous about whether her provings were blinded or not, so I've taken the liberty of editing her words slightly to make clear that they *were,* as she reassured me when I asked her: "Neither provers nor supervisors know what the substance is."[47] Her views differ most significantly from Rajan's in the area of supervision. Here are her own words on the matter:

Up to twenty volunteers, preferably students or colleagues, but not patients or anyone unfamiliar with homeopathy. *I trust homeopaths to record symptoms accurately and in detail, especially about mental and emotional states. Provers who are homeopaths decide if they want a supervisor, and if so I will provide one. Non-homeopaths must have a supervisor,* who also takes their case beforehand.

Provers get a vial of 30C and a booklet to record symptoms. 3 weeks after the dose they record in detail all symptoms that differ from their usual state. The supervisors call to review physical symptoms, experiences, and state of mind. Dreams, emotional states, and unusual events such as acute illness or crises are important. If they have no symptoms, they repeat the remedy twice more, two days apart. If their symptoms are slight, they repeat it once more after they've gone. If they are strong, they wait and watch.

After three weeks a group meeting is held in a quiet room where we will not be interrupted. Provers are asked not to discuss symptoms or their state with anyone before that. The session is videotaped, but anyone may choose not to be filmed. All provers read their booklets, summarize their experiences, and elaborate as seems appropriate. Then I reveal the name of the substance, and we conclude.[48] [Italics mine: R. M.]

As I wrote in my own review of her book, I have my doubts about allowing provers to decide for themselves whether they need a supervisor or not.[49] Exactly analogous to that of taking the case of a patient, the supervisory role is likewise no more to be left to the provers' discretion, it seems to me, than we give our patients the option of taking their own cases. But these are practical guidelines that cannot and should not be written in stone. Nancy simply chooses to take advantage of the special trust she clearly enjoys with her own students and colleagues, by giving higher priority to positive feelings of love and communication than to "checking up" on or surveillance over them. To that I say, more power to her. But while I'm willing to give her the benefit of the doubt, I'm not convinced.

A related issue is her conducting the supervision by telephone, which I distrust in the same way and to the same extent as for patient interviews, although like everyone else I often have to do them that way. Without in-person contact and the non-verbal communication that helps me to ask or reframe questions in ways I'd never have thought of, the phone interview reduces to merely taking down information, and the quality of the data is likely to suffer from that impoverishment.

As for the alleged "anthropomorphizing" that so bothered Julian and others, it is not an issue for me. As I've already said on the subject of signatures and other non-proving data, these are simply metaphors or learning tools that we use to describe animal behavior as best we can, and Nancy's versions are not at all wild, extreme, or out of the mainstream of how animal biologists do natural history today.

For Julian, another bone of contention is her choice of remedies, which in the past has always been left to the discretion of the master-prover. Thus Swan and a few of his contemporaries were inspired almost simultaneously to make attenuations of pus, which became *Pyrogenium* and *Sepsin,* both marvelous remedies, while Hahnemann's interest in non-material energies led him to prove such *imponderabilia* as the magnet and its poles, while Caspari went for electricity, and Rajan was drawn to rat's blood, the main reservoir of bubonic plague, which still survives in India, and also to plastic, that ubiquitous, non-degradable symbol of the human race befouling our own nest.

Most of Nancy's book is taken up with the milks of important mammals, which are obvious and welcome additions. Easily her two most quixotic choices were the butterfly, among the most ephemeral of living animals, which perhaps explains why the Hopi still dance an annual ritual in its honor, and the fossilized bone of a dinosaur that has been extinct for millions of years, about the symptoms of which I can only say, good luck and God bless her for trying.

What struck Julian as her most egregious innovation, her attempt to identify "themes" on the basis of group discussion rather than simply letting the data speak for themselves, also strikes me as far less threatening and certainly no cause for alarm or ridicule. As I said in my review, her aim is simply to find the essence, which she wins my admiration just for daring to attempt, because it's difficult and risky, and nobody else will touch it with a ten-foot pole. My beef with her themes is just the opposite, that they're too vague and general, maybe because of her laid-back attitude to supervision, and offer no really controversial interpretations, revealing little more than the sort of topical headings that Sankaran uses to organize his data, which is to say, a lot less radical and threatening than Julian feared, but also far less interesting and useful than they would need to be.

Jeremy Sherr has also made several fine provings, the main critic of which is Vithoulkas, but chiefly it seems to me on flimsy *ad hominem* grounds, such as 1) that "no case in my life ever needed *Hydrogen* or *Chocolate,*" i.e., these are remedies we don't really need; and 2) that George got very different symptoms when he gave *Hydrogen* to attendees at one of his own seminars, which led him to disparage the integrity of Jeremy's work. In any case, the result was a few lame and perfunctory assumptions about where Jeremy went wrong. But I'll come back to Vithoulkas presently. First listen to what Jeremy says, because it seems to me he gets it exactly right on the very same issues that we've been discussing:

> It has been my experience that "echo" symptoms highly consistent with the proving have often occurred in those in close proximity who did not actually take the remedy, namely, supervisors, placebo controls, class members, or close

relatives. I've not included them, but the phenomenon is interesting, and raises questions about the validity of giving placebo.

Good supervision is the key to quality provings. Ideally supervisors should be experienced homeopaths and should take no more than two supervisees, since they must take their cases every day; and it's best if they are well acquainted with them already, if they are already their patients, or at least in geographical proximity. It's essential to take provers' cases beforehand, to compare their symptoms before and after the proving.

Inadequate supervision is the main reason for poor results. Provers *become* the proving, as if "infected" by the remedy, and cannot perceive that they are changing. Quite a few report that nothing has happened. So I send them back to investigate more thoroughly, and they return saying things like "I hadn't noticed this was happening," or "the prover didn't realize these were proving symptoms." The surprising thing was that these unnoticed symptoms were all unusual, and so they recorded many symptoms which were omitted.[50]

For Jeremy the need for supervision has less to do with trust or the lack of it than the built-in tendency for the best and most distinctive symptoms to remain hidden from the patient's conscious awareness and thus go unreported with even the best of intentions. He also makes some highy pertinent comments on themes or essences that resolve this issue along the same lines that Habich et al. proposed, namely, that such formulations should be withheld from the proving itself, but may be published as opinion in later articles for teaching purposes, leaving ample room for others to do the same in their own fashion, which is exactly the way the *Materia medica* and our understanding of particular remedies have developed over the years:

I decided not to venture any of my private ideas concerning the "image" of the remedy. My opinion is that a proving should be a pure document, without prejudice or interpretation. It should be left to each individual homeopath to weave the symptoms into a meaningful and coherent picture. Any early attempt to sum up the elaborate proving symptoms carries the price of sacrificing the totality of symptoms. It is much easier for the student to hang onto a few simple lines of "essence," which would be fine if the totality were also studied. But the mind always grasps the convenient, short-term solution.

The master prover will have perceived many hidden threads running through the proving, and these can be explained in a general way or published in future articles to facilitate the work of the student. But provings themselves should be in the format of the *Materia Medica Pura* and not diluted to mere essences, which can cause so much damage to homeopathy.[51]

This Solomonic judgment offers a sensible compromise that could satisfy innovators and fundamentalists alike, giving each side their due, acknowledging the validity and usefulness of formulating the essence, but leaving that task for each practitioner, while adhering to the traditional format for the proving itself.

Innovation and Fundamentalism in Our History.

As I reconsider all the arguments and counter-arguments, I can feel these same controversies reverberating from the depths of our history, in which contentious and internecine quasi-theological disputation has figured prominently almost from the beginning. Here is Hahnemann himself railing against the "half-homeopaths" of Leipzig, and torpedoing his own pet project for a homeopathic hospital in the same breath:

> *Some who pretend to be homeopaths allow their patients to choose whether to be treated homeopathically or not.* Whether they are not yet sufficiently well-grounded in the new doctrine, or lack due benevolence to their species, or dishonor their profession for gain, they should not expect me to recognize them as disciples! Combined with the use of our remedies, such quackeries as bloodletting, mustard plasters, salves, emetics, purgatives, etc., identify these crypto-homeopaths as surely as a lion is known by his claws. Either practice honorably as an allopath, as yet ignorant of anything better, or as a homeopath for the welfare of mankind. But as long as you wear this double mask, you will be a contemptible hybrid of a physician, of all the most pernicious. Should any false doctrine be taught in the name of homeopathy, or patients be treated with any imitation of allopathic practice, I will raise my voice to warn against such treachery.[51] [Italics mine: R. M.]

To that extent, André is only doing his duty, as set forth in no uncertain terms by his master Hahnemann and his mentor Lippe before him:

> Possibly some of the twenty-one signed mainly to protest against censorship or dogmatism, for liberty of opinion and the freedom to investigate. But while everyone is free to practice medicine as they choose, nobody has the license to call Homeopathy what is not Homeopathy! In 1870 Lippe warned, "There are true and good men among us who erroneously believe that anyone professing to be a homeopath must be allowed full freedom of opinion and action, to do

whatever he has a mind to do. But the liberty to accept homeopathy does not include the freedom to reject, alter, or modify its fundamental principles."

Some want us to believe that the method of Hahnemann is a thing of the past, that we must evolve from it. But his inductive method is what brought the medical profession out of its chaos. If the basic principles of homeopathy were true yesterday, they will continue to be true until the end of time. Others want to combine both methods, homeopathy with a speculative approach. But it is impossible to advocate both: they are as opposite as day and night, as truth and falsehood.[53]

And in one sense he is perfectly right. Since the laws of homeopathy do indeed have the shine of the eternal and immutable about them, it seems as though they can only be added to, not changed in any significant way, so that almost by definition the method is incompatible with innovation *per se,* with any possibility of meaningful change. It is truly a *philosophy* in that sense, a coherent system of principles about health and disease that all follow logically from a few simple axioms, like the vital force, the totality of symptoms, and the "Law of Similars," which cannot themselves be proved or disproved in the same way that ordinary scientific hypotheses are expected to be.[54] In any case, the method which Hahnemann left us remains practical and serviceable even today, having stood the test of time, such that we who carry on his work are quite content and even proud to acknowledge our greatest achievements as mere footnotes to the books he wrote and the principles he enunciated so long ago.

But homeopathy has also grown and developed over the years in important ways, some developed by the master himself, and others that the master did not and could not have foreseen, less by the addition of new remedies than in the depth of how we understand the ones we already know. As André has said so often and so well, it is the fixed and seemingly unalterable character of our principles that effectively assures every innovation of being opposed and rejected, just as is happening now.

Perhaps less well known is the coincidence that the innovators of yesterday are apt to become the fundamentalists of tomorrow. Just as Kent in later life took up the cudgels against mongrels and backsliders even more zealously than had Lippe before him, so the great Vithoulkas, the much-maligned "illuminist" of his own time, now dishes it out to Rajan, Jan Scholten, and Jeremy in much the same casserole of curmudgeonly rant and seasoned wisdom that Künzli once served up to him, and sounding a lot like Julian, André, and Habich in the process, as if no more innovations could be possible or tolerable after his own:

> You can separate what is serious from what is not. If I give a remedy and the placebo group has the same dream as the ones who took it, and I say the dream belongs to the remedy anyway, it's not to be taken seriously. Why not potentize a stanza or a piece of music? Put the powder here, play the music, and make a proving with the powder: do you believe it can make a proving, can make you sick? If you put remedies in the same chemical group, like lead with antimony, what's the use? First of all, it's a fantasy. Second, it doesn't prove anything. If you prove a substance correctly, OK, I have no problem. But to imagine that *Diamond* will be a hard person because the diamond is very hard, that's ridiculous. Sankaran and Scholten have done more harm to homeopathy than all our enemies put together.
>
> People go crazy over hearing that a patient looks like an animal or a flower, yet claim to be classical homeopaths. I gave *Hydrogen* to some Italian doctors, and the results were totally different from Jeremy's. No case in my life ever needed *Hydrogen* or *Chocolate.* Yes, *Scorpion* is a remedy, but prove it right, so that the information you give out is correct. First, take people who are poisoned. Only those sensitive to a remedy develop clear, reliable symptoms. You can't just give a dose of 30C to fifty people and expect them to develop symptoms. To record all the euphoria, fantasy, and group nonsense as provings of the remedy is killing homeopathy.[55]

So the wheel has come full circle, from which I conclude that both innovators and fundamentalists are permanent features of our landscape, equally important if not inseparable parts of the legacy that Hahnemann left us, each needing the other. Simply acknowledging the validity of our principles lends to everything that follows the force of absolute truth, so that every disagreement easily becomes a holy war. Yet failing to honor them will indeed undermine the elegant system and incomparable method that we all hold dear. Maybe we just need to agree to disagree, and leave it to our cured patients to decide the question on its merits, as they always do, no matter what we say.

NOTES.

1. Moskowitz, R., "Innovation and Fundamentalism in Homeopathy," *American Journal of Homeopathic Medicine* 95:91, Summer 2002.
2. Winston, J., "But Is It Homeopathy?" *Homeopathy Today,* December 2000.
3. Winston, J., Book Review, loc. cit., December 2000.
4. Habich, K., et al., "Controversy in Homeopathy: Magic or Science?" *American Journal of Homeopathic Medicine* 96:82, Summer 2003.
5. Jacobs, J., and Crothers, D., Letter, 'The Emperor Has No Clothes," *Homeopathy Today,* July-August 2001.
6. Saine, A., "Drawing a Line in the Sand: Homeopathy or Not Homeopathy?" *American Journal of Homeopathic Medicine* 95:69, Summer 2002.
7. Winston, J., "Back to Basics," *Homeopathy Today,* April 2001.
8. Künzli, J., "Impressions of Homeopathy in the United States," *Journal of the American Institute of Homeopathy* 75:42, March 1982.
9. Saine, op. cit., 2002.
10. Habich, op. cit. , 2003.
11. Saine, op.cit., 2002.
12. Habich, op. cit., 2003.
13. Morrison, R., et al., Letter, "Against Divisiveness," *Homeopathy Today,* May 2001.
14. Saine, "Homeopathy vs. Speculative Medicine: a Call to Action," *Homeopathy Today,* September 2001.
15. Declaration, *American Journal of Homeopathic Medicine* 96:91, Summer 2003.
16. Preamble and Resolutions, International Hahnemannian Association, Adopted 1881, *IHA Transactions,* 1881-83, pp. 10-11 and 14-15, passim.
17. Hahnemann, S., *Organon of Medicine,* 5th Edition, with Additions from the 6th, R. E. Dudgeon and W. Boericke, trans., B. Jain, New Delhi, 1992, ¶9,10, 12, *passim.*
18. Ibid., ¶108, 119, 144, *passim.*
19. Farrington, E. A., *Clinical Materia Medica,* 2nd Ed., Hahnemann Publishing House, Philadelphia, 1890, pp. 20-21.
20. Lippe, A., *Textbook of Materia Medica,* L. H., Tafel, trans., A. H. Tafel, Philadelphia, 1866, pp. 294, 299, *passim.*
21. Kent, J. T., *Lectures on Homeopathic Materia Medica,* 4th Ed., Boericke & Tafel, Philadelphia, 1956, pp. 574-576, *passim.*
22. Vithoulkas, G., *Essence of Materia Medica,* 2nd Ed., B. Jain, New Delhi, 2011, pp. 88-90, *passim.*
23. Moskowitz, *Resonance: the Homeopathic Point of View,* Xlibris, Philadelphia 2001, p. 86.

24. Ibid., p. 85.

25. Ibid., pp. 87, 117, 119, passim.

26. Sankaran, R., *An Insight into Plants,* vol. 2, Homeopathic Medical Publishers, Mumbai, 2002, pp. 569-570, 576.

27. Moskowitz, *Resonance,* pp. 196-197.

28. Farrington, op. cit., 1890, pp. 23-24, *passim.*

29. Mangialavori, M., NCH Summer School Handout, 1995.

30. Moskowitz, *Resonance,* pp. 162-163.

31. Ibid.,pp. 125-128.

32. Scholten, J., *Homeopathy and Minerals,* Stichting Alonissos, Utrecht, 1993, p. 23.

33. Moskowitz, *Resonance,* p. 200.

34. Hering, C., "The Pathogenetic Power of the Snake Venom," *The Homœopath* (UK) 12:155, March 1992, and Knerr, C. B., *Life of Hering,* p. 197.

35. Moskowitz, *Resonance,* pp. 183-187.

36. Ibid., p. 106.

37. Ibid., p. 189.

38. Ibid., pp. 170-171.

39. Ibid., p.l51.

40. Ibid., pp. 168-169.

41. Hahnemann, *Chronic Diseases,* vol. 1, L. H. Tafel, trans., Boericke & Tafel, Philadelphia, 1896, pp. 4-9, *passim.*

42. Vithoulkas, *The Science of Homeopathy: a Modern Textbook,* Grove Press, New York, 1980, p. 130.

43. Moskowitz, *Resonance,* pp. 327-329.

44. Hahnemann, *Organon,* ¶123-144, passim.

45. Sankaran, *Provings,* Homeopathic Medical Publishers, Mumbai, 1998, pp. 2-4.

46. Hahnemann, *Organon,* ¶293.

47. Herrick, N., *Animal Mind, Human Voices,* Hahnemann Clinic Publishing, Nevada City, CA, 1998, pp. xii-xiv, *passim.*

48. Ibid.

49. Moskowitz, Book Review, *Homeopathy Today,* January 1999.

50. Sherr, J., *Dynamics and Methodology of Homeopathic Provings,* Dynamis Books, Malvern, UK, pp. 33,46,47, passim.

51. Ibid., pp. 79-80.

52. Hahnemann, "To the Half-Homeopaths of Leipzig," in Bradford, T. L., *Life and Letters of Hahnemann,* Boericke & Tafel, Philadelphia, 1895, p. 300.

53. Saine, op.cit., 2001.

54. Moskowitz, "Hahnemann' s Achievement and Legacy, *American Homeopath,* 6:65, 2000.

55. Vithoulkas, Interview, C. Hiwat and H. van der Zee, *Homeopathic Links* 12:202, Winter 1999, *passim..*

For Homeopathy: A Practicing Physician's Perspective*

I am writing in response to "Against Homeopathy: a Utilitarian Perspective,"[1] by Kevin Smith, Ph. D., whom I commend for the clarity of his writing and the thoroughness of his logic. I suppose I should also derive some comfort from the fact that, contrary to the advice he gives to his readers, he takes homeopathy at least seriously enough to go to such trouble to denounce it.

Long familiar to every homeopath, his main argument that homeopathic remedies are nothing but placebos was already current in Hahnemann's time, decades before Oliver Wendell Holmes made it famous 150 years ago,[2] and has since been incorporated into the conventional wisdom. When I was in medical school, the term "homeopathic dose" was used almost affectionately to signify an amount of medicine far too small to have any noticeable effect whatsoever; and even today, as various modalities of alternative and complementary medicine enter the mainstream, and many American physicians aspire to broaden their outlook in order to accommodate them, most would probably still agree with Dr. Smith, at least in private, that homeopathy defies common sense, ordinary logic, and some basic laws of chemistry.

Indeed, even I feel a little uneasy with patients who can swallow the whole concept without hesitation, utterly untroubled by the profound mysteries at the center of it. Hahnemann's Law of Similars, for example, "Let likes be cured by likes," the founding principle of homeopathy, is still far from intuitively obvious, even to those of us who use it every day, and remains essentially a *postulate,* by definition not amenable to conclusive proof or disproof as a scientific hypothesis must be. Still less satisfactorily has anyone ever explained how medicines diluted beyond the level of Avogadro's number could possibly have *any* effect on a patient, let alone a curative one.

* "For Homeopathy: a Practicing Physician's Perspective," *American Journal of Homeopathic Medicine* 104:125, Autumn 2011.

But the mere fact that homeopathy is based on a conundrum as yet opaque and unfathomable to the science we have now is by no means sufficient to prove that it is a nullity, a fake, and thus a false belief, indeed a delusion, on the part of anyone who takes it seriously enough even to entertain the possibility that there might just be something to it. It almost embarrasses me to have to say that Dr. Smith's entire argument, like that of the distinguished Dr. Holmes before him, boils down to one defective syllogism, that because homeopathy *can't* work, it therefore *doesn't* work.

Once that premise is accepted, to be sure, his reasoning sounds persuasive enough. For if it could be shown that the homeopathic phenomenon does not exist, that medicines do *not* in fact have the po\ wer to elicit or provoke the same symptoms that they help to cure, and that remedies diluted beyond the level of Avogadro's number are simply inert and have no effect of any kind, then he would be entirely right to insist that such beliefs are utterly groundless, that those who persist in them are mired in wishful thinking, and that public funds should not be provided for the medical care of indigent people based on them, or even for further research as to their efficacy, since more than enough would already have been carried out to disprove the need or value of proceeding any further along this path. As if all that were not enough, and saving the best for last, he adds the novel *tour de force* that homeopathy is not only ineffective, but *immoral* as well, according to the utilitarian standard of doing the greatest good for the greatest number, mainly to the extent that it dissuades people from seeking the kind of heavy artillery that really *does* work.

Such a virtuoso display of logical reasoning might have been more persuasive had he not named as authorities on the subject the likes of Wallace Sampson[3] and Stephen Barrett,[4] both professional 'quackbusters' who have made discrediting homeopathy their life's work, and who automatically offer the most damning possible interpretations of anything pertaining to it. Proudly acknowledging Prof. Sampson as his chief mentor and source of information,[5] and falling back on the seeming absurdity of infinitesimals, he sheds all pretense at even-handedness, making quick work of the alleged benefits of the method, and deducing a litany of serious faults *ex cathedra* without any knowledge of or interest in the actual practice, like how the interview is conducted, how various possible reactions to the remedy are identified, and the like.

In any case, all his excellent reasoning goes for naught, because the postulates that it is built upon, the implausibility of the Law of Similars, and the common assumption that the remedies are nothing but blanks, turn out to be simply and demonstrably false. The basic "law" of homeopathy, for example, the phenomenon that medicines tend to elicit or provoke the same symptoms that they are meant to relieve, is widely familiar even in allopathic circles, where "paradoxical" effects, such as antihypertensives raising blood pressure, antidepressants making depression worse to the point of suicide, and so on, are commonplace and well-documented in standard reference texts like the *Physicians' Desk Reference*,[6] albeit not yet proclaimed as a general rule.

As for those notorious infinitesimal doses, experiments have repeatedly shown that highly diluted remedies are capable of both stimulating and inhibiting colony growth in bacterial cultures,[7] *in vitro* enzymatic activity in tissue culture and cell-free extracts,[8] seed germination and growth in various plant species,[9] and various global properties of higher animals.[10] While equally unambiguous results are naturally much more difficult to attain with human subjects in clinical situations, it is nevertheless irrefutably clear that highly diluted homeopathic preparations are capable of significant biological activity.

No matter how these mysteries are best understood, the fact remains that dedicated physicians have continued to follow homeopathic principles and to practice medicine on the basis of them for more than two hundred years, and now do so on every continent and in most countries of the world. In the face of determined opposition, general ridicule, and the sacrifice of more prominent and lucrative careers for their sake, the mere fact that homeopathic medicine has managed to survive intact for so long and even continued to grow and develop under such adverse conditions is sufficient answer to the unexamined faith of Dr. Smith and the quackbusters that it is a delusion and nothing more, and indeed suggests precisely the opposite conclusion. Its singular propensity to attract qualified doctors from almost every country at a time when allopathic medicine has become the dominant model of health care in the world represents not only a significant historical achievement in its own right, but also a persuasive argument for the validity of the Law of Similars, the efficacy of Hahnemann's infinitesimal doses, and the ultimate authenticity of the homeopathic phenomenon itself.

I have practiced general and family medicine for 44 years. No matter what type of treatment we prefer to use, all physicians are obliged to know and live by what Dr. Smith seems to have overlooked, that our reputations and livelihoods depend on the extent to which our patients are benefited by our efforts on their behalf. For the past 37 years, I have treated mine with homeopathic remedies exclusively, not because I believe that pharmaceutical drugs have no value; I often refer patients whom I've not been able to help to my allopathic colleagues, and am more than grateful for what they do. I choose to practice homeopathy in part because I prefer to try a gentler and safer approach first, whenever possible, but mainly because matching the treatment to the individuality of the patient allows and encourages a deeper and more comprehensive level of healing than is possible with drugs that merely counteract a specific symptom or correct a particular abnormality by applying superior chemical force at that strategic point.

I will give a few examples from the early years of my practice. The first was an eight-pound baby girl who was born covered with thick, green meconium, took one gasp, and then breathed no more. Brisk suctioning produced only more of the same sticky material. At this point the child lay limp, white, and motionless with a heartbeat of 40 per minute, responding feebly to mouth-to-mouth resuscitation but incapable of breathing on her own. I put a few tiny granules of *Arsenicum album* 200C on her tongue,[11] and almost instantaneously she awoke with a jolt, crying and flailing, her heart pounding at 140 per minute, her skin glowing pink with the flame of new life. The whole evolution took no more than a few seconds. After a night in the hospital to be on the safe side, mother and baby went home in the morning with no outward sign that anything untoward had happened. Experiences like these are imprinted for life in every practitioner's mind.[12]

Of course, since the child was well-formed and appeared normal in every other respect, I am well aware that this could have happened spontaneously without any remedies at all; and anyway, she was just one patient, a mere "anecdote," utterly without statistical significance.

But all of us who were present, including my nurse, the baby's mother and father, and I daresay the child herself, by now fully-grown and undoubtedly steeped in the legend of her birth, know as surely as we can know anything that the conjunction of the infinitesimal dose and her abrupt awakening was no mere coincidence.

My second case was that of a 34-year-old R. N. who had been plagued with severe endometriosis since her teens. Already a veteran of four surgeries to remove large blood-filled cysts from her bladder and pelvic organs, and several courses of male hormones to suppress the condition, she came seeking only to restore her menstrual cycle, having long since abandoned any hopes of childbearing. While intensely painful at first, her periods had become "dead," dark-brown, and scanty from so many years of surgery and hormonal treatments in the past.

After a few remedies, her menstrual flow became fuller and richer, and within six months she was pregnant. By the next time I saw her for a different ailment nearly eight years later, she had given birth to two healthy children after uncomplicated pregnancies and normal vaginal deliveries, and had remained in good health ever since.[13] While no one can attribute such an outcome to a homeopathic remedy or any other agency in precise, linear fashion, my patient has never stopped thanking me for it, which is reason enough to be grateful for a process that is inherently catalytic and persuasive, rather than forcible or compulsory.

Still less can these happy endings be imputed to any unusual skill of mine, since they are entirely comparable to what every competent prescriber has seen or could easily duplicate, and I could just as well have cited other patients whose conditions were far from hopeless, who believed in the remedies and in me, but whom I was nevertheless unable to help.

As Dr. Smith is at pains to insist, homeopathic remedies are safe, economical, simple to use, and gentle in their action, with notably few serious or prolonged ill effects. What he does not say and clearly does not know is that they are also capable of acting thoroughly, deeply, and for a very long time, requiring only infrequent repetition of the dose, and posing minimal risks of chronic dependence. Patients, friends, and loved ones alike often notice a general improvement in vitality and a sense of well-being, such that recurrence seems less frightening and indeed less likely.

To be sure, it is far from a panacea for all ills. Homeopathy is a difficult and exacting art, and even after years of study and practice a skilled prescriber may need to try several remedies before obvious benefit is obtained, while in some cases, in spite of the most devoted efforts, there is little or no benefit at all. But if the ultradilute remedies can be seen to have worked well and often enough to sustain me in a general practice for 45 years, like so many others over the past two centuries, that too is more than enough to refute Dr. Smith's bland assumptions that they are no treatment at all. Although of course deeply flattered by his insinuation that we heal our patients solely by some kind of magic or shamanic spell that we cast over them unawares, I continue to believe what my experience has taught me, that the "placebo effect," that starved and tattered remnant of the innate self-healing capacity, is an essential component of *all* healing, even with pharmaceuticals, even though by no means the whole of it.

For medicinal substances, the reigning standard of efficacy is the Random Controlled Trial, or RCT, in which subjects are randomized into two groups, one receiving the drug, the other only a placebo or inert imitation, with both patients and doctors kept blinded as to who gets which. In these experiments, the causal power of any drug against a particular symptom or abnormality equals the extent to which patients actually taking it outperform their placebo controls; and rather than an optimal *qualitative* fit with the illness of each patient as a whole, as homeopaths aspire to, the best drugs and the ones most diligently sought after are simply the most *potent* ones, those with the most chemical power to compel the organism to function in whatever minutely targeted ways the profession decrees that they should.

Thus modern physicians are duly equipped with the latest chemical weapons to attack a vast array of diseases and abnormalities as if they were enemies on a battlefield: *anti*biotics to kill bacteria, *anti*hypertensives to lower the blood pressure, *anti*convulsants to control seizure activity, *anti*metabolites to destroy cancer cells, *anti*histamines to suppress the allergic response, and so forth, all developed to act as selectively as possible, with little or no regard for the individuality of the patient. In advanced cases, such drugs may indeed save life, give miraculous relief, buy valuable time, or do the best that can be done under adverse or extreme circumstances.

Leaving aside the bottom-line question, whether most patients taking such drugs will actually feel better, live longer, and suffer fewer complications as a result of taking them, I am prepared to stipulate what is not always true in practice, that many of the drugs in common use do indeed have the power to accomplish at least some of what we ask and expect of them, in the hope that those more subjective and personal goals will eventually follow. But the high price that we have to pay for such seemingly precise and overriding causal power includes three enormous and largely hidden cost and risk centers that are each well-known on a general level, but rarely considered together or taken seriously as systemic issues that could be, should be, and indeed must be resolved.

First, when a drug really works to suppress or counteract the target symptom or abnormality, the condition is likely to reappear with equal or greater intensity as soon as the drug wears off. Using chemicals in this fashion, to force the issue rather than simply to assist whatever self-healing processes are already under way, cannot fail to pose the major risk of needing to *continue* using them for long periods of time, if not indefinitely, and thus transforming what is often an idiomatic *episode* in the patient's life into an ongoing if not permanent chronic illness with the power to propagate itself through time.

Second, narrowly targeting drug treatment to specific chemical abnormalities and abstract pathological "entities" without rebalancing the energy dysfunction of the patient as an integrated whole naturally and inevitably leads to *polypharmacy,* the need for still other drugs to correct or control whatever other diseases and abnormalities we are able to identify in the future.

Third, drugs powerful enough to do what we expect them to do are also capable of acting coercively on various other physiological functions, although these usually undesirable "side effects" may vary quite a lot, according to each patient's unique tendencies and predispositions, and will therefore be rather more difficult to attribute unequivocally to the action of the drug.

The ubiquity and relative invisibility of such adverse reactions make it a lot easier to understand why homeopathy has become so popular with patients caught in the tentacles of the medical system on the one hand, yet so easily dismissed by those who administer that system as ineffective, impossible, or unworthy of serious study on the other. In pointed contrast to allopathic drugs, which are developed solely for their power to force the organism to do what it has no natural inclination to do, homeopathy seeks rather to assist and even enhance the innate self-healing capacity that is synonymous with life, continually at work in every patient, and encompasses precisely those same individualizing tendencies, sensitivities, and predispositions which as physicians we are expected to ignore in our diagnoses, outperform in our research, and override in our treatment.

That is also the reason why, even when homeopathic remedies do act curatively, the results are simply dismissed or written off as isolated cases, perhaps "miraculous" at times, but in any case merely "anecdotal evidence" without scientific import, and therefore always located on the placebo side of the ledger, because medical science as presently constituted restricts the term "cause" to those interventions that *force* things to happen, and measures that power against the idiomatic and somewhat unpredictable tendency of every individual patient to recover without it.

Even in the case of well-designed RCT's that demonstrate a statistically significant benefit from homeopathic treatment, the result still "feels" unscientific and unpersuasive to most people, simply because no such chemical force had to be exerted and no such resistance overcome, while to trained scientists its looser interpretation of causality and its emphasis on subjective and individual variables both disqualify it from serious consideration as a force potent, measurable, and consistent enough to count as "hard science."

But the standard argument that homeopathic remedies are merely placebos actually cuts both ways. In the first place, it's simply *wrong;* homeopathic treatment has an impressive track record in the treatment of animals, newborn babies, and comatose patients, in whom the influence of suggestion is clearly minimal. In the second place, giving placebo, natural remedies, and nothing at all have often been shown to achieve clinical results comparable to those obtainable with suppressive drugs or crippling surgery, making it only fair to ask why anyone of sound mind would not prefer the cheaper, gentler, and safer alternative, at least to begin with.

Finally, when homeopathic remedies do act curatively, our patients rightly feel the "delicious quandary" of having healed themselves, and even wondering if they might have done so without our help. To all those skeptics and quackbusters still inclined to ridicule or dismiss such tales, I would issue the following challenge, to imagine a higher compliment to pay to a medicine than that its action cannot be readily distinguished from a gentle, spontaneous, and long-lasting cure requiring no further treatment.

Indeed it strikes me that the irony runs in precisely the opposite direction, that this optimal response is relegated to the placebo half of the equation, while pharmaceutical drugs are valued and considered effective only to the extent that they can overpower the physiology of as many patients and for as long a time as possible. I find it absurd and contemptible to boast of standards that prize brute force over elegance of fit, and that subordinate healing the sick to manipulating life functions artificially in the name of science, ambition, mastery over nature, or some equally abstract, hypothetical goal that we are obliged to take on faith.

That is why, for the present at least, I am thankful that our cures tend to remain snugly ensconced on the placebo side of things, because until we develop a kinder, more accurate, and inclusive model of causality, and a workable notion of the unified life energy of the patient as a whole, that is precisely where they belong. What the nuclear physicist J. R. Oppenheimer once told a group of psychologists thus seems even more apposite for the medical community as a whole:

> We inherited at the beginning of the Twentieth Century a notion of the physical world as a causal one, in which every event could be accounted for if we were ingenious, a world characterized by *number*, where everything interesting could be measured, and anything that went on could be broken down and analyzed. This extremely rigid picture left out a great deal of common sense which we can now understand with a complete lack of ambiguity and phenomenal technical success. One [such idea] is that the world is not completely determinate. There are technical predictions you can make about it, but they are purely statistical. Every event has in it the nature of a surprise, a *miracle*, something you could not figure out. Every pair of observations taking the form "we know this and can predict that" is global and cannot be broken down. Every atomic event is individual: it is not in its essentials reproducible.[14]

For all of these reasons, instead of competing with the placebo effect in order to defeat and discredit it, I have come to realize that the highest goal of medicinal treatment, whether homeopathic or otherwise, is precisely to assist and optimize it, by doing everything to promote healing in its most global sense, not just correct abnormalities, and by cultivating a deeper and more thorough knowledge of our patients, not ignoring, circumventing, or overriding what they have to teach us. To that end, while admiring the ingenuity and dedication of my colleagues who design and conduct RCT's to demonstrate the effectiveness of homeopathic treatment in the usual way, I offer an alternative model for clinical research, based on the inescapable bottom line of self-healing, which is equally applicable to allopathic medicine as well:

Nobody is blinded: all subjects know whether they are receiving homeopathic or allopathic treatment, having chosen it beforehand precisely because of their interest, belief, or faith in it.

Nobody gets placebo: everyone gets the treatment they select, while the doctors giving it out are matched to them by *their* beliefs, and encouraged to use prayer, suggestion, exhortation, shamanic incantation, or whatever they or their subjects believe will most effectively assist them on their healing path. In other words, *each group will serve as the control of the other.*

Using the totality of signs and symptoms over time, including both subjective and objective criteria, and reports of family, friends, teachers, employers, etc., *both homeopathic and allopathic subjects will be followed for a period of months or years,* depending on the condition, and extending beyond the acute phase to include the chronic dimension. *Both groups will then be evaluated as to how well or badly they are measuring up in their own lives, by their own standards and those of their community, and also with respect to appropriate clinical and pathological criteria.*

Qualified judges not exclusively or doctrinally committed to either point of view will then determine which form of treatment proves more beneficial in which respects, and will publish the results in a friendly, fair, and unbiased journal of good repute, to be selected and agreed upon in advance.[15]

For myself and my colleagues, homeopathy has stood the test of time as a *philosophy,* a coherent, logical system of thought, derived from the self-evident unity of the life force, a simple truism, and the "Law of Similars," a bold postulate, neither of which follows logically from anything else, or is therefore subject to experimental proof or disproof, like ordinary scientific hypotheses, as in Bertrand Russell's whimsical definition:

... the point of philosophy is to start with something so obvious as not to seem worth stating, and to end with something so paradoxical that no one will believe it.[16]

I freely admit, as I think even Dr. Smith would heartily agree, that homeopathy fits this description perfectly. Yet the authenticity of the homeopathic phenomenon, the enduring relevance of the point of view it offers, and the obvious effectiveness of minute doses when competently used, all imply the existence of a bioenergetic science that is still in its infancy, and will undoubtedly add to the atomic theory of matter and the laws of chemistry, many of which we already know, a further set of rules, laws, hypotheses, and predictions as it develops in the future, just as Dr. Smith has foretold. In that sense, homeopathy also looks beyond itself, to a more open and inclusive conceptual scheme that can accommodate both points of view, as well as perhaps others as yet unknown to us. Helping to envision, identify, and elaborate this new synthesis thus becomes our highest mission, which we share with like-minded physicians and healers of all persuasions and in every part of the world.

NOTES.

1. Smith, K., "Against Homeopathy -- A Utilitarian Perspective," *Bioethics,* 14 February 2011, pp. 1-12.
2. Holmes, O. W., "Homeopathy and Its Kindred Delusions," 1847, *Medical Essays,* Houghton Mifflin, Boston, 1895, pp. 1-102, *passim.*
3. Cf. Sampson, W., *The Braid of Alternative Medicine,* Prometheus, New York, pp. 21-31, and "Homeopathy Does Not Work," *Alternative Therapies in Health and Medicine* 1:48-52, 1995. Cf. also the **Health Care Reality Check** website, www.hcrc.org: "Dr. Sampson is Professor of Medicine (Emeritus) at Stanford, Editor-in-Chief of *Scientific Review of Alternative Medicine,* and teaches about unscientific and aberrant medical claims. He sits on the Board of Directors of the National Council Against Health Fraud, and is affiliated with other organizations that protect consumers from bogus healthcare claims and products."
4. Cf. Barrett, S.,"Homeopathy's Law of Similars" and "Homeopathy's Law of Infinitesimals," *Homeowatch* Home Page, www.homeowatch.org, posted March 20, 2002; and "Homeopathy: the Ultimate Fake," *Quackwatch* Home Page, www.quackwatch.org,, revised August 23, 2009.

5. Smith, op. cit., p. 12, *Acknowledgement:* "The author would like to thank Wallace Sampson, M. D., for valuable comments and criticism."

6. *Physicians Desk Reference,* 63rd Edition, 2009, Montvale, NJ. Cf., for example, "Catapres, *Overdosage,*" p. 842: "Hypertension may develop early . . ."; and "Prozac, *Warnings: Clinical Worsening and Suicide Risk,*" p. 1854: "Patients with major depressive disorder may experience worsening of their depression and/or the emergence of suicidal ideation and behavior . . ."; *et passim.*

7. Cf., for example, Noiret, P., "Activity of several dilutions of copper sulfate in different microbial species," *Proceedings* of 31st Congress, International League of Homeopathic Physicians, Athens, 1976, pp. 137-147; and Brack, A., et al., "Effect of ultra-high dilutions of 3,5-dichlorophenol on luminescence of the bacterium *Vibrio fischeri,* in *Biochimica et Biophysica Acta* 1621:253-260.

8. Cf., for example, Davenas, E., et al., "Effect on mouse peritoneal macrophages of orally-administered, very high dilutions of *Silica,*" in *European Journal of Pharmacology* 135:313-319; Petit, C., "Effect of homeopathic dilutions on subcellular enzymatic activity," *Human Toxicology* 8:125-129; and Shabir, S., et al., "Effect of homeopathic drugs on *in vitro* activity of alpha-amylase from human saliva," *Indian Journal of Homeopathic Medicine* 31:93-98.

9. Betti, L., et al., "Effect of high dilutions of *Arsenicum album* on wheat seedlings from seeds poisoned with the same substance," *British Homeopathic Journal* 86:86-89, 1997; and Binder, M., et al., "Effects of *Arsenicum album* 45X on wheat seedling growth," *Forschende Komplementärmedizin und Klassische Natur heilkunde* 12: 284-291.

10. Banerjee, P., "Comparative efficacy of two dilutions of *Arsenicum album* to ameliorate toxicity by repeated sublethal injections of arsenious trioxide in mice," *Pathobiology* 75:156, 2008; Fisher, P., "The influence of the homeopathic remedy *Plumbum metallicum* on the excretion kinetics of lead in the rat," *Human Toxicology* 6:321, 1987; and Doutremepuich, C., et al., "Aspirin at ultra-low dosage in healthy volunteers: effects on bleeding time, platelet aggregation, and coagulation, *Hemostasis* 20:99-105.

11. The 200C, or 200th centesimal dilution, means a dilution on a scale of 1:100, carried out 200 times, for a concentration on the order of 10^{-400}!

12. Cited in Moskowitz, R., *Resonance: the Homeopathic Point of View,* Xlibris, Philadelphia, 2001, pp. 14-15.

13. Ibid., p. 15.

14. Oppenheimer, J. R., "Analogy in Science," *The American Psychologist* 2:134, March 1956.

15. Moskowitz, op. cit., p. 342.

16. Russell, B., "The Philosophy of Logical Atomism," in *Logic and Knowledge: Essays, 1901-1950,* Allen & Unwin, London, 1968, p. 193.

V. Writings on the Philosophy of Medicine

"Some Thoughts on the Malpractice Crisis"

"Plain Doctoring"

"Diagnosis"

"Vaccines, Drugs, and Other Causes: a Homeopath Looks at the Medical System"

Some Thoughts on the Malpractice Crisis*

Malpractice as a Subset of Medical Risk.

The legal term "malpractice" applies only to those cases of patient injury for which individual or group liability can be attributed to human error, in the form of specific acts or failures to act, such as negligence, incompetence, poor judgment, or simple oversight on the part of physicians, hospitals, and often other health professionals as well. A verdict of malpractice further implies that reasonable standards of care exist for the procedures and situations in question, are generally well known and adhered to by the profession, and were violated in the particular instance.

Malpractice tends to be difficult to prove in court, because medicine remains to a large extent an art, with standards that must be infinitely adaptable to each new situation and therefore often cannot be formulated rigorously or agreed upon in advance. But in many cases the chief reason is simply that no definite *mistake* can be found, that the patient fell victim to a drug or procedure that is inherently dangerous, even when used appropriately.

Unfortunately, injured patients have no other redress than this difficult, prolonged, and expensive legal action, which attempts to assign specific liability for damages to the doctors, hospitals, and any other professionals involved. While patients thus assume an enormous burden of proof, doctors need only establish that they acted more or less as their peers would have acted under similar circumstances, such that patients' suffering and disability come to be reframed as a *misfortune,* in which nobody was specifically at fault and for which nobody in particular can be held responsible.

This old and cumbersome machinery is also stacked against the patient in another important sense. As in most other legal proceedings, malpractice cases are highly ritualized controversies in which the key roles and arguments are largely predetermined, and the often impassioned

---

* "Some Thoughts on the Malpractice Crisis," **British Homœopathic Journal** 77:17, January 1988.

disagreements between them are reduced to the narrowly technical questions of whether malpractice occurred and how much compensation should be awarded to the victim. No relief whatsoever is available to those who cannot or may not even want to restrict themselves to these issues, but are nevertheless genuine victims of the medical system, with a need and a right to be heard.

Consider a few common examples. If a gynecologist performs a hysterectomy and severs a ureter or leaves a sponge or hemostat in the abdomen, a finding of malpractice is assured, and the woman will receive major compensation for damages, if she survives and can still afford an attorney. But if the surgery is performed competently and the patient dies of an anaphylactic reaction to the anesthetic, or becomes chronically disabled from thrombophlebitis or a pelvic infection acquired during her hospital stay, the individual liabilities of the doctors and nurses attending her and the hospital where the events took place are likely to be far from clear. If the case is dismissed or decided in favor of the defendant(s), as so often happens, the victim receives no compensation of any kind, and the doctors, the hospital, and the entire medical system escape any burden of responsibility for the outcome.

Many other cases fall somewhere between these prototypes. Often a diligent and skillful attorney can find evidence of laxness in obtaining informed consent, careless record-keeping, or simple inattentiveness under the strain of a busy schedule or a contemptuous attitude. Under such circumstances, insurance companies may well decide to settle out of court, even if their clients are innocent of more serious wrongdoing, rather than incur the trouble and expense of further litigation. In either case, by focusing on the narrower question of individual responsibility, malpractice effectively conceals the broader institutional and deeper systemic issues posed by these vastly more common and important types of injury.

The largely hidden bulk of this gigantic iceberg is also the main reason why skyrocketing liability insurance premiums cannot be blamed primarily on unscrupulous attorneys looking for work. Even if nobody was specifically at fault, a malpractice case could not even be brought to trial, let alone settled, without grievous harm having been suffered by a patient. In my experience the vast majority of patients injured by the medical system never attempt to sue. It cannot be the fault of either patients or their lawyers for attempting to redress their grievances, when their only available recourse is to enter the great malpractice sweepstakes or forever hold their peace.

Expensive though it may be, malpractice insurance continues to buy for physicians the privileged assurance that most lawsuits brought against them will fail, and that the few exceptions will tend to be settled without further loss of income or disciplinary action, thereby allowing their business to continue more or less undisturbed, and thus protecting the basic features of medical practice from outside scrutiny or change.

In exchange for these guarantees, however, malpractice litigation has had a chilling and largely destructive effect on the practice of medicine and the doctor-patient relationship. By exaggerating the risk of injury due to individual human error, at times sensational but to a great extent unavoidable, it overlooks the more fundamental and correctable risks posed by the medical system as a whole, even when it is practiced conscientiously, with reasonable skill, and with genuinely informed consent.

In 1981 the nature and extent of iatrogenic illness and injury were investigated by Knight Steel and his team, who followed 815 consecutive admissions to a university hospital medical service over a five-month period.[1] Of those admitted to the 80-bed unit, the authors found

1) that 36% suffered at least one iatrogenic complication during their stay;

2) that one-fourth of these, or 9% of the total, developed complications that were seriously disabling, or potentially fatal, or both; and

3) that 2% actually died as a result of such complications while still in the unit.[2]

In addition, as they pointed out, these figures were in fact considerably lower than they would have been if they had counted

4) iatrogenic events suffered by the same population over the same time period, but before their admission or transfer into the unit, or after their discharge or transfer out of it, and

5) other episodes not attributable to any specific drug or procedure, such as seizures or falls in heavily medicated patients, which were written off as "incident reports," even though their medications clearly made such events more likely.[3]

In any case, their findings were more than adequate proof that, regardless of the personnel who happen to administer it, the medical system is inherently dangerous to everybody seeking its help, or in other words, to *everybody.*

In the latter part of the study, the authors tried to determine which drugs or procedures posed the greatest risk of serious and fatal complications. Even more to their surprise, they discovered that the risk depended much less on *which* diagnostic tests were ordered, *which* drugs were prescribed, or *which* surgical procedures were performed, than simply on *how many,* on the total number of transactions with the medical system, regardless of their specific content.[4] Although Dr. Steel and his team were understandably reluctant to spell it out, the obvious implication of their data is that patients are harmed much less by how well or badly medicine is practiced than by *how much* it is practiced.

The Principal Sources of Medical Risk.

Although its practitioners habitually regard modern medicine as a purely empirical science, with no general philosophy of health and disease, and no desire for any, it would be truer to say that its fundamental principles are *methodological,* consisting of the experimental rules and procedures of anatomy, physiology, biochemistry, pathology, microbiology, and the like, which specify how to acquire valid scientific knowledge about human ailments, and how to devise practical technologies for controlling them. We of today are so accustomed to its achievements that we seldom appreciate the profound shift in thought that was required to bring them about. Consider the following passage, written in 1833, and sounding almost quaint today:

The physician's high and only mission is to restore the sick to health, to *cure,* as it is termed. The highest ideal of cure is rapid, gentle, and permanent restoration of health, in the shortest, most reliable, and most harmless way, on easily comprehensible principles.[5]

287

These are the opening lines of Hahnemann's *Organon* of Medicine, the original homeopathic text, which was considered a radical and even heretical work in its own time. But compare them with another passage, written only a few decades later, and already we are in a different world, much more like our own:

> What we call the immediate cause of a phenomenon is nothing but the physical and material conditions in which it exists or appears. The object of the experimental method, and the limit of every scientific research, is therefore the same for living as for inanimate bodies. It consists in finding the relations which connect every phenomenon with its immediate cause, in defining the conditions necessary for the appearance of the phenomenon. *When the experimenter succeeds in learning the necessary causes of a phenomenon, he is in some sense its master. He can predict its course and appearance; he can promote or prevent it at will.*
>
> Neither physiologists nor physicians must imagine it their task to seek the cause of life or the essence of disease. That would be entirely wasting one's time in pursuing a phantom. The words "life," "death," "health," and "disease" have no objective reality. *Only the vital phenomenon exists, with its material conditions. That is the one thing that they can study and know.* [Italics mine: R. M.] [6]

In these words, which still ring true today, the great Claude Bernard perfectly captured the spirit that has ruled medical science for the past hundred and fifty years. Discarding the absolute, metaphysical unity of the "vital force," and the existential unity of the living patient, modern medicine prefers the defective but objectifiable unity of the *disease process*, e.g., TB, cancer, or hypertension, which can be defined on the basis of measurable abnormalities (TB bacilli, cancer cells, elevated blood pressure, etc.), and studied in the abstract, independently of the patient who happens to exhibit them. Such disease "entities" can then be used to group and even help *explain* the clinical signs and symptoms, to the extent that the corresponding abnormalities would tend to produce them, like cough and hemoptysis for TB, headache and neurological deficits for brain tumor, or heart disease and stroke complicating high blood pressure.

No longer content simply to "heal the sick," contemporary medicine is driven mainly to achieve effective control and dominion over every identifiable aspect of the life process. What Bernard so clearly envisioned, and what modern medicine routinely seeks to accomplish, is to acquire the knowledge and devise the means to regulate biological phenomena artificially, more or less at will. In his formulation, the experimental method in human biology consists of

characterizing the phenomenon to be studied;
identifying its component parts;
isolating its physicochemical "causes;" and
devising appropriate technologies for manipulating them, with as little disturbance as possible to the remainder of the organism.

Furthermore, what cannot be subdivided or objectified in this way need not and indeed should not be studied at all, since it cannot as yet be defined rigorously or thereby understood in any useful or meaningful sense. But this technological requirement is also inherently dangerous to the patient, not only because it makes human error more serious and more likely, or because it may well fail or fall short, but also and especially when its immediate objectives are successfully attained. However worthwhile its purposes, and regardless of their outcome, the attempt to control life processes by force creates insoluble theoretical and practical dilemmas for the profession that underlie and help explain the major crisis in our so-called "health care system."

First, the diagnostic process whereby living patients are assigned to abstract pathological categories deliberately ignores and distorts how they subjectively feel and even objectively function according to their own *personal* criteria, such as job record, school performance, ability to cope with stress, and the like, in favor of whatever generic norms and statistical averages happen to be calculated for them. Thus many patients with X-rays showing advanced osteoarthritis of the spine experience no pain, stiffness, or functional impairment to speak of, while others suffer extreme impairment and disability without any detectable pathology at all, and perhaps the largest group lie somewhere uneasily in between. Yet crucial life decisions, such as whether to undergo surgery, radiation, or drug therapy, continue to be made largely on the basis of X-ray shadows, statistical abnormalities, and what biopsied cells look like under a microscope, despite the poor and at best inconsistent correlation between *any* test result and how well or badly any given patient feels or functions, then or later.

The hypothetically important technical question of whether or not the test or its interpretation is accurate thus tends to obscure its equally important tendency in either case to prod or bully the patient in the direction of undergoing still more diagnostic and treatment procedures in the future, all of which help in turn to exacerbate or bring about the reality, the suspicion, or at least the fear that at least in retrospect seems to justify the intervention. Always in the name of greater precision, this obsessive reliance on diagnostic testing generates an unending cycle of ever more uncertainty, fear, and confusion in doctor and patient alike that multiplies exponentially and across the board both the probability and the risk of still further interventions within the system.

Perhaps even more dangerous is the concerted effort of medical science not only to avoid, obscure, and discredit, but also in fact to *weaken* the innate self-healing capacity of the patient, which by modern standards seems at once too crude to define or measure and too unpredictable to control. Thus illness is diagnosed primarily on the basis of objective abnormalities, that is, physical signs, structural lesions, and increasingly, simple deviations from statistical norms, while older terms like pain, nausea, vertigo, etc., which denote purely subjective states of *feeling,* tend to be given lesser value, or dispensed with entirely.

In this fashion, the concept of the disease process reduces the actual experience of illness to a mere automatism, a self-propelling chain of necessary causes preprogrammed to *worsen,* and thus silently ignores the equivalent tendency of every illness in every patient to *recover.* To accept any pathology as *given,* to surrender ourselves to what we imagine or are told to be *its* laws, is to forget that every illness must also be *received* and expressed by every patient in his or her own way, and that whatever individual factors may have played a role in our falling ill in the first place may well help us recover in the future.

The total eclipse of the natural self-healing capacity at the hands of modern science is regularly celebrated and even *sanctified* in the famous "double-blind" experiment, in which drugs and procedures are officially pronounced as effective if and only if they can wield enough force to outperform and thus supersede the now naked and merely sentimental hope of all patients to recover, and of their doctors to help them recover. Like the starved and tattered remnant of the ancient *vis medicatrix naturæ,* heretofore thought indispensable in maintaining the health and well-being of every patient, this so-called "placebo effect" is carefully minimized by keeping both doctors and patients ignorant of whether the drug or procedure in question was actually used, or only a passable imitation.

Much as in a bullfight, the superior technical resources of modern civilization are thus ritualistically pitted against the primitive forces of nature in an absurdly unequal contest, in which the latter is hobbled in advance and almost always defeated. Seemingly so precise and useful in other respects, the double-blind experiment ironically obliges the medical system to resurrect the self-healing capacity just long enough to vanquish it again and again, and thus to eliminate what most urgently needs to be studied. For if they cannot ultimately help sick people to heal themselves, even the most powerful technologies must remain doubly-blinded forever, with the blind leading the blind along a perpetually sightless path.

Finally, as an important corollary, the abstract concept of the disease process also distorts and trivializes both prognosis and case management, by reducing the whole art of treatment to simply correcting the abnormalities used to define it, namely, killing the TB bacilli, destroying cancer cells, lowering blood pressure, and the like. Just as histologically "cured" cancer patients with aplastic anemia or dementia are often at least as sick as before, these crude oversimplifications leave a profound ambiguity in the assessment of improvement and worsening, and even in the taxonomy of disease itself.

Thus patients developing a severe or intractable illness following apparently successful treatment of another illness pose a major practical dilemma that cannot be resolved within the theory of the disease process. For even if we say that the two conditions are related, the patient will still require diagnosis and treatment for each of them, while if we say that they are not, then there is no meaningful way to address the individual patient as a whole, as a unified bioenergetic system evolving through time. In either case, the net effect of medical science as a conceptual system is still to multiply non-specifically the number of technical interventions that are called for within it, by virtue of its awesome power to subdivide the living organism into ever more identifiable, subdividable, and potentially controllable phenomena.

Given their own fears and hesitations on the one hand, and the immense knowledge and power of the medical system on the other, our patients themselves provide a fitting epilogue in their profound desire, need, curiosity, and endless fascination to try to match up and integrate their own uniquely lived experience with the independent and often profoundly alien version of the body as a machine, so blissfully or horribly anonymous and neutral.

In precisely analogous fashion, these considerable perils involving diagnosis and case management are then further intensified and even consummated in the sphere of treatment, where something more or less drastic is *done to* the patient, and its stated purpose virtually guarantees that potentially destructive force will be required to achieve it.

Modern surgery, for example, the epitome of technical mastery in medicine, could not reliably succeed without the ability to control pain, bleeding, and infection by purely artificial means, or the precise and systematic identification of the structure and function of the parts of the human body, a truly heroic achievement. Without consummate skill and effective moment-to-moment control at every point, our surgical patients would regularly die or suffer crippling impairment on the operating table.

But the surgical ideal of technical control is also inherently dangerous, quite apart from the innumerable ways in which it may fail. Surgical procedures often seem irresistibly attractive, because they conjure up the prospect of immediate, profound, and permanent relief, and because wounds tend to heal automatically, whereas diseases have to be slowly, laboriously, and often painfully cured. By converting diseases into wounds, surgery more than any other branch of medicine ironically relies on its patients to heal themselves, to summon their optimal self-healing capacity just in order to survive. In emergency situations, such as a ruptured spleen or gallbladder, tubal pregnancy, or overwhelming pelvic infection, surgical intervention may be the only way to save life, and often miraculously achieves a complete recovery.

But the act of cutting into a living body also means that something momentous and perhaps irreversible has been done: certain parts have been removed, bypassed, repaired, or replaced; the seamless integrity of the organism has been interrupted or interfered with; and the experience and functioning of the patient has been disfigured or altered in some way that requires a series of artful decisions in every case, and the long-term consequences of which can never be precisely foreseen.

As a way of assisting the natural healing process, of repairing the body when it is already broken or removing a part when it is already dead, modern surgery must surely be ranked among the supreme technical achievements in human history. But as the preferred method of curing illness, and indeed the ruling paradigm or conceptual model of the medical enterprise as a whole, it is a cruel travesty, a quasi-military decision to cut and burn in lieu of gentler, safer, and more authentic modes of healing. A telling indictment that never shows up in our statistics, the burden of suffering and disability cheerfully borne by our "cured" patients furnishes a true measure of the risk that such procedures will continue to succeed in the future.

A very similar calculus applies to treatment with pharmaceutical drugs, which are also designed to correct specific abnormalities, as we saw. While physicians certainly *assume,* for example, that most hypertensive patients will feel better, live longer, and suffer fewer heart attacks and strokes as a result of their treatment, its proximate goal remains simply to normalize the blood pressure, hoping that the other purely derivative and statistical goals will eventually follow. In analogous fashion, modern doctors routinely use antibiotics to kill or inhibit bacteria, anticonvulsants to control seizure activity, corticosteroids to suppress inflammation, antithyroid drugs to block excessive secretion of thyroid hormone, bronchodilators to open constricted air passages, diuretics to force the kidneys to excrete more urine, insulin to substitute for a diabetic pancreas, and so forth. In advanced cases, such drugs may indeed give miraculous relief, buy valuable time, or at least do the best that can be done under adverse circumstances.

But because such abnormalities represent only a limited aspect of all that our patients are struggling to overcome, drugs potent enough to counteract them are also capable of overriding other unique, individualizing features at work in the case, and thus of weakening the total self-healing capacity in some manner and to an ever-increasing extent, as larger and larger doses are required, and the "margin of safety" between the therapeutic and toxic doses becomes smaller and smaller. What used to be called the "art" of medicine has long since been reduced to simply walking this tightrope as adroitly and with as generous an allotment of good luck as possible.

Just as with surgery, the risk of iatrogenic complications is far more serious when the drugs "work" than when they don't. Any reasonably experienced, attentive physician is able to suspect and willing to make the proper adjustment when the prescribed dose is excessive or insufficient, and to identify and discontinue medicines that are ineffective or produce serious toxicity in the form of "side effects." But when the drug effectively suppresses or counteracts the abnormality in question, the latter either reappears with equal or even greater force when the drug wears off, or disappears entirely, in which case some deeper and more serious condition often arises in its place. Either way, using drugs to force the issue in this manner entails the readiness to continue using them for long periods of time, perhaps for life, with the clear expectation that the original complaint, or worse, will reappear as soon as they are discontinued. A pretty fair definition of "addiction" in its original sense, a deep and prolonged chemical dependence of this type follows reliably and more or less automatically from our habit of using drugs to control abnormalities, rather than assist and enhance the patient's innate self-healing capacity. It is also the fitting conclusion to the self-fulfilling prophecy already implicit in the theory of the disease process, that chronic diseases are by definition incurable in any case, and must therefore be controlled with drugs throughout life, removed surgically, or simply borne in silence.

In this way, what began in most cases as an episodic illness, idiosyncratically programmed, readily and insidiously becomes a chronic and indeed less and less curable process, *chemically* programmed, in exchange for temporary palliation of symptoms, quasi-mechanical "correction" of abnormalities, and long-term perpetuation of the original energy dysfunction. Insofar as all drugs tend to become less and less effective over time, increasingly large doses will often be required, as we saw, and the already slim margin of safety eliminated entirely in sensitive cases.

Finally, effective suppression of symptoms or abnormalities for long periods of time may itself lead to more serious ailments in the future, as previously shown. Thus asthma appearing after suppression of eczema or hay fever, endometriosis or ovarian cysts after a course of oral contraceptives, and Crohn's disease following years of anti-inflammatory drug treatment for irritable bowel syndrome all exemplify a problem that cannot even be meaningfully stated without going beyond the theory of the disease process to consider the patient as a unified bioenergetic system that grows and develops through time.

Thus several orders of magnitude beyond that of its deviant youth, our society as a whole is itself built on an almost insatiable drug habit of truly colossal proportions. Without accurate statistics of the hundreds of millions of patients maintained for years on officially sanctioned drug dependencies, it is impossible to give true weight and measure to the mistakes, overdoses, side effects, and allergic, idiosyncratic, and toxic reactions that inevitably follow in their wake. By providing formidable biological weapons with the power to kill, maim, or at least keep patients effectively trapped within their orbit, the medical system makes it seem possible and even attractive to ignore, circumvent, or supersede the natural self-healing capacity and the practical understanding of life that alone could guide or restrain us in their use. Much more dangerous than our sophisticated methods of diagnosis and treatment *per se,* in themselves capable of much good as well as harm, is the idolatrous worship of biotechnology for its own sake, and the mindless but hugely profitable substitution of technical imperatives for authentic human problems requiring art and caring and individualized attention.

Healing the Doctor-Patient Relationship.

Since all of these risks are ultimately realized or dispelled through actual relationships with physicians and other health professionals, they cannot be readily distinguished from the risk of the disease itself, or from that impending sense of danger that motivates a patient to seek such help in the first place. Whether for good or ill, the awesome power vested in the doctor-patient relationship arises from the basic human need to comprehend the mystery of illness and contain it within the familiar parameters of a personal encounter. Arising from a request for help and a hope for change, the interaction is poignant and fraught with the nearness of suffering. Even in the face of such pressures, a relationship based on mutual trust and respect can help even gravely ill patients to heal what can be healed, and to accept what cannot be changed, while a breakdown in communication can transform even a minor illness into a nightmare of anguish and betrayal. Not by skill and training alone, the prominence and high estate of physicians in society must also be earned through diligent and reliable *service*.

If doctors and patients can agree to make all decisions jointly, and to share responsibility for both the process and the outcome, the risk of drugs and procedures is minimized by the sober realization that both parties are committed to doing the best they can, without expectation of cure or guarantee of benefit, such that death and failure to recover are always possible, and therefore in themselves no cause for personal or moral blame on either side. But by substituting its own primarily technical priorities for the give-and-take of human relationships, the runaway growth of the medical system threatens to dissolve the therapeutic alliance, the indispensable glue which cannot itself be measured, yet holds the system together at every point and makes it *work*. In no small part, this divergence is attributable to the fact that the goods and services of the health care *industry* – the diagnostic equipment, the surgical instruments, the pharmaceutical drugs, and the techniques and policies governing their use – are controlled by the companies that produce them, the research institutions and training hospitals that house and maintain them, and the physicians and other health professionals that prescribe and use them.

Whether sold to the patient for profit, or made available on some other basis, these major commodities are doled out on a highly restricted basis, dictated almost entirely by their owners, in accordance with their own corporate, institutional, and professional values, and having at most secondarily to do with the felt needs and expressed wishes of the individuals about to be subjected to them. In addition, the rampant specialization of medical care obliges patients to seek out and maintain relationships with an ever-wide network of physicians and allied health professionals, whose diverse roles and areas of expertise are likewise ruled by institutional, guild, or team criteria that are minimally responsive to criticism or negotiation from outside.

Finally, as we saw, conventional medicine and surgery are explicitly designed to identify the chief abnormalities and diseased parts, and to correct and at times literally remove them from the body. Reduced to a specimen of his or her disease, the patient becomes the passive recipient of various procedures, with residual power to give or withhold consent, but few opportunities to negotiate diagnostic or treatment plans, or to alter or modify them once begun. In short, the patient stands essentially alone, isolated, and defenseless against the entire medical system, with compelling reasons to fear it, no effective check on its power, and no realistic alternative but to submit to at least some of its offerings, and to bring a malpractice suit after the fact for actual damages done.

Extending well beyond the narrowly technical and legal question of malpractice, the so-called "malpractice crisis" of our time actually represents the spontaneous and mostly leaderless insurrection of millions of patients against the harsh restrictions and impositions of the medical system as a whole. By far the most prevalent and dangerous of these is the pervasive sense of fear, rage, powerlessness, and distrust that have come to be shared by doctors and patients alike, poisoning their ability to work together in harmony, and twisting their very different experiences of illness and disease into an obsessional neurosis of calculated risks and hidden meanings. By no means accidental, or attributable solely to prejudice or fault on either side, the adversarial relationship now prevailing between doctors and patients follows logically and inexorably from the dominant conception of chronic disease as a sequence of abnormal mechanisms predestined to worsen and therefore always in need of artificial correction.

Under these circumstances, the idea of malpractice insurance does seem compelling, to the extent that physicians are allowed and even expected to assume effective responsibility for the lives of their patients, many of whom truly believe that medical science understands their needs better than they do themselves, and should therefore be authorized to decide when and how they live or die, recover or fail to recover. The incalculable risk to which malpractice insurance does in fact address itself is the infinite liability that doctors incur once death and worsening come to resemble failure in their Sisyphean quest for purely technical solutions to disease and all other human problems.

Because no amount of insurance could ever adequately indemnify a risk of such proportions, to most doctors the idea seems almost too good to be true, no matter what it costs. It not only protects them from catastrophic loss of income if a claim against them proves successful, but could also become a profitable investment in its own right, since the initial outlay is made up many times over by the ever-increasing volume of procedures that it underwrites, and the ever-higher fees that can be charged for them. In physician-owned companies, the combined premiums actually resemble a tax-free mutual fund that could also generate major dividends, if the claims made against it can be kept sufficiently small.

In either case, the bottom line is that, by deciding which doctors to insure and how much to charge them, which practices to defend, and which to settle out of court for, liability insurance companies have in effect substituted their own technical, actuarial, and simple herd criteria for the independent and inescapably artful clinical judgment of practicing physicians, based to a large extent on unique individual variables at work in each situation. Consulted for what appears to be a simple tension headache, for example, a conscientious physician could well decide to hospitalize the patient, consult a neurologist, and obtain a CAT scan, just to make sure, without the slightest reason to suspect a brain tumor, except for our technical capacity to find it, and thus a potentially serious legal liability for *not* finding it.

While physicians thereby limit their own exposure by sharing it liberally with colleagues, their patients incur a tremendous added expense and receive nothing but the same old treatment, which most often merely palliates the symptoms in any case. In this fashion, both the patient's overall risk and the physicians' total liability for even this routine indisposition are compounded again and again over a long period of time, rather like a home mortgage loan.

Similarly, gynecologists regularly advocate hysterectomy for uterine fibroids, even without pain or bleeding, and although the chances of malignancy are vanishingly small, merely because surgery is what they know how to do superbly well, and the insurance company can more readily defend a recognized procedure, even one that is ineffective or unsafe, than doing nothing, and simply admitting that we do not understand tumor formation well enough to help our patients heal it naturally and in a timely fashion.

Although what we call "the medical system" is in fact merely a heterogeneous assortment of techniques with only a restrictive methodology to unite them, both the constant threat of litigation and the breakdown of the doctor-patient relationship exert intense and powerful pressure on every physician to practice in conformity with

300

the real or imagined standards of their insurors. In effect the lowest common denominator of what our least imaginative colleagues are doing, such standards often amount to little more than *doing something,* that is, filling the void with a definite action or procedure, whatever the outcome, leaving no plausible diagnosis unlooked for, and no possibly corrective treatment untried. Thus awkwardly and inadvertently, the law of malpractice teaches doctors to fear their patients, to sacrifice their own personal enjoyment of and fulfillment in their work, and to restrain the temptation to follow the intuitive or creative impulse of the moment, so apt to seem meaningless and indefensible outside of that unique and never-to-be-repeated situation.

Ironically, when a doctor is sued, the insuror may well choose to settle out of court, even when no mistake was made, or try to secure an acquittal for wrongs that were in fact committed, purely on the basis of their own corporate needs. In other words, malpractice insurance protects doctors and hospitals solely for playing by the rules of high-cost, high-tech, high-risk medicine. The standard argument that it also protects the patient overlooks the inconvenient truth that the victims of medical malpractice are people who have already been maimed or killed by their doctors, that the kind of protection they needed was precisely the kind they *didn't* get.

Indeed, by promoting fear and suspicion on both sides, and thus multiplying immeasurably the total number of diagnostic and treatment procedures, as we saw, both malpractice insurance and the law that it underwrites must be reckoned as liability risks of enormous proportions in their own right. By singling out a few egregious mistakes, they allow the main business of the medical system to continue without interruption, and leave its radical distortion of health and illness both unexamined and unchanged. Far from protecting patients, the malpractice system is the principal reason why the vast majority of medically injured patients will never have to be compensated or even heard.

From these simple truths, it follows that malpractice insurance alone cannot solve or even meaningfully address the present crisis in health care, and that the imperative of rebuilding the doctor-patient relationship and the level of trust required to sustain it will never be possible without a serious commitment on both sides. For patients to become equal partners in their health decisions, both parties will need to affirm as a fundamental political, legal, and moral right that birth, death, health, and illness are core experiences belonging primarily to the people undergoing them, and that nobody has the right to manipulate or control them without their explicit request, or that of someone duly authorized by them to act on their behalf.

For the physician, the duty to serve begins and ends with being attentive to and respectful of patients' expressed needs and wishes, enlisting their active participation whenever possible, making no decisions without their approval, and being ready and willing to advise and learn from them in a manner congruent with their own life experience. Most of all, it calls for a deep and abiding commitment to the relationship itself as the most precious resource, and the basis of all genuine healing work. As set forth in the policy guidelines of two prominent consumer organizations, these minimal standards actually correspond fairly closely to what most patients are really asking for.[7] As a sign of good faith, it makes practical sense for doctors to make public acknowledgement of these duties, or something like them, as some of what is owed to patients. In like manner, it costs us very little to allow and encourage our patients to invite friends and relatives to attend their consultations, both to bear witness, and to serve as advocate or intermediary if necessary. Finally, patients have every right to form their own political organizations and interest groups to represent them, just as they are already doing, and to use them to negotiate with doctors, hospitals, insurors, legislators, and government agencies, and to appear in court on their behalf.

Far from limiting their freedom of action, physicians committed to these basic rights for their patients are entitled to expect certain responsibilities from them in return:

1) to learn as much as possible about their condition and what they can do to promote and assist in their healing work;

2) to be familiar with and mindful of all rules and policies governing their care, and to honor and carry out all agreements freely entered into; and

3) to make their needs and wishes known as clearly as possible, and to give feedback and constructive criticism when they feel dissatisfied or unheard.[8]

302

But healing the doctor-patient relationship is only the beginning. Even if these guidelines are honored in good faith and carried out to the letter, malpractice and the larger problem of iatrogenic illness and injury will not simply disappear. Patients will still be injured by what doctors do or fail to do, and some way will have to be found for society as a whole to acknowledge and indemnify the large majority of instances where no individuals were specifically at fault. But it is undeniably true that doctors who are attentive to their patients, respectful of their wishes, and sensitive to the needs of the relationship between them are much less likely to be sued. For doctors and patients alike, their relationship itself provides the best possible insurance against harm, and ultimately there need be and can be no other.

Healing the Medical System.

As we saw, malpractice and the other forms of medical risk originate in our fundamental concepts of health and disease, and the often inarticulate and unspoken assumptions that underlie them, such that reducing them substantially will require major changes in how both physicians and the lay public are taught to think about illness and disease, as well as diagnosing and treating them in practice.

One simple and effective initiative would be to provide comprehensive and universal health education to the general public, beginning in elementary school and continuing throughout life. With a basic core of good habits built into the curriculum at every level, children of all ages can readily grasp that good health is not solely or primarily the absence and prevention of diagnosable diseases and abnormalities, that it must also develop and cultivate a general sense of physical, mental, and spiritual well-being, by learning and teaching how we humans maintain and repair ourselves, recover from acute illness, and seek out compatible health professionals to guide us through more serious complaints.

Already prominent in Hippocratic medicine, the enduring idea of the natural self-healing capacity is beautifully expressed in these classic aphorisms of Paracelsus, the great Renaissance physician and alchemist:

The art of healing comes from Nature, not the physician . . .
Every illness has its own remedy within itself . . .

A man could not be born alive and healthy were there not already a Physician hidden in him.[9]

Evoking a venerable philosophy of ancient lineage, these simple maxims may be interpreted roughly as follows:

Healing implies wholeness.

Derived from the same root as "whole," the English verb "to heal" literally means to make whole [again], and represents a fundamental property of all living systems, as evident in wound healing, for example, and represents a concerted effort of the entire organism that cannot be achieved by any part in isolation.

All healing is self-healing.

As an intrinsic function of the organism, healing occurs automatically and continuously throughout life, with or without outside help. In other words, all healing is self-healing, such that the proper role of drugs, surgery, and professional or other designated healers is simply to facilitate or assist the natural process that is already under way, and not to alter, interfere, or substitute for it.

Healing applies only to individuals.

Healing is always possible, but also inherently problematic, even risky, and may always fail to occur. That is because it pertains solely to living individuals in concrete, unique, here-and-now situations, rather than to abstract "diseases" or principles. In other words, healing is also inescapably an *art,* which can never be and should never be reduced to any formula or technique, however powerful it may be, and however scientific its foundation.

I envision a basic health and self-care curriculum for everyone, beginning in primary school, and offering physical training, nutrition, and regular spiritual practice, in order to assist students in understanding and coping with ordinary life stress, and to provide simple, safe, and effective techniques that are readily accessible to everyone and applicable throughout life. A corps of part-time community health workers, analogous to China's "barefoot doctors," could be recruited from a pool of qualified applicants, offered a brief but rigorous training program, and employed to teach and supervise others in the areas of self-care, health maintenance, triage, and first aid of simple domestic ailments.

At the level of full-time licensed providers of primary health care -- Nurses, Physician-Assistants, Nurse-Practitioners, Certified Nurse-Midwives, and Family Physicians -- graded and certified programs would be offered in yoga, nutrition, acupuncture homeopathic and herbal medicine, midwifery, counseling, meditation, and the like, to promote and facilitate self-healing and supervise the self-care of patients with common functional ailments in which anatomical lesions and tissue damage are minimal or insignificant. By reserving the most advanced medical and surgical facilities for severe, intractable, or emergency cases, these primary-care providers could offer safe and effective health services inexpensively to millions, and help restore them to optimal health and well-being at modest expense and with minimal risk.

Even at the most advanced levels of subspecialty and tertiary hospital care, a self-healing orientation would teach surgeons, cardiologists, and other highly-skilled specialists to make the proper diagnosis but then set it aside, at least for long enough to allow the unique, individualizing features of the case to assist and guide them in healing it, trying gentler methods first, and resorting to conventional drugs and surgery only when they fail, in urgent or desperate cases, or where nothing else will serve.

By helping people to keep themselves sane and fit, a self-healing philosophy would also create new possibilities at every level of the system. Developing and perfecting non-invasive methods of diagnosis and treatment will require new clinical training facilities for teaching and practicing them. Keeping the concept of separate abnormalities and disease entities in reserve for when they are clinically necessary or useful rather than as the default setting for every transaction will suggest new research protocols for studying patients as unified bioenergetic systems growing and developing through time. In addition to acupuncture, homeopathy, Kirlian photography, radionics, and other methods already in use, this simple but crucial paradigm shift will naturally tend to promote new, experimental health technologies that are more advanced and sensitive than any now available.

Once supported in this way, and made to feel secure in their helping and facilitating rôles as educators, counselors, advocates, and healers, physicians and other health professionals will learn to feel appreciated and rewarded not solely or primarily for what they *do to* their patients, but equally for *being there for them,* for helping them heal themselves, each in his or her own way. Conversely, once confident that they will truly be cared for on a personal level, patients will be that much more willing to trust themselves and their caregivers to make the hardest decisions when that time comes.

In a system modeled on self-care, it is very likely that the risk of malpractice and other forms of iatrogenic illness would become tiny fractions of what they are now, such that injured patients could be compensated from the same insurance plan that covers their regular health and medical expenses, and that the latter would also cost much less than it does now, because society as a whole would be underwriting it, so that health care would be recognized as a basic human right, rather than a privilege available only to the wealthy. In the simplest and most efficient "single-payer" model, the same government-sponsored insurance plan, similar to MEDICARE, would pay all primary-care physicians and other health providers directly for basic health and wellness care, simple triage, diagnostic work, emergency care when necessary, and specialty care as authorized by referral at the time. All services would be covered and paid for by the plan, which like MEDICARE would function as a huge HMO for basic health services, with the whole population as subscribers, and all licensed health professionals as providers. Patients made ill or injured by their care would still be entitled to legal redress, and to receive compensation from the plan if their claims were upheld.

Additional private insurance could still be made available for "big-ticket" items, such as elective surgery or specialty care desired by patients or doctors more often than the plan would cover. In any case, as we saw, providing safe and effective preventive, wellness, and holistic medical care would hopefully keep the need for conventional drugs and surgery to a minimum. Surely there can be no higher praise for a doctor or a health-care system than that patients regularly heal themselves without needing drugs or surgery, and continue to do so in the future. In the words of Lao-tse,

A leader is best when people barely know he exists,
Not so good when they obey and acclaim him,
Worst when they despise him.
Of a good leader, when his work is done and his aim fulfilled,
The people will say, "We did this ourselves."[10]

NOTES.

1. Steel, K., et al., "Iatrogenic Illness on a General Medical Service at a University Hospital," *New England Journal of Medicine* 304:638, 12 March 1981.
2. Ibid., p. 638.
3. Ibid., pp. 638-639.
4. Ibid., pp. 640-641.
5. Hahnemann, S. *Organon of Medicine*, 6th Ed., trans. Boericke & Dudgeon, Boericke & Tafel, Philadelphia, 1935, ¶1,2.
6. Bernard, C., *Introduction to the Study of Experimental Medicine,* trans. H. C. Greene, Dover, New York, 1957, pp. 65-67, *passim.*
7. Cf. "Code of Practice," People's Medical Society, Emmaus, PA; and Haire, D., "The Pregnant Patient's Bill of Rights," International Childbirth Education Association (ICEA), Minneapolis.
8. Cf. "The Pregnant Patient's Responsibilities," ICEA, Minneapolis.
9. Paracelsus, *Selected Writings*, trans. N. Guterman, ed. J. Jacobi, Bollingen Series, Pantheon, New York, 1958, pp. 50, 76.
10. Lao Tzu, *The Way of Life,* trans. W. Bynner, Putnam, New York, 1944, pp. 34-35.

Plain Doctoring*

For years I've wanted to write something with this title without any clear idea of what I meant by it, until recently the phrase came back to me as an apt metaphor for what I do, and for some broader issues pertaining to the medical profession in general.

Often used as a title, the common noun "doctor" comes from the Latin verb *docere,* to teach, and is applicable to an advanced level of academic attainment in any field, such as Doctor of Philosophy, Doctor of Laws, "Doctor of the Church," and so forth. A Doctor of Medicine is thus first of all essentially a teacher or educator, one qualified through training and experience to inform, advise, and instruct about matters of health and illness, both to individuals and the general public.

Although educating about health is one of the most important things that practicing physicians do, it is by no means the only thing, nor even the most common or important meaning of the word "Doctor" as applied to physicians today, when teaching and learning are regularly upstaged by the urgent requests of sick people to be "fixed" or "done to" in some way.

Indeed, the familiar conception of the medical doctor in contemporary life is precisely the opposite, as a "doer" or performer of specialized diagnostic and therapeutic procedures. This is our sense of the word "doctor" when it is used as a verb, meaning roughly to "tinker" or "fool around with," to make careful adjustments and readjustments until we get the thing more or less the way we want it, contingent to a great extent on our skill and experience, on the art and craft of the profession. In this vein, we might speak of doctoring a salad or an automobile engine, always with the implication of risk-taking, of the possibility of ruining it beyond repair, of making some mistake that cannot be undone, in exchange for the estimable benefit to be enjoyed if it is done perfectly, or at least well enough. Doctoring in this activist sense implies the existence of some standard, goal, or desired endpoint, and here too we can distinguish two

---

* *"Plain Doctoring,"* **Resonance,** Journal of the International Foundation for Homeopathy 19:30, March-April 1997

subtypes which coexist in practice but differ fundamentally and often compete with each other.

One is older and more primitive, comparable to doctoring the salad, which is judged according to its taste, freshness, and nutritional value. In this most basic kind of doctoring, the goal of doctors and patients alike is simply to improve how we feel or function according to our own individual standards. This huge, all-purpose category begins with subjective feelings, such as happiness or well-being, energy or vitality, equanimity, freedom from pain and suffering, and the like. But it also includes measured observations by family members, friends, employers, and teachers, as well as the patients themselves, as to their performance in work, career, school, marriage, relationships, and family life. Collectively these variables encompass the rather vague and imprecise but indispensable human criteria that doctors and patients have always used to evaluate their work together since the earliest times.

Corresponding more closely to our second example of the car mechanic, the other aspect of doctoring is distinctly modern in being more objectively and even quantitatively defined, and in regarding the human organism as a machine with separate and more or less exchangeable parts. In mechanical doctoring, the narrower goal of identifying and removing obstacles to health is achieved primarily by developing performance criteria as precise and unambiguous as possible, in order to be equally applicable to and measurable in other patients with similar conditions. Morphological and statistical deviations such as abnormal cells, pathogenic bacteria, X-ray shadows, elevated blood pressure, serum cholesterol, etc., can then be substituted for all the subjective and idiosyncratic elements of illness, which tend to be too crude to define or measure and too unpredictable to control.

Modern doctoring employs both of these styles simultaneously and cannot be carried out effectively with either of them alone. But in practice they are often rivals, each representing a distinct conceptual language that is supple and powerful within its own sphere, but utilizing methods and purposes that cannot always be reconciled, and appealing to standards that are often untranslatable. I shall call the first the ordinary or "human" language of lived experience, and the second the technical language of abnormalities.

309

While demonstrably more precise and accurate for certain specialized purposes, the newer technical language of medicine nevertheless ultimately derives its own meanings and values from the older human or ethical standard. The only conceivable rationale for giving drugs to lower the blood pressure and prevent strokes and heart attacks is that such a life will be fuller, richer, and happier than otherwise.

The same is true of surgery, which would succeed far less often without the language of abnormalities, and its extraordinary ability to identify and regulate critical life functions on a moment-to-moment basis, a truly magnificent achievement. Even for surgeons, the ultimate test of diagnosis and treatment is the same one that doctors and patients have always used, namely, do they help? Do they relieve suffering and disability? Do they promote the health of the patient as a whole? Do they minimize our long-term dependency on the medical system? Such questions cannot be asked or answered meaningfully from any viewpoint except that of the patients who are subjected to them.

In short, the technical language of the physician is a derivative language and should only be used to facilitate or clarify the awareness of the patient, not substitute for it. The older phenomenological language arises directly from our personal awareness of ourselves and our bodies as sensed, imagined, thought, and felt. With all its limitations, the subjective awareness of how we feel and function is still the bottom line for what doctoring is ultimately about.

Especially in a profession dominated by science and technology, it provides our best assurance that health and illness, improvement and worsening, and the success or failure of our work as physicians will be judged according to the patient's own standards, rather than others imposed arbitrarily or coercively by and for the profession itself. Our failure to keep these priorities straight is a lot of what I hear from patients about what they think is wrong with medical system today, and it is difficult not to agree with them.

I'll also say it the other way: the excesses and deficiencies of the present medical system are intelligible and predictable to the extent to which we have reversed these priorities. By subordinating the ordinary language of the patient to the technical jargon of the physician, we have replaced our sacred and noble calling of healing the sick with the purely

310

technical imperative of acquiring the knowledge and devising the means to manipulate and control biological processes artificially and more or less at will.

This brings me to the adjective "plain," the first word of my title, which I can now understand why I chose even before I knew what I wanted to write about. To me, "plain doctoring" means simply reaffirming the ordinary language and thought of our patients as the truest standard for evaluating our sophisticated diagnostic and therapeutic interventions, the basic human wisdom that alone can guide or restrain us in their use.

The word "plain" also means "generic" rather than specialized, and refers to those aspects of health and illness that are universal and fall within the province of every physician and every patient. Such would naturally include the experience of falling ill, worsening, and recovering, with their attendant lessons of pain, suffering, disability, and the proximity of death, as well as the gifts of giving birth and being born, of health and vitality, of tranquility and joy, of healing and being healed. None of these can be understood outside the context of actual human life, and all of them are part of the life experience of every human being.

Finally, plain doctoring is blissfully neutral with respect to the Cartesian riddles and rivalries of mind and body, for the simple reason that the seamless biological integrity of each living creature must take precedence over the mental or physical subcategories we learn to make use of in our study and practice. When we see our patients, we encounter physical, mental, and emotional symptoms, all in the soup together: neither making the diagnosis nor instituting the treatment need impose on us any prior metaphysical commitment to any particular subset of them as having "caused" the others. Our job is simply to taste the soup.

In addition to these general remarks that most of my readers can identify and perhaps even agree with, I retain my own personal version of plain doctoring that I try to live by in my practice. Though far from perfect, and everywhere subject to my own full share of limitations and failings, it works well enough for me and my patients alike that I can write these lines without shame and practice medicine credibly in their sight. I hope that simply talking about it publicly in this fashion will stimulate and encourage others to come forward and articulate what plain doctoring means for them.

My basic text is from Paracelsus, the great Renaissance physician, who prophetically formulated a great deal of what modern medicine seems to have contrived to ignore:

> The art of healing comes from Nature, not the physician . . .
> Every illness has its own remedy within itself . . .
> A man could not be born alive and healthy were there not already a Physician hidden in him . . .[1]

I interpret them roughly as follows:

1. Healing implies wholeness.

Etymologically, the English verb "to heal" comes from the same root as "whole," meaning essentially to make whole [again], and refers to a basic attribute of all living systems, which is evident both in wound healing and in spontaneous recovery from illness, but presupposed even in effective medical and surgical treatment, our standard Operating-Room alibi "poor protoplasm" signifying the relative deficiency of it. Like the metastatic cancer patient who pulls off a regression against every expectation or probability, healing represents a concerted response of the entire organism, cannot be achieved by or ascribed to any part in isolation, and implies a deeper level of integration than could be defined or approximated by any mere assemblage of parts.

2. All healing is self-healing.

As a fundamental property of all living systems, healing proceeds continuously throughout life and tends to complete itself spontaneously, with or without external assistance. This means that all healing is ultimately self-healing, and the role of physicians and other professional or designated healers must be essentially to assist and enhance the natural healing process that is already under way. However useful and necessary it may be, merely correcting abnormalities will also have to be judged in relation to that fundamental standard. Finally, a self-healing orientation transforms the doctor-patient relationship itself, from a hierarchy of knowledge and command into a partnership of consensus and trust.

312

3. Healing pertains solely to individuals.

Always possible but also inherently problematic and even risky, healing applies only to individuals, to flesh-and-blood creatures in unique, here-and-now situations, rather than to abstract "diseases," abnormalities, principles, or categories. In other words, whatever else it may be, it is inescapably an art, and should never be and can never be reduced to a mere technique or procedure, however scientific its foundation.

To these three aphorisms I would add a fourth of my own, arising directly out of what I hear patients complaining about, which may need to be affirmed as a basic moral, legal, and political right of what it means to be a patient:

> Health, illness, birth, and death are inalienable life experiences belonging wholly to the people undergoing them, which nobody else has the right to manipulate or control without their explicit request, or that of somebody duly authorized by them to act on their behalf.

My concluding text is from Lao-Tse, supplying an appropriate bottom-line criterion:

> A leader is best when people barely know he exists,
> Not so good when they obey and acclaim him,
> Worst when they despise him.
> Of a good leader, when his work is done and his aim fulfilled,
> The people will say, "We did this ourselves."[2]

NOTES.

1. *Selected Writings of Paracelsus,* Ed. N. Guterman, Trans. J. Jacobi, Pantheon, Bollingen Series, New York, 1958, pp. 50, 76, *passim.*
2. Lao Tzu, *The Way of Life,* trans. W. Bynner, Perigee, New York, p. 46.

Diagnosis*

The physician's task is to make sense of the patient's story in the generally accepted terms and concepts of the scientific world. Yet the two narratives, the physician's account and the patient's story out of which it was made, continue to exist side by side. Although the patient's story is contained in and explicated by the physician's, it has not been replaced by it. Nor are the two narratives simple translations of each other. They are incommensurable: neither can be comprehended in or simply reduced to the other's terms.

The medical interpretation of the patient's story bears great power for healing. As the location of the malady in the social universe, a diagnosis relieves suffering in itself, as well as in the guidance it provides for therapeutic action. Like all power, it must be exercised with care.

-- Kathryn Montgomery Hunter, *Doctors' Stories*

1. Illness and Disease.

The art of caring for the sick transcends merely assembling information and doling out treatment, which may not work or even be chosen properly until an appropriate setting and healing relationship are created for them. As much as whatever we *do to* them, those afflicted with pain, suffering, and disability seek relationships of trust with friends, loved ones, and professionals,

1) to help them make sense out of what is happening to them;
2) to help them construct a working mythology of their illness;
3) to help them discover and navigate a safe passage through it; and
4) to help them envision a life beyond it, insofar as possible.

But how do physicians accomplish these purposes, and how faithfully do our words and actions reflect what our patients actually feel and are bothered by? Like my colleagues, I take "illness" to refer to what people actually *complain* of, encompassing both the particular symptoms and the

---

* "Diagnosis," *American Journal of Homeopathic Medicine* 102:7, Spring 2009, and 102:56, Summer 2009.

general malaise that prompt them to seek (or avoid) our help. But these felt complaints can only hint at or approximate the full extent of their condition, and our endeavor to understand that totality raises a still more basic problem, namely, how we know that someone is truly sick.

This is by no means a silly or rhetorical question, for if we stipulate that being sick is merely a *sensation* or awareness of feeling ill in some way, then we ignore the obvious possibility that the patient, the doctor, or both could be *mistaken,* that we might only suspect or fear an illness that does not actually materialize, as with anxious patients who keep imagining the worst, even when no other evidence turns up. Virtually every practice attracts its share of devoted followers for whom definite confirmation of a disease long feared or suspected brings a perverse yet genuine relief. Although some might well argue that obsessiveness of such high degree is itself a kind of sickness, both physicians and patients rightly search for outwardly perceptible signs to confirm the reality of what they feel.

Yet if, on the other hand, we suppose that an adequate definition is possible with nothing but such objective evidence, we are even more likely to fall into the opposite error, by singling out an abnormal but harmless variant, say, which the patient has lived with happily for years or even decades, and might never be bothered by in the future. The obvious solution would be to postulate that illness should include *both* elements, i. e., both an inner awareness of feeling unwell, and some manifest interference with normal functioning that could be witnessed and attested to by other observers, such as one's spouse, family members, friends, employers, colleagues, teachers, doctors, and the like.

But what is perhaps most striking about this formula is the extent to which modern medicine has managed to *ignore* it, by concealing the subjective elements of illness within the vastness of the seemingly more objective and precise term "disease" wherever possible. Reducing illness to disease enables modern physicians to sidestep the metaphysical question of whether or not a person is really *ill,* in favor of the more practical task of organizing the myriad forms and manifestations of disease into a taxonomy or classification scheme that assists both diagnosis and treatment. After several notable attempts in ancient times, such as Greco-Roman theories of the four humors, the tripartite Hindu or Ayurvedic system, the Five-Element disciplines of China, Japan, and Tibet, and the innumerably diverse oral traditions of tribal and folk medicine, many of which are still in use, the concept of disease in contemporary Western medicine is distinctly modern, and radically different from all of these.

As we know it today, the science of pathology grew out of the systematic dissection of human corpses, beginning with grave-robbing painters and anatomists of the Italian Renaissance, and reaching a peak of achievement in the middle and late Nineteenth Century, based on surgical specimens from the living and autopsy specimens of the dead. Making use of unimaginably detailed and painstaking observations, these early pioneers of what we now know as scientific medicine succeeded in

1) tracing the signs and symptoms of living patients back to anatomic and microscopic structures first identified in the cadaver;

2) refining the physical examination itself, on the basis of these correspondences; and

3) developing new diagnostic instruments and tests that could likewise be defined in wholly objective terms, independently of the patient's lived experience.

Two inventions of this kind, the stethoscope and mercury sphygmo-manometer, or blood pressure machine, were introduced in the first and second halves of that remarkable period, and taught physicians how to distinguish normal and abnormal sounds in the heart and lungs, such as murmurs, arrhythmias, wheezes, râles, rhonchi, and so forth; how to measure and standardize the blood pressure; and ultimately to identify diseases, complications, and sequelæ both old and new, like mitral stenosis, pneumonia, bronchitis, asthma, hypotension, and high blood pressure, among many others.

Flushed with the power of such discoveries, the modernists perhaps too easily phased out the "vital force" or unitary life principle of ages past, in favor of the limited but seemingly more precise unity of separate "disease processes," such as "cancer," "hypertension," and "tuberculosis," which could also be defined solely on the basis of objective, measurable abnormalities -- cancer cells, high blood pressure, and TB bacilli -- and thus diagnosed and studied in the abstract, as concatenated sequences of mechanical causes and effects, quite independently of the patients who happened to exhibit them. Such pathological "entities" could then be used to group and ultimately explain the clinical signs and symptoms, insofar as the diagnostic abnormalities would naturally tend to produce them, like headache and neurological deficits in the case of brain tumors, heart disease and stroke for hypertension, or cough and hemoptysis for TB.

This elegant sleight-of-hand is still famously celebrated in the weekly or monthly spectacle of "Grand Rounds," also known as the Clinical Pathological Conference, or CPC, wherein the medical history, physical examination, and laboratory tests of a selected patient are reviewed and discussed by the Attending Physician to explain how the clinical diagnosis was arrived at, and then confirmed or refuted by the pathologist, who climaxes a series of anatomic and microscopic views of the surgical or autopsy specimen with the long-awaited announcement of what the patient *really* had. The subtext and ulterior purpose of these ceremonies is to uphold the final authority of the disease process as the most accurate version of the patient's underlying condition, whatever the clinical signs and symptoms, and thus in every respect superior to them in explanatory value.

2. The Disease Process as Explanation.

Although long accustomed to the practical advantages of this viewpoint, and to rejoicing in its accomplishments, we seldom appreciate the profound revolution in human thought that was needed to bring them about. Modern surgery, for example, presupposes the exact and detailed identification of the parts of the human body, their gross and microscopic structure, and their physiological functions, a truly monumental achievement, which would not have been possible without the uninterrupted collaboration of dedicated scientists in all parts of the world, extending over many generations, and indeed continuing right up to the present, and beyond.

Although the new paradigm did not become dominant until the introduction of microscopic pathology and analytic chemistry in the latter half of the Nineteenth Century, its essence was clearly discernible in the work of the Renaissance anatomists, and immortalized in Rembrandt's masterpiece, *Dr. Tulp's Anatomy Lesson,* which celebrates the same genre of causal thinking that modern physicians still use in diagnosis today. After carefully dissecting and exposing the forearm muscles of the cadaver, the eminent Professor places his clamp on the common sheath of the flexor tendons, and ceremoniously pulls back on it, sharing the thrill on the faces of his adoring students, as the stone-cold fingers obediently rise again, Lazarus-like, to contract in response. The notion of mechanical causality implicit in these discoveries was elegantly formulated two centuries later by Claude Bernard, the great French physiologist, who not only designed and carried out some of the first quantitative experiments in medical research, but also envisioned and helped bring about a lot of what scientific medicine has since become:

> What we call the immediate cause of a phenomenon is nothing but the physical and material conditions in which it exists or appears. The object consists in finding the relations that connect every phenomenon with its immediate cause, in defining the conditions necessary for the appearance of the phenomenon. When the experimenter succeeds in learning the necessary causes of a phenomenon, he is in some sense its master. He can predict its course and appearance; he can promote or prevent it at will.

> As a corollary to the above, neither physiologists nor physicians must imagine it their task to seek the cause of life or the essence of disease. That would be entirely wasting one's time in pursuing a phantom. The words "life," "death," "health," and "disease" have no objective reality. When a physiologist invokes the "vital force," he likewise does not see it: he merely pronounces a word. Only the vital phenomenon exists, with its material conditions: that is the one thing that he can study and know.[1]

His search for mathematical models led Bernard to reinterpret the ancient concepts of health and disease, hitherto regarded as polar opposites, as relative and therefore measurable quantities along the same continuum, differing solely in *degree* rather than kind:

> Health and disease are not two essentially different modes, as the ancient practitioners believed. These are obsolete medical ideas. In reality, between these two modes there are differences only of degree: exaggeration, disproportion, and discordance of normal phenomena constitute the diseased state.[2]

In the spirit of William Harvey, the Seventeenth-Century physician who discovered the extent and direction of the circulation of the blood, as well as the arterial and venous compartments and the capillary network that separates them, physicians today draw on much the same reasoning to suspect acute cholecystitis, for instance, as the most likely explanation for attacks of fever and pain in the right upper quadrant of the abdomen that radiates to the right shoulder or shoulder blade, and to confirm the diagnosis by ultrasound of the gallbladder, in conjunction with other tests. The train of reasoning proceeds "backwards," so to speak, from the signs and symptoms of the patient to the pathognomonic features of the known disease process, which lead us to the anatomical structures that would have to be affected in order to produce them, in much the same way that a plumber or auto mechanic locates the offending valve or pipe in a closed system of human manufacture.

Diagnosing acute diseases of this sort, such as heart attack, stroke, pneumonia, yellow fever, stomach ulcer, appendicitis, and so forth, regularly proves its worth not only by identifying and confirming, but also in large part *explaining* the illnesses that patients are actually complaining of. Perhaps because these pathological "entities" explain the "how" or *pattern,* as much as the "why" or precipitating cause or circumstances of illness, acute diseases tend to exhibit a consistent natural history across the whole range of various possible reactions to them, and thus yield an approximate standard or average against which variations in severity, duration, clinical course, prognosis, and outcome can all be assessed and even predicted with some accuracy. This ever-growing body of clinical experience may then be offered to the patient as a model of the healing work that remains to be done, as well as what to expect in the aftermath. Further proof of the relevance and accuracy of these diagnostic categories lies in the remarkably high degree of congruence between the clinical and the pathological data, as recapitulated in the Grand Rounds or CPC ritual just described.

More or less the same is true of subacute and intermittent conditions, such as rheumatic fever, pleurisy, nephritis, migraine, sciatica, asthma, malaria, and the like, even if chronic traces of these illnesses remain behind, since both their defining characteristics and the patient's overriding concerns still refer back to the acute episode or flareup, in which subjective and objective elements again coincide quite closely, and thus invite deeper levels of understanding. In other words, they too may fairly be called "diseases" in the modern sense, precisely because they are also *illnesses,* such that the patient's signs and symptoms can be comprehended and at least in part explained as pathological mechanisms, which have in turn been elucidated by observation and experiment.

In relatively well-defined diseases of this kind, the patient's lived experience of illness remains distinct from the pathological knowledge that was acquired in order to explain it, and continues to exist side by side with it, such that the "disease" perspective, which applies equally to all patients with the same diagnosis, and the "illness" perspective, which seeks out those features which are peculiar to and characteristic of each individual, tend to complement and enrich each other, to achieve the optimal "fit." Thus the modern physician is trained to anticipate conduction abnormalities in heart attack patients, uses routine electrocardiography to detect them as early as possible, and can often prevent fatal arrhythmias by treating them promptly at this stage, but also knows, or should know, that the fear and depression so often encountered in these same patients can easily hamper their recovery, even if the electrical picture stabilizes. In diagnosis as well as treatment, successful practitioners learn how to use both of these perspectives idiomatically and synergistically in each case.

3. Vague, Uncertain, Long-Term Diagnosis: the "Nocebo" Effect.

Diagnosis tends to be much less reliable, however, and often misleading or even harmful, when disease is allowed to take precedence over illness, to the extent that details of the patient's history are ignored, discounted, reduced, or subordinated to the purely technical and objective data of the physical and laboratory examination, and the physician's time and energy come to be monopolized by the endless search for abnormalities to explain the most ordinary complaints, as students today are routinely trained to do. This kind of oversimplification was and still remains a chief lament of master clinicians, like the gastroenterologist Howard Spiro, recognized as an authority on the most advanced diagnostic techniques of his time, who nevertheless regarded medical science itself as a major threat to the core humanistic values of the profession, which have hardly changed since ancient times:

Physicians have been trained to think of themselves as scientists, and to search for a biologically detectable reason for every complaint, partly in the fear that they may be sued for missing something. The explicit teaching at many medical schools is that every clinical problem is reducible to some detectable abnormality that can be captured on a screen, be given a number by a laboratory test, or otherwise quantified. Specialists see their main task as ruling out potential structural alterations in some segment of the body. As the diagnostic approaches multiply, so do the tests that patients undergo.

There must be a middle ground between mindless ordering of tests and foolish ignoring of disease. Does every complaint need a workup [and] a diagnosis? We need to revise our concepts of health and disease, and begin to think about restraining the percentage of the gross national product that medical care entails. We need more public discussion, and not simply external financial restraint.[3]

The same quest for wholly objective and impersonal diagnostic criteria also underlies the concept of "preventive medicine" as we know it today, and earns considerable prestige for the effort, even when it fails or falls short. As chronic illnesses are reframed as ongoing disease processes, it seems feasible and even irresistibly tempting to try to identify their microscopic, microchemical, and microbiological precursors, to devise methods for detecting them as early as possible, and to abort them before they become real illnesses by correcting the abnormalities wherever they can be found.

A familiar early example is "essential," primary, or "idiopathic" hypertension, that is, simple "high blood pressure" in patients without kidney disease, pheochromocytoma, or other organ pathology to explain it. All denoting a purely statistical abnormality, these terms are applied more or less interchangeably to readings above a predetermined normal range, based on studies linking them with higher rates of stroke, heart attack, and cardiac failure years and even decades later. During my student years, pressures in the 140/90 range were considered mild or "borderline," and earmarked for observation, while those of 150/100 or higher were said to be "moderate," and recommended for treatment.

But just as Claude Bernard had proclaimed, modern disease differs from health only in degree, and later studies have placed the threshold lower and lower, to the point that physicians today are exhorted to treat an ever-larger population of asymptomatic patients, including those with pressures of 130/80 and above, and the elderly with purely systolic or calcific hypertension, who had always been exempted in the past. Commenting on a 2008 study in the *New England Journal of Medicine,* an editorial in the same issue considered all those with blood pressures over 115/75 to be at higher risk for the complications, and therefore recommended antihypertensive treatment for them, in a pep talk that stopped just short of advocating a lifetime of medication for the entire adult population:

> Hypertension is prevalent and accounts for a large proportion of cardiovascular morbidity and mortality worldwide. The level of blood pressure is related to the risk of stroke, ischemic heart disease, heart failure, and death in a continuous and consistent fashion for values as low as the optimal blood pressure of 115/75.
>
> In 1937 the eminent cardiologist Paul Dudley White wrote that "for aught we know, hypertension [even] in advanced cases may be an important compensatory mechanism which should not be tampered with." Our knowledge has advanced a lot since then. In 1967 treatment was shown to confer clinical benefit in patients with severe hypertension (diastolic BP 115 to 130). Since then clinical trials have shown benefit in treating less severe degrees of diastolic and even systolic hypertension in older persons. An overview of such trials involving 160,000 patients indicates that any common regimen to lower pressure reduces the risk of major cardiovascular events, and larger reductions even more so. In a study of patients 80 and older, active treatment achieved a 21% lower risk of death from any cause, a 64% lower risk of heart failure, and a 30% lower risk of stroke. These results prove that it is never too late to start treatment in old people.[4]

The vague, uncertain, long-term diagnostic category "hypertension," which has no precise definition, extends far into the future, and is related to illness only statistically, exemplifies what has been called the "nocebo" effect, the tendency of merely *bestowing* such a diagnosis to sicken and harm patients, both by imprinting the fear and expectation of developing a serious illness in the future, and by providing a compelling rationale for treatment with powerful and dangerous drugs for decades, and indeed for life:

What greater anxiety can a patient suffer than to be told that he is likely to develop a serious or fatal disease unless he agrees to take powerful drugs for the rest of his life, and possibly even then? What doctor is courageous or foolhardy enough *not* to diagnose hypertension, or not to tell his patients that they have it? What patient would be willing *not* to know if he had it, or be less anxious for not knowing? The diagnosis of hypertension is anxiety-provoking by its very existence, because it causes every patient to *wonder* if he has it, even if he never goes to the doctor. Our system rests on the validity of pathological diagnosis in providing accurate information about the objective reality of a disease (abnormal physiology, natural history, and prognosis), apart from the lived experience of the patient. The assumption is untestable within the system, and functions like a religious commandment: obey it without question, and ignore it at your peril.

Yet pathological evidence is a relatively poor guide to whether our patients will recover, worsen, or die, and what their lives will be like, when measured against what nobody dares measure, namely, what would happen if the exam was not done and the patient merely sent home without treatment. When is pathological diagnosis useful? It can be life-saving in acute diseases, where it helps doctor and patient to know what they are up against and what they have to do next. It is often injurious when the patient presents with no symptoms, is told that he has a disease on the basis of some test that has no correlation with his actual experience, and must be kept on a regimen of drugs throughout life. The anxiety provoked by making these diagnoses will pressure patient and doctor to discover the disease they seek to prevent.

The placebo effect denotes the healing power of giving our patients blank pills and passing them off as real. But don't forget its opposite, the *nocebo* effect (literally, "I will harm") to signify the damaging effect of telling a patient what he "really" has, of redefining his reality in such a way that he must forever live in its shadow, by substituting its law (i.e., *ours*) for his own.[5]

For better or worse, preventive screening of this type has long since become the main focus and rationale of the famous "annual physical," in which the conscientious physician is expected to conduct a thorough, head-to-toe search at frequent intervals for the slightest traces, hints, and harbingers of diagnosable pathology, both present and future. To be sure, doubts and scruples about the wisdom of such open-ended fishing expeditions continue to be raised from time to time. Twenty-five years ago, a British physician calculated that even those whose high blood pressure, high serum cholesterol, and regular tobacco use put them in

323

the most serious risk category for coronary disease and stroke still ran a 60% chance of *not* developing these conditions during their productive years (ages 40 to 64), and a much better chance if only one such factor was present.[6] These still rather favorable odds led him to entertain seriously for once the bottom-line question that is rarely given so much as lip service:

> Are we entitled to expose patients who have identified risk factors but are otherwise healthy to long-term administration of drugs for prevention of a disease that most of them will never have?[7]

Apart from these occasional caveats, quibbles, and nitpickings, however, the preventive strategy continues to thrive as if it embodied the highest ideals of the medical enterprise, largely unchallenged by the public despite fundamental deficiencies in the concept. Apart from the risk of human error, which is significant but to some extent unavoidable, one equally important and obvious problem is the subjective bias that is inherent in the interpretation of many tests, and in some cases in the nature of the testing medium.

As an example of the second type, a retrospective study of mammograms in women previously biopsied revealed surprisingly large discrepancies in the readings of board-certified radiologists and their recommendations for treatment, discrepancies that were significant enough to cast serious doubt on the efficacy of the procedure as a tool for detecting breast cancer and its precursors.[8] For 150 women diagnosed with cancer, the radiologists' blinded recommendations for further workup varied from 74% to 96% of the total, a discrepancy of nearly one-fourth, while for 123 women with negative biopsies over a period of 3 years the variation was much larger, from 11% to 65%, depending on the radiologist.[9]

In this instance, one major problem was the inherent subjectivity of the X-ray medium, coupled with the intricate, arcane, and exacting skill set required for interpreting it. But even more prevalent, more important, and more difficult to detect are errors embedded deeply in the *concept* of the test, especially in the significant possibility that what it measures is and will prove irrelevant or misleading as a predictor of serious illness. The widely felt urgency about early detection of breast cancer again provides a classic example, based on the traditional breast exam and the identification of "fibrocystic disease" as a pre-cancerous lesion meriting biopsy and closer surveillance. In 1982 this reigning mythology was authoritatively discredited by Susan Love, the esteemed breast surgeon, in a landmark article entitled "Fibrocystic Disease of the Breast: a Non-Disease?"

Fibrocystic disease is defined as a condition in which there are palpable lumps in the breast, usually associated with pain and tenderness, that fluctuate with the menstrual cycle and become progressively worse until menopause. This description applies to the majority of women of reproductive age. Most of these lumps represent a physiologic nodularity that is under hormonal control.

Physiologic nodularity is clinically important because of the difficulty of distinguishing it from a "dominant" lump, which requires aspiration and biopsy. Autopsy studies have shown that 58% of patients of all ages had histological changes associated with fibrocystic disease, and that 89% of women over 70 without breast disease also had them. Other studies have concluded that the differences between normal breasts and those with clinical features of cystic mastitis are only of degree, not of quality. Yet a diagnosis of normal breast tissue almost never appears on a surgical pathology report. Is it reasonable to define as a disease a process that occurs clinically in 50% and histologically in 90% of women?

The real problem is that this nebulous disease has been said to impart a two- to four-fold increase in the risk of breast cancer. But many studies show no greater incidence of it in cancerous than in non-cancerous breasts at autopsy. In fact it was found in 58% of non-cancerous breasts at autopsy, but only 26% of breasts with cancer. *What a review of previous studies does suggest is a roughly two-fold increase in the risk of cancer following breast biopsy. This increase applies to all patients who have had a biopsy, whatever the reason for it, and regardless of the outcome.*

Although it could be argued that surgery itself stimulates a neoplastic change, the cancer is often on the side opposite to the biopsy specimen, so any carcinogenicity must be systemic. A more obvious explanation is the change in the criteria used to make a histologic diagnosis. The decision to perform a biopsy is subjective, based on clinical judgment of the relative risk of cancer. Since having had a biopsy makes one more likely to have another, closer surveillance may simply increase detection without increasing the actual incidence of breast cancer.[10]

In this case, the universal dread of the disease was aggravated by both the screening program and the biopsy that it increasingly led to, which further magnified the doctors' already considerable fears, even when the biopsy itself was negative, and was therefore likely to prejudice their subsequent readings, thus adding to the already large total of false-positive diagnoses in women who were not ill and might never have become so if the biopsy had not been performed in the first place.

Such ambiguities are unavoidable, even with actual illness and confirmatory laboratory or X-ray findings, because no test by itself is sufficient to explain what patients feel or experience. Every practicing physician knows substantial numbers of patients with spinal films that look like Swiss cheese, indicating degenerative osteoarthritis, advanced osteoporosis, and the like, who nevertheless experience no pain, stiffness, or functional impairment to speak of, as well as another group at least as large who suffer excruciating pain and/or serious disability with no detectable pathology whatsoever, while by far the largest group, and maybe the hardest to be clear about, inhabit the vast, uncharted territory in between. Yet no matter which point along this spectrum a given patient happens to occupy at a given moment, crucial life decisions, such as whether or not to undergo surgery, chemotherapy, or still more invasive tests and punishing treatments, continue to be made largely on the basis of X-ray shadows, statistical averages, what biopsied cells look like under a microscope, and so forth, despite the inconsistent and often unreliable correlation between *any* test and how well or badly a particular patient actually feels or functions, either then or later.

But these already major difficulties are compounded exponentially when the patient is not ill, and the "disease" to be tested or screened for is merely a technical abnormality, a hypothetical risk of developing a serious illness perhaps years or decades in the future. Even if the test makes sense, and is performed competently, read accurately, interpreted according to the best available standards, and improbably faithful to the natural history of the disease process, it will necessarily include substantial quotas of both false-positive and false-negative results, and still leave us in the dark about what we really need to know, namely, which cases of the disease so defined will prove to be serious clinically, and which will not. Thoroughly steeped in the exalted scientific ideals of objectivity and precision that undoubtedly inspire such exercises, most physicians tend to accept and shrug off these ambiguities as unavoidable consequences of medical practice, of doing no more nor less than what we were trained to do, as indeed they are.

But particularly in the case of chronic disease, these knotty conceptual tangles tend to deepen and multiply to the extent of casting doubt on the integrity of the disease process itself. Like any other ailment, the term "cancer," for example, encompasses a broad spectrum of possible outcomes, including

1) an incidental finding, with no symptoms whatsoever;

2) spontaneous remission or cure of an actual illness;

3) widespread regional, lymphatic, or blood-borne metastasis;

4) severe, life-threatening systemic disease; and

5) death.

Such a distribution is easier to accommodate within our general conception of acute, subacute, and intermittent diseases, as we saw, because they occur now and then, as discrete episodes or flare-ups, scattered throughout the course of patients' lives. For a disease to be defined as "chronic," on the other hand, means that it has become essentially co-extensive with the "normal" life of the patient, such that it can no longer be readily distinguished from it, and therefore cannot and must not be thought of as a *thing* or "entity" existing on its own, with a well-defined path or natural history that is intelligible and makes useful sense apart from the patient's own experience of it.

This conundrum is well illustrated by the debate surrounding prostate cancer, which is defined by microscopic changes that almost all adult males will eventually develop if they live long enough, and that in the vast majority of cases will produce no symptoms and no functional impairment and has no clinical significance whatsoever. It is nevertheless a major problem for the *imagination,* 1) because some men will become seriously ill and die with it; 2) because almost everyone dreads suffering and death; and 3) because nobody knows or *can* know who will fall ill, who will recover, who will live, and who will not.

327

Resolving these genuine and intractable dilemmas is the estimable mission of the Prostate-Specific Antigen or PSA test, which measures a glycoprotein constituent of seminal fluid that is secreted by the prostate, spills over into the blood to some extent, and is used to detect prostate cancer at its earliest and presumably most curable stage. The PSA level rises substantially with age, after ejaculation, and in men with benign prostatic hypertrophy and prostatitis, tends to fall in parallel with low testosterone levels, and unfortunately also varies significantly from day to day in normal life.[11]

According to the *Harvard Medical School Guide to Men's Health,* blood levels of 0-4 ng. per ml. are generally read as normal, levels of 4-10 ng. as "borderline," and those above 10 ng. as unambiguously abnormal.[12] But as is widely acknowledged, these thresholds are arbitrary and inexact, with no clear or fixed boundary between levels that are clinically unimportant and those that accompany or predict serious illness, as well as including the inevitable percentage of false positives and false negatives, as above, which in this instance tend to vary inversely with each other, no matter which threshold is chosen. The current rule of thumb considers levels below 10 ng. to indicate early disease confined to the gland, levels of 10-20 ng. to signify local spread beyond the capsule, and levels above 50 ng. as highly suggestive of metastatic cancer involving lymph nodes, bones, and other tissues.[13]

There is some limited consensus that the PSA does provide a quick, easy, safe, and economical way to monitor the progress of the disease and the effectiveness of the treatment in men who are significantly ill, with a biopsy-confirmed diagnosis. But routine PSA screening for all men above a certain age is still hotly debated, and rightly so, since even if it were 80% effective in detecting cancer, as alleged, it would still miss 20% of the cases, as well as subjecting millions of healthy men to expensive and potentially harmful biopsies and treatment that they didn't need and would never have needed. While advocates of the test point to a steady reduction in the death rate from prostate cancer since 1992,[14] that result cannot be attributed to PSA screening, since a comparable decline has been reported in England and Wales, where the test has not been in general use.[15] Just as with hypertension and breast cancer, once the abnormality is permitted to define the ailment, the same set of facts leads to exactly the opposite conclusion, that there is no minimum threshold that guarantees freedom from disease, just as Claude Bernard foresaw so long ago.

As if to prove the point, another study using the same microscopic criteria found "prostate cancer" in

6.6% of men with PSA's of 0.5 ng. or lower;
10.1% " " " " " 0.6-1.0 ng.;
17.0% " " " " " 1.1-2.0 ng.;
23.9% " " " " " 2.1-3.0 ng.; and
26.9% " " " " " 3.1-4.0 ng.,[16]

as well as "high-grade" cancers, with Gleeson scores of 7 or higher, in

12.5% " " " " " 0.5 ng. or less, and
25.0% " " " " " 3.1-4.0 ng.[17]

While the authors of the study spoke out against doing so, these data lend added support for lowering the upper limit of normal still further, to catch these large numbers of false negatives as well. Just as with mammograms, breast biopsies, "high blood pressure," and many other tests, the net effect of preventive screening for specific diseases is often increasingly hypochondriacal versions of the same basic dilemma that we started with, always in the name of greater precision, which in this case clearly measures *something* relevant to prostate function, yet in the end still leaves us hanging on nothing more than a risky wager on the outcome for you or me. Once again, our genuine and inevitable fear, doubt, and uncertainty are simply papered over with statistics and a blind faith in "preventive medicine" for its own sake, and bullied by our own obsessive need and ambition to diagnose as many diseases and abnormalities as possible, as far in advance of actual illness as possible, and regardless of the significant probability that they will never materialize or become actual health problems at all.

4. Endless Diagnoses and the Need for Restraint.

Screening for subclinical abnormalities can be perfectly legitimate and useful in some cases, because medicine involves art as well as science, and requires *ad hoc* decisions on behalf of real people in concrete, here-and-now situations, while the range of our sense-perception is limited and therefore always amenable to extension and improvement. As we saw, the PSA test can be helpful in monitoring the treatment of patients who are actually sick with prostate cancer. Screening tests may also be useful in retrospect, as in an update of the celebrated Framingham Study, in which routine electrocardiograms taken at six-month intervals uncovered a surprisingly high percentage of subclinical myocardial infarctions, roughly half of which were completely asymptomatic, half exhibited symptoms but remained undiagnosed, and the total of both groups, amounting to almost 25% of the total number of heart attacks in the study, were just as likely as the rest to result in heart failure, stroke, or other major complications, including death.[18] Nor would I hesitate to perform targeted screening of selected individuals at their own request, or with strongly-positive family histories, or on an *ad hoc* basis for *any* reason, even a hunch. Introducing subjective or personal factors, like the patient's fear of illness, or the doctor's gut-level intuition of unseen forces at work, lends real meaning to the procedure, by providing an unequivocal, up-or-down criterion for interpreting it.

As a general rule, then, I propose nothing more radical or outlandish than simply taking seriously what every medical student is piously taught, and what experienced clinicians observe every day, that pathological diagnosis, the identification and classification of disease, works best when it includes both subjective and objective elements side by side, as we saw, that is, a *Gestalt* or ensemble of symptoms complained of by a patient, together with manifest signs elicited by the physician, such that the clinical diagnosis based on the history and physical examination can then be confirmed or refuted by laboratory evidence that would be imperceptible otherwise.

When pathology is diagnosed solely on the basis of an abnormality in a lab test, an X-ray shadow, or a biopsy specimen, with no clinical information to complement it, narrowly technical questions as to whether the test is relevant or its interpretation accurate tend to upstage the well-nigh irresistible tendency in either case to bully both doctor and patient into ever more numerous diagnostic and treatment procedures in the future, all of which conspire to bring about the reality, the suspicion, or at least the fear, that in retrospect appears to justify the concern. Always in the name of greater precision, obsessive reliance on diagnostic testing in reality tends to propagate an unending cycle of further doubt, uncertainty, fear, and confusion in everyone concerned, that multiplies exponentially and across the board both the probability and the risk of still further interventions within the system.

This preconscious and virtually automatic response also proceeds in tandem with the proliferation of medical specialties and subspecialties, each with its own full complement of diseases, some old, some new, and many overlapping with those of various colleagues, as the finite amount of physiological space is assigned and parceled out among them. Once fields are mapped out, and a limited degree of mastery attained, disproportionate attention is similarly paid to early signs and harbingers of disease, as we have seen, and our seemingly limitless fixation on normalizing them.

Thus endocrinologists, internists, and family physicians all frequently or semi-routinely check for "subclinical hypothyroidism," high TSH levels indicating diminished thyroid function, despite normal T_4 and other thyroid hormone levels, and no signs and symptoms of overt illness, although they may differ considerably about the threshold of such abnormality and the need to correct it. In the *American Family Physician,* for example, the official journal of the AAFP, or American Academy of Family Practice, the article "Subclinical Hypothyroidism: Deciding When to Treat" began with what seemed like a judicious compromise, but effortlessly morphed into a typical exhortation:

> While screening for thyroid disease, physicians often find increased TSH levels in patients whose free thyroxine (T_4) levels are normal. Termed "subclinical hypothyroidism," this state is most often an early stage of [clinical] hypothyroidism. Although the condition may resolve or remain unchanged, in some patients overt disease develops within a few years. The likelihood that this will happen increases with greater TSH levels and detectable antithyroid antibodies. Because patients with subclinical hypothyroidism sometimes have subtle symptoms and mild abnormalities of cardiac function and serum lipoproteins, patients with definite and persistent TSH elevation should be considered for thyroid treatment.[19]

Another gynecological application is the familiar Papanicolau or "Pap" smear, based on the common observation that cervical dysplasia may sometimes progress to carcinoma *in situ,* and even to invasive cancer of the cervix. The prompt and predictable result of this disarmingly simple and seemingly innocuous procedure has been a schedule of frequent, routine repetitions, leading to epidemics of colposcopies, cone biopsies, and a spectrum of even more invasive treatments, for a disease that was already a major cause of death and morbidity, but with the labeling of dysplasia as a pre-cancerous state, began to loom even larger. It required decades of such aggressive surveillance for cooler heads to acknowledge that, even though the U. S. death rate from cervical cancer declined by 62% between 1965 and 1988,[20] this laudable result was achieved at the expense of subjecting tens of millions of healthy women with mild and moderate dysplasia to colposcopy, cone biopsy, and hysterectomy, in spite of the fact that such pathology reverted to normal in most cases if simply allowed to do so,[21] a largely unpublicized fact which disproved the assumption that it was a pre-cancerous lesion to begin with. Here again, a similar pattern is discernible:

1) the identification of a subclinical abnormality as a hypothetical precursor of overt disease in the future;

2) the adoption of a preventive strategy of close surveillance and aggressive treatment of the abnormality; and

3) the long-delayed finding, requiring the most painstaking scholarship and the courage to speak out against the tide, that the abnormality in question represents essentially a normal variant, such that the true risk factor must be a concomitant variable, either invisible or in some cases an artifact of the surveillance itself.

A Disease for Every Pill.

It is no longer surprising, mysterious, or unknown to the public that the relentless pressure and at times fanatical zeal for preventive screening and the early detection of subclinical abnormalities has been assiduously cultivated by the pharmaceutical industry, has proceeded in parallel with the development of new drugs designed to correct them, and thus provides a built-in marketing strategy both before and after the fact.

This was already evident in the decades-old crusade against high blood pressure, beginning with the introduction of thiazide drugs on a large scale in the 1950's.

As several new generations of drugs were developed, the disease itself has been redefined, including lower and lower thresholds of abnormal diastolic pressure, as we saw. New and ever more aggressive treatment protocols, directed against even mildly elevated or borderline pressures, have required subjecting an ever increasing proportion of the entire adult population to lifetime drug maintenance, with the result, according to some studies, of somewhat lower incidence and morbidity of heart attacks and strokes, but also the exact opposite in many cases, where the drop in blood pressure proved excessive,[22] and with no clear or fixed boundary between therapeutic and dangerously low levels.

Once again, the felt need for more and more aggressive treatment, in this case largely generated by the drug industry, subliminally persuaded doctors to broaden their definition of the disease itself. Notwithstanding the measured scruples and conscientious warnings of senior clinicians, the impetus for preventive screening today enjoys almost unchallenged supremacy in medicine, recognizing few if any restrictions beyond the limits of the drug industry's own fevered and well-funded imagination.

How far afield it can lead is illustrated by the current fashion of routine cholesterol screening in young children, partly inspired by a legitimate concern about widespread obesity both before and after puberty, and promoted to lower the risk of atherosclerosis, heart attacks, and strokes in their mature years. In a disclaimer issued by a joint task force of the AMA, the AAFP, and the American Academy of Pediatrics, the American medical establishment stopped just short of mandating such tests for all children, but did recommend targeted screening for many tens of millions with "high-risk" parents, according to the same criteria that have long been part of the conventional wisdom for adults:

> Of the leading risk factors for coronary heart disease, 25% of children have total serum cholesterol levels above 170 mg./dl. Autopsies of children dying from other causes have found that aortic fatty streaks correlate with total cholesterol and LDL levels. Children with high cholesterol are also at risk of having high levels as adults. Many children with high cholesterol do not maintain high levels as adults, and the safety and effectiveness of treating

high cholesterol has not been established. We therefore do not recommend universal cholesterol screening in children.

But children older than 2 years with a parent whose total cholesterol is 240 or higher should be screened, as should those with a parent or grandparent who had a documented MI, angina, peripheral or cerebrovascular disease, sudden cardiac death, or atherosclerosis at 55 or younger, or had coronary bypass surgery or angioplasty. Screening may also be indicated if the family history is unobtainable and risk factors are present. The Canadian Task Force holds that there is insufficient evidence to recommend routine screening in children and adolescents and that individual judgment should be exercised.[23]

Although further doubts continue to be raised about the validity of cholesterol screening even for adults, statins and other cholesterol-lowering drugs still hit the jackpot among the top-selling drugs in history. Yet an article in *Medical World News* many years ago reported serious and even fatal consequences from lowering the serum cholesterol below 160 mg./dl., a level previously thought optimal:

Some leading heart researchers are calling for a change in the nation's cholesterol policy, including a retreat from universal screening and treatment of high cholesterol to prevent heart disease. In an editorial in the journal *Circulation,* Dr. Stephen Hulley and his colleagues at UCSF wrote that the 6% of middle-aged adults with cholesterol below 160 mg./dl. are at increased risk of dying from lung and other non-colon cancer, respiratory and digestive disease, trauma, hemorrhagic stroke, and other causes, and concluded, "The overriding ethical obligation is to do no harm. Especially when considering the long-term use of drugs for people in good health, the burden of proof falls on the proponents of intervention.[24]

As diseases are broadened, multiplied, and redefined in accordance with the drug industry's commercial priorities, even normal physiological processes become fair game for manipulation, as new abnormalities are identified, new drugs developed to correct them, and new "diseases" created after the fact as an appropriate marketing strategy. One of the best-known examples is the exploitation of menopause, beginning innocuously with the short-term use of estrogens to relieve hot flashes and other symptoms, but quickly progressing to X-ray detection of osteoporosis and "osteopenia," or low bone density at an earlier stage, and ultimately to prescribing estrogenic hormones routinely and for many years to countless millions of women, in order to prevent hip and spinal fractures, cardiovascular disease, dementia, and a host of other common ailments of middle and later life.

The unprecedented scale of this sales pitch, and the new diagnosis that appeared to justify it, goaded Susan Love into writing another eloquent and timely dissent, "Sometimes Mother Nature Knows Best," in which she spoke out clearly and forcefully against the practice of long-term hormone replacement therapy, and the commodification of the female life cycle itself, as a fit target for the drug industry, and its self-serving redefinition of menopause, as if it were a disease requiring treatment:

> The pharmaceutical industry and the medical profession have discovered a new disease: menopause, or estrogen-deficiency disease. Women with hysterectomies may want to take hormones until the natural age of menopause, while others have troubling symptoms like hot flashes and insomnia that warrant treatment. No one argues that short-term use is dangerous. But the push is on to use these drugs long-term, in the name of "disease prevention." The American College of Obstetrics and Gynecology (ACOG) recommends that every post-menopausal woman should be on hormones for life unless she has a compelling reason not to be.
>
> This sweeping recommendation is based on inadequate evidence. Menopause is no disease, but a normal part of life. A woman's ovaries don't shut down: they continue to produce hormones well into her 80's. Synthetic hormones don't replace something that is missing, but add something that is not naturally there. Pharmaceutical companies realize that for marketing it is smarter to emphasize diseases than hormones. In this they are helped by the medical profession, which has recently redefined osteoporosis. The term once referred only to actual fractures caused by the thin bones of old women, but now it is defined as low bone density. This is like telling someone with high cholesterol that they have heart disease.
>
> Women are encouraged to have bone density tests just the same as mammograms or Pap smears. The result is an epidemic of healthy 50-year-old women being diagnosed with osteoporosis, even though women on average don't have hip fractures until they turn 79. Someone once said that if you're healthy, you haven't hadenough tests done yet. We need accurate information, and must be on guard, lest vested interests sell us a bill of goods.[25]

It is noteworthy that Dr. Love wrote this article solely on methodological grounds, years before the extra cases of breast cancer finally discredited long-term estrogen therapy and confirmed what many had long suspected but did not oppose publicly. Unfortunately, her arguments went unheeded for so long that the manufacturers' enormous profits were unaffected, and when hormone-replacement therapy finally did go out of fashion, the conquest of menopause continued uninterruptedly, according to a thoroughly predictable sequence. By then the industry had already produced and marketed a new generation of even more potent and dangerous drugs, the biphosphonates, with the aid of which it similarly claims to prevent fractures by increasing the bone density, but this time by playing with the critical and still poorly-understood mechanism of bone formation, and with calcium and phosphorus metabolism in particular, which influence and therefore potentially threaten the structural integrity of the body as a whole. It would of course be unfair to deny or fail to mention that much of scientific value is learned along the way.

The wholesale repetition of this entirely predictable sequence led Bernard Lown, the prominent cardiologist and Nobel Prize-winning humanitarian, to question the need for early diagnosis in all its forms, and the almost limitless multiplication of diseases that it entails:

> Medicine has expanded into almost all facets of human existence, including conditions that do not cause symptoms or impair life, but indicate potential illness in the future, such as high blood pressure, blood sugar, cholesterol, osteoporosis, colon polyps, heart murmurs, carotid artery narrowing, memory loss, and sun exposure: the list is constantly expanding. One may reasonably anticipate that such risk factors will be recognized even earlier in life, at birth, *in utero,* or even before conception. Should everyone be screened? Everyone is tied to the medical establishment from birth, resulting in preoccupation with survival, rather than the challenge of creative living.[26]

One unavoidable by-product of this tendency is some kind of compendium of officially recognized diseases and subtypes, such as the prodigious ICD-9 Classification, a book and software database, which runs to hundreds of densely-packed pages, lists tens of thousands of pathological diagnoses, each one numerically coded, and is updated annually, as new diseases are identified, and old ones renamed or eliminated. Even the most cursory examination of this monstrosity leaves no doubt that most of the entries are merely technical abnormalities, adopted purely for administrative and taxonomic purposes, without the slightest pretense of referring to a dynamic process that could help us understand the lived experience of our patients.

6. The Patient as Pathological Specimen.

Reducing illness to disease also harms patients in an indirect but even more fundamental way, which I have not directly addressed, but is implicit in what I have already said. Without regard for the individuals who suffer from it, studying a disease process in the abstract tends to reduce the patient to a mere specimen, and his or her actual experience to an *automatism,* a self-propelling chain of necessary causes, which also seems pre-programmed to *worsen,* because the corresponding tendency of every patient with every illness to *recover* depends upon idiosyncratic variables within the individual that are rendered invisible, mysterious, or simply irrelevant by the disease concept, and simply fall through the cracks, rarely if ever to be seen or thought of again.

By thus ignoring and indeed obscuring the self-healing capacity of the patient, modern medicine repeatedly undermines and defeats the seamless integrity, resilience, and restorative power of life itself, whatever we choose to call it, precisely because it is global, indivisible, and therefore resistant to definition, quantification, or analysis into separate parts, even when we remember to look for it. Once we fall ill, or are labeled as a specimen of a disease, whether in the present or the future, it is difficult not to feel overawed, intimidated, and even compelled to accept such pathology as *given,* to surrender ourselves to what we suppose or are told to be *its* laws, and to forget that every illness must also be *received* by the patient, and expressed by each of us in our own way, such that whatever factors may have influenced our getting sick in the first place are just as likely to help us recover in the future. Because the reality and even the concept of self-healing have been largely hidden from view, and are therefore unfamiliar to most people in most situations, the idea of chronic disease, in particular, includes nothing but its tendency to persist and get *worse,* and hence seems to require an aggressive strategy of treatment, to control it insofar as possible.

The concept of objectified or reified disease processes similarly distorts and trivializes both case management and prognosis, by reducing the difficult art of treatment to the technology of forcibly correcting the abnormalities used to define them, by killing the TB bacilli, selectively destroying the cancer cells, normalizing the blood pressure, and so forth. In the same way that histologically "cured" cancer patients who develop cachexia and aplastic anemia as a result of their chemotherapy may be at least as sick as before, these crude oversimplifications leave a dangerous ambiguity in the assessment of improvement and worsening, indeed in the definition of the disease itself.

Thus patients who develop a severe or intractable illness following apparently successful treatment of another illness pose a critical dilemma that cannot be solved or even meaningfully stated within the concept of the disease process. For whether or not the two conditions are said to be *related* to each other, the patient will still require a separate diagnosis and treatment for each of them, and there is still no meaningful way to address the condition of the individual as a living whole, an integrated bioenergetic system that evolves and develops through time. In either case, the net effect of medical science as a *philosophy* or conceptual system is always simply to multiply exponentially and across the board the number of diseases, abnormalities, and diagnostic and treatment procedures to be comprehended within it, through its awesome power to subdivide the living patient into ever more numerous identifiable and potentially controllable phenomena.

7. Diagnosis as Truth and Falsehood.

It would of course be unjust to dwell on the authentic defects and limitations of routine screening tests without also acknowledging the numerous instances where our patients would have died or suffered far worse had they *not* been done. Just such a patient came to see me recently, as I was finishing up this article, and congratulating myself on having demolished the established concept of preventing various specific diseases in healthy patients without illness or symptoms.

An attractive divorcée with two young children who had been my patient for several years arrived one day, quite distraught and sobbing uncontrollably, after a routine Pap smear found a large number of what

338

her gynecologist described as "highly abnormal and suspicious cells," and for which the latter recommended complete hysterectomy -- removal of the uterus, ovaries, Fallopian tubes, and even the vagina and regional lymph nodes -- even though and indeed precisely because she felt entirely well, had no other complaints or symptoms, and ultrasound, colposcopy, and endometrial biopsy had all failed to detect a localized tumor mass to account for them.

Consulting another gynecologist for a second opinion at my request, she learned that the original smear actually read "adenocarcinoma, type undetermined," which explained why immediate action was called for, as well as why her own doctor had lied that she *didn't* have cancer, and had urgently insisted on the surgery as a 100% effective way of preventing the near-certainty of it in the future.

In short, hers seemed to be precisely the test case I had envisioned earlier, a life-changing decision made solely on the basis of what cells looked like under a microscope, with as yet no symptoms or illness for them to explain. Yet whatever the differences among us as to the exact interpretation of these findings, or what we thought the wisest course for her to follow, all of us, her two specialists, the patient herself, and even I, seemingly contrary to what I had just written, accepted the provisional *truth* of this report as signifying a very high probability of serious, life-threatening illness in the near future, and agreed on the urgency for some kind of active and timely intervention to try to save her life, or at least to buy her as much time as possible for continuing to parent her twins as she sees fit. By that calculus, neither she nor I had the slightest doubt that her diagnosis was accurate, useful, and indeed supremely valuable to her, however grim and terrible the news it brought, and although the action it called for will almost certainly be disfiguring or worse.

As this by no means rare example makes clear, preventive screening tests and procedures continue to earn a central place in modern diagnosis, and cannot be dismissed *a priori* on purely ideological grounds, even when no signs and symptoms of illness are manifest. As to when they are most likely to be helpful, harmful, or merely distracting, the doubts and scruples I have just cited may help to redefine the circumstances under which the added information they provide may be judged as true, false, or uncertain, and even what we mean by these heavily loaded words.

The example of my patient is especially instructive in an additional sense, because the Pap smear is widely regarded as inadequate for detecting frank or invasive cancer, so that the presence of unequivocally malignant cells was already sufficiently unusual to alarm every doctor and technician who saw them, while the absence of well-differentiated cell types left open the possibility of ovarian cancer, statistically the most dangerous kind, and called for immediate action just to rule it out. Under these ominous circumstances, not least because she felt well and had no symptoms, the test helped to convince my patient that she already had or would soon develop a life-threatening illness, and that drastic action was imperative to arrest or forestall it.

Finally, the rather high degree of integrity of the various possible disease processes, that is, of vaginal, cervical, endometrial, tubal, ovarian, and bladder cancer, respectively, was also an important component of the urgency for further diagnostic and surgical procedures to differentiate them, so that the only disagreements between the various players involved the ever-present issue of how best to balance the need for effective diagnosis and treatment with the patient's optimal comfort and quality of life. In short, the only ambiguity remaining in her case was the standard policy of screening all adult women.

But that is the whole point. Pap smears are done routinely to screen the entire adult female population, involving the detection of cervical dysplasia and other cellular abnormalities as risk factors for cancer of the cervix in the relatively distant future. Even its most zealous proponents would hesitate to advocate the procedure solely to catch the very few exceptional cases like my patient, and it is now widely known, as we saw, that mild and moderate dysplasia, while sometimes progressing to cancer after periods of months or years, most often revert to normal if simply left alone and allowed to do so. Charting a path somewhere between these two essentially uncontested truths suggests the reasonable and increasingly popular compromise of doing the test, yes, but then simply watching, waiting, and taking no further action unless the morphology spreads and worsens.

At least on the face of it, a similar strategy seems equally applicable to mass screening for cholesterol, blood pressure, bone density, and so forth, which are likewise designed to assess risk factors for particular

340

diseases and illnesses, for the most part in the relatively distant future. As with the Pap smear, the main problem with routine screening is not so much the discomfort of the procedure itself, but rather the pain, suffering, disability, and expense incurred by the further diagnostic tests and treatment procedures that they seem to make necessary. No competent physician would hesitate to recommend further testing and corrective action for those with abnormalities lying well outside the normal range, and thus indicative of something in the *present,* some illness as yet unsuspected and unperceived by either the patient or the doctor, but which a more detailed and extensive workup would probably reveal, and which the patient would want, expect, and be grateful to know about. Given a blood pressure of 180/110, a cholesterol over 300, a TSH of 15 or 20, a liver transaminase in the 400's, or a PSA of 20, few doctors would be content to dole out the usual drug without first trying to get to the bottom of these findings, to establish a more definite and comprehensive diagnosis, because all of them indicate authentic disease processes and indeed actual illnesses that are already under way, so that the pathology is very likely to illuminate, explain, and indeed to predict them. In this situation, such striking abnormalities and the diseases that they represent may both be considered real and true, in the same sense and to the same extent as the acute, subacute, and intermittent diseases we discussed earlier.

With "borderline" result, on the other hand, a slight deviation with at most possible significance in the distant future, it seems completely excessive and amounts to cruel and unusual punishment to inflict these largely arbitrary and ever-changing standards on otherwise healthy patients for years and decades of their lives, artificially forcing their test results back into line and holding them there, without compelling evidence of benefit to their general health and well-being from doing so, let alone due regard for the predictably adverse effects of the coercion itself. Simply being less zealous about *enforcing* such dubious diagnoses would save enormous sums in follow-up visits, drug costs, and the tests to monitor them, to say nothing of the anxiety that sustains them all, and would thereby help to reduce the size and weight of our famously bloated medical enterprise to a more nearly human scale.

Meanwhile, on the receiving end, so to speak, confronted by their own fear and hesitation on the one hand, and the vast knowledge and formidable power of the medical system on the other, our patients themselves provide a fitting epilogue in their profound desire, need, curiosity, and fascination to match up and integrate their own unique lived experience with the independent and profoundly alien version of the body as a machine, so blissfully or horribly anonymous and neutral. That is why it makes good sense, for medical as well as social, political, and ethical reasons, to order such tests for those patients who *want* them, whether we recommend them or not, and to build a patient-centered criterion into the system, even if it costs a little more, to allow patients to screen themselves, to allow their physicians to try to dissuade them when it seems appropriate, and thus to facilitate an ongoing negotiation about fine-tuning their care.

The high value and awesome power of a proper diagnosis for individual patients are nowhere more evident than in the remarkable growth and diversity of charities and support groups for those afflicted with diseases of every description, many recruiting informally through the Internet, and achieving major status and political clout through conferences, publications, fund drives, and research sponsorship. Although many individuals find it distasteful to be thus lumped together with people having little else in common, or to dwell on their diseases to the exclusion of pleasanter or more edifying topics, many others who suffer most intensely tend to find comfort, solidarity, and even personal truth in the company and fellowship of others similarly affected, at times attaining a level of peace and equanimity that would have hardly been possible otherwise. Still others are moved to social action, such as lobbying Congress to call attention to diseases that are new, controversial, or poorly understood, like Autism Spectrum and Asperger's Syndrome disorders, or to right a perceived wrong, such as the side effects of drugs, vaccines, toxins, chemicals, and additives. Precisely because they empower patients to find and speak their truth, however unreasonable or unpalatable it may seem to others, and thereby to participate more actively in a health care system that seems increasingly disinclined to listen, such groups deserve encouragement and support from physicians, no less than the public at large.

For all of these reasons, I can think of no wiser rule for our profession to live by than the one proclaimed by Hippocrates almost twenty-five hundred years ago:

Declare the past, diagnose the present, and foretell the future;
But as to diseases, let us try to help, or at least to do no harm.[27]

NOTES.

1. Bernard, Claude, *An Introduction to the Study of Experimental Medicine,* trans. H. C. Greene., Dover, New York, 1957, pp. 63-65, *passim.*
2. Bernard, *Principes de medicine expérimentale,* Paris, Presses Universitaires de France, 1947, p. 391, quoted in Canguilhem, Georges, *The Normal and the Pathological,* trans. C. Fawcett, Zone Books, New York, 1991, p. 71.
3. Spiro, H., "Delayed Diagnosis of Disease," *Journal of the AMA* 253:2258, 1985.
4. Kostis, J., "Treating Hypertension in the Very Old," *New England Journal of Medicine* 358:1958, 2008.
5. Moskowitz, R., "Vague, Long-Term Diagnosis: the *Nocebo* Effect," *Journal of the American Institute of Homeopathy* 76:26, 1983.
6. Oliver, M., "Risks of Correcting the Risks of Coronary Disease and Strokes with Drugs," *NEJM* 306:297, 1982.
7. Ibid.
8. Feinstein, A., et al., "Variability in Radiologists' Interpretations of Mammograms," *NEJM* 331:1493, 1994.
9. Ibid.
10. Love, Susan, "Fibrocystic 'Disease' of the Breast: a Non-Disease?" *NEJM* 307:1010, 1982.
11. Simon, H., "Diagnosing Prostate Cancer: the PSA," *The Harvard Medical School Guide to Men's Health,* Free Press, New York, 2002, p. 364.
12. Ibid.
13. Ibid., p. 365.
14. Ibid., p. 366.
15. Ibid.
16. Thompson, I., et al., "Prevalence of Prostate Cancer Among Men with a PSA Level at or below 4.0 ng. per Milliliter," *NEJM* 350:2239, 2004.
17. Ibid.
18. Kannell, W., and Abbott, R., "Incidence and Prognosis of Unrecognized Myocardial Infarction," *NEJM* 311:1144, 1984.
19. Adlin, V., "Subclinical Hypothyroidism: Deciding When to Treat," *American Family Physician,* February 1998, p. 776.
20. *Medical Tribune,* April 1992, p. 4.

21. Ibid.
22. *Medical World News,* August 1988, p. 51.
23. "Cholesterol Screening in Children," U. S. Public Health Service, *American Family Physician,* June 1995, p. 1923.
24. "Lipid Controversy Builds Up," *Medical World News,* October 1992, p. 15.
25. Love, Susan, "Sometimes Mother Nature Knows Best," *New York Times,* March 20, 1997, reprinted in the *Public Citizen Health Letter* 13:1, 1997.
26. Lown, Bernard, "The Commodification of Health Care," *Hastings Center Report,* September-October 2006, p. 42.
27. Hippocrates, *Epidemics,* Book I, Section 2, ¶xi.

Vaccines, Drugs, and Other Causes: A Homeopath Looks at the Medical System*

Today I want to speak about allopathic medicine, the kind we all grew up with and were trained in, a subject that homeopaths tend to find distasteful, having sacrificed more prominent and lucrative careers by rejecting major parts of it. Nevertheless, if only as moth to flame, I am irresistibly drawn to the subject for two main reasons. The first is personal, and has to do with why I became a homeopath in the first place, which was no dramatic cure that I witnessed or benefited from, but simply glaring inconsistencies in my medical training that troubled me on an intuitive level long before I could identify them. Practical dilemmas encountered on the wards of a large city hospital led me to question the values I was being taught, and to study philosophy before going into practice, bad habits that have shaped my career ever since, and deepened my sense of estrangement from the profession I still call my own. Well before I ever saw it work in a patient, I clung to homeopathy as to a life-preserver, because it gave me a method for doing what I was already trying to do, a coherent system of thought that still works and makes sense, and a practice of medicine that I could at last be proud of.

Thirty-six years of studying and applying it have only further convinced me that the homeopathic point of view and its systematic critique of medicine are even more pertinent today than when Hahnemann thought them through, a durability in pointed contrast to the system that nearly killed it, which gorges itself on a high-powered diet of rapid and constant change. Within a generation after the master's death, the allopathic school had already evolved into something that he would scarcely have recognized, while since World War II it has risen to become the dominant form of medicine and indeed the model of health care throughout the world.

---

* "Vaccines, Drugs, and Other Causes: a Homeopath Looks at the Medical System," *American Journal of Homeopathic Medicine* 103:214, Winter 2010, and 104:13, Spring 2011.

That is why I think we make a huge mistake in attributing our defeat and inferior status to some combination of allopathic persecution, our own internal divisions, and the public's inability to grasp our higher truths, however relevant these factors may have been. The elephant in the room that dwarfs them all is the mighty revolution in human thought that created medical science as we know it today, a transformation so stunning in its impact and so radical in its implications that "conventional medicine," our own tame, sanitized, and condescending term for it, is a mere euphemism for trivializing that achievement, if not the exact opposite of the truth.

This brings me to philosophy, the second reason for my talk, the purpose of which is to help us identify and articulate what we used to know but have somehow forgotten, and what we think we know but have never bothered to question. Here I use the term both in its ordinary meaning, that is, an inquiry into the most fundamental principles of a subject, and also in its narrower, more technical sense, of a methodology for fitting them together into a coherent system of thought, logically derived from a few simple axioms and postulates that cannot be proven or disproven within it, quite in the spirit of Bertrand Russell's whimsical definition:

> . . . the point of philosophy is to start with something so obvious as not to seem worth stating, and to end with something so paradoxical that no one will believe it.[1]

Classical homeopathy fits this description admirably, since its basic principles are all neatly laid out for us, beginning with the vital force and the totality of symptoms, both of which are essentially *truisms,* and the Law of Similars, which even Hahnemann admits is not wholly amenable to scientific proof,[2] but then giving rise to the single remedy, the minimum dose, the concept of miasm, and the Laws of Cure, all of which seem outlandish and even incredible to most people, yet follow from the first three as irresistibly as the night the day.

Allopathic medicine I find compelling for precisely the opposite reason, that it looks like and even purports to be a *non-system,* a bewildering array and profusion of techniques and procedures with an avowedly *anti*-philosophical stance, as if conspiring to keep its basic conceptual scheme

346

hidden from view and resistant to straightforward formulation. My task is thus to convince you of what its own practitioners are apt to deny, that allopathic medicine likewise rests upon an elaborate, pervasive, and well-defined conceptual system, but one so limiting in its methodology that we must look elsewhere for the tools to excavate and reconstruct it. That is why we owe it to *ourselves* as much as our allopathic colleagues to understand what they do and how they think, and to identify the underlying principles and assumptions that they themselves are reluctant to acknowledge.

Since the allopathic system has also contributed so much of lasting value, and in any case is clearly here to stay, my subject also looks far beyond itself, to a more open and inclusive conceptual scheme that can accommodate both points of view, and maybe even others as yet unknown to us. Helping to envision, identify, and elaborate this new synthesis is therefore our highest mission, which we share with like-minded physicians and healers of all persuasions, and in every part of the world.

1. Is It Really a *System?*

Attempting to identify and characterize the philosophy of allopathic medicine as a whole begins with the obvious question, whether this vast enterprise, which has no general philosophy of health and disease, and no *desire* for any, can fairly be thought of as a system at all. Among the clearest and most emphatic declarations that it cannot and should not be we owe to Claude Bernard, the great French physiologist of the Nineteenth Century, who clearly envisioned and helped bring about so much of what modern medicine has since become:

> Neither physiologists nor physicians must imagine it their task to seek the cause of life or the essence of disease. That would be entirely wasting one's time in pursuing a phantom. *The words '"life," "death," "health," and "disease" have no objective reality.* When a physiologist invokes the "vital force," he does not see it; he merely pronounces a word. *Only the vital phenomenon exists, with its material conditions: that is the one thing that he can study and know* [Italics mine: R.M.].[3]

Since medicine has indeed become an empirical science based largely on experiment, it sounds reasonable enough to suppose that it would have no further need of any fixed dogma, ideology, or philosophy to adhere

347

to, and would forfeit nothing of value by their absence. Yet today both homeopaths and allopaths, doctors and patients alike, ordinarily think and speak of medicine as if it *did* constitute a system of some kind, while a broad, informal consensus does appear to exist at all levels of society about what sorts of things belong to it, and what others, including various forms of "alternative medicine," lie beyond the pale, although the boundary between them keeps changing all the time.

A similar demarcation is evident in the existence of the "medical underground," that extensive, thriving counter-culture, with its own industries and even a black market to support it, populated by those suffering from various conditions and the innumerable patient advocacy groups created on their behalf, and extensively promoted over the Internet and elsewhere. All of these evidently spontaneous developments point to a clear or at least commonly accepted distinction between the diagnostic and treatment procedures, drugs, surgeries, and other technologies that are endorsed by the medical "establishment," and the almost equally populous and elaborate universe of everything else which is *not*.

But the most conclusive evidence is the nature and extent of the medical community itself, those numberless legions of students, physicians-in-training, teachers and mentors, practicing and attending physicians, specialists, physician-assistants, nurse-practitioners, nurses, hospital employees, lab assistants, technicians, and research scientists, backed up by the vast medical-industrial complex of institutions and corporations that serve them by developing new procedures and manufacturing drugs and equipment, all of which occupy such an inordinate share of our economic and cultural life, and continue to grow and multiply exponentially, without effective regulation or restraint. Like a colossal ant colony, with satellites, branches, and spin-offs on a global scale, this self-replicating nexus of goods and services could not continue to function, let alone propagate itself down through the generations, if its diverse members did not know how to perform their assigned rôles, and understand their relationships with superiors, colleagues, and subordinates. The mere existence of a collective enterprise on such a scale clearly presupposes a basic conceptual scheme to hold it all together, to define these rôles, create these positions, and train the individuals who will eventually fill them.

If we think of the medical system as an elaborate, interlocking institutional structure, it is much easier to grasp that the conceptual glue holding it all together has less to do with its particular *content,* which varies considerably from one part of the system to another, than its shared *methodology,* the rules, techniques, and procedures governing the basic sciences of anatomy, physiology, biochemistry, microbiology, pathology, and the like, with their applications to the various clinical specialties. Taken together, these guidelines specify how we can acquire valid and useful scientific knowledge about living beings, and what other kinds of investigation are to be avoided.

Although our modern paradigm did not become dominant until the emergence of microscopic anatomy and analytic chemistry in the latter half of the Nineteenth Century, its essence was already clearly discernible in the work of the Renaissance anatomists, and immortalized in Rembrandt's masterpiece, *Dr. Tulp's Anatomy Lesson,*[4] which celebrates the same genre of causal thinking that modern physicians still use in diagnosis today.

After dissecting and exposing the forearm muscles of the cadaver, the noted Professor places his clamp on the common sheath of the flexor tendons and savors the anticipation on the faces of his students at the moment before he pulls back on the clamp, and the stone-cold fingers obediently rise again in response to it.

The revolutionary concept of mechanical causality exemplified by these discoveries, which inspired great painters like Leonardo and Michelangelo to traffic in stolen bodies in order to explore them first-hand, received perhaps its classic formulation two centuries later, once again in the words of Claude Bernard, who elegantly summarizes the scientific truths we still live by in medicine today:

> What we call the immediate cause of a phenomenon is nothing but the physical and material condition in which it exists or appears. The object of the experimental method, and the limit of every scientific research, is therefore the same for living as for inanimate bodies: it consists in finding the relations which connect a phenomenon with its immediate cause, or, to put it differently, in defining the conditions necessary to the appearance of the phenomenon. *When the experimenter succeeds in learning the necessary conditions of a phenomenon, he is in some sense its master: he can predict its course and appearance; he can promote or prevent it at will.* We shall

therefore define physiology as the science whose object is to study the phenomena of living beings, and to determine the material conditions in which they appear [Italics mine: R. M.].[5]

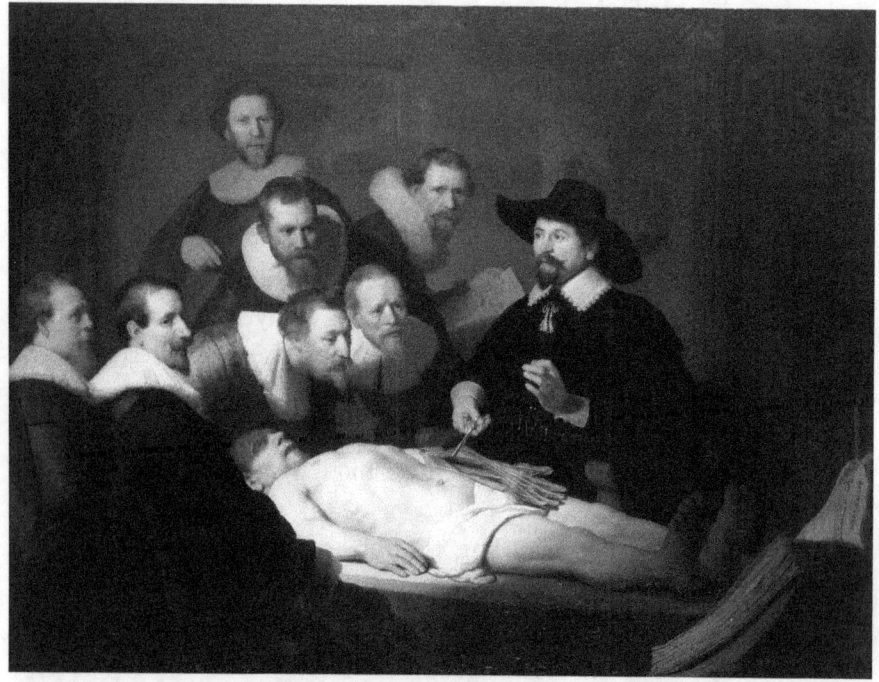

Rembrandt van Rijn, Dr. Tulp's Anatomy Lesson, 1632, Mauritshuis, The Hague, Netherlands.

No longer content merely to heal the sick, contemporary medicine is driven above all to achieve effective dominion and control over every identifiable aspect of the life process. What Bernard foresaw and his successors still routinely seek to accomplish is to acquire the knowledge and devise the means to regulate biological phenomena artificially and more or less at will, on the assumption that our prior, more subjective goals will eventually follow. Now as then, the experimental method in human biology still consists of the same simple steps:

1) characterizing the phenomenon to be studied;

2) identifying its component parts;

3) isolating its physicochemical "causes;" and

4) devising appropriate technologies for manipulating them,

5) with as little disturbance as possible to the remainder of the organism.

In another brilliant passage, Bernard understood with perfect clarity that the path to scientific knowledge in medicine lies in number, quantification, and measurement, no less than in physics and chemistry:

> Health and disease are not two essentially different modes, as the ancient practitioners believed. These are obsolete medical ideas. *In reality, between these two modes there are differences only of degree: exaggeration, disproportion, and discordance of normal phenomena constitute the diseased state.* [Italics mine: R. M.][6]

Easily overlooked in these statements is their important subtext, that whatever *cannot* be subdivided, objectified, and quantified in such ways need not and should not be studied at all, since it cannot as yet be defined rigorously or thus understood in any useful or meaningful sense. I now realize that I became a homeopath in part to reinstate the subjective aspects of human experience that have been demoted and largely banished from medical practice. Much as I admire and still try to achieve the careful reasoning and yogic discipline that experimental science requires, I cannot accept a philosophy of healing the sick that seeks to override the individuality of the patient and the beauty and richness of human life that emanate from it.

In what follows, I will argue that this sin of omission is also inherently dangerous to the patient, not only because it makes human error more likely and more serious, and is very likely to fail or fall short, but also and especially when its prized objectives are successfully attained. For no matter how noble its motives and how favorable its outcome, the ambition to control life processes by force automatically creates insoluble ethical and practical dilemmas that go a long way toward explaining the current crisis in our embattled, dysfunctional, and badly mis-named "health-care" system.

2. Hidden in Plain Sight: Adverse Reactions to Vaccines.

I will start with the example of vaccines, a subject which I have thought about for most of my career, not least because the United States *requires* them of all children to an extent that is unparalleled in the developed world, a circumstance that dramatizes and gives real immediacy to the same problem I have been speaking of. The vague unease I have always felt about mandating them began to make more sense when I became interested in homeopathic medicine, which reminded me of the obvious but unremembered truth that medicines have the power to elicit a totality or *array* of symptoms, not just the one we happen to be interested in at the moment. In contrast, vaccines need achieve just two limited and predefined goals to be deemed effective, namely,

1) a significant reduction in the incidence of the corresponding natural disease, and

2) a measurable titer of specific antibodies in the blood.

But *how* they achieve these results -- their actual mechanism of action -- and whatever *else* they do along the way, are not thought to be interesting questions, or in any case are rarely talked about. How much this simple schema leaves out is evident in the tale of a 10-year-old boy who developed the nephrotic syndrome soon after his MMR vaccination. One of the clearest and most obvious examples of an adverse reaction that I am personally acquainted with, it was nevertheless adamantly denied to be so by every one of the doubtless sincere and well-meaning physicians who cared for him. Although he lived nearly a thousand miles away, and I know of him solely from his mother's letter, her words were so heartfelt and so congruent with the rest of my experience that I cannot imagine them to be anything but the honest truth:

My son Adam was healthy until his first MMR at 15 months. Within 2 weeks he had flu and cold symptoms, which persisted for 6 weeks, at which point his eyes became puffy, he was hospitalized with nephrotic syndrome, and a renal biopsy showed "focal sclerosing glomerulonephritis." When it didn't respond to steroids, I asked if it could be related to the vaccine, but they told me it couldn't, and we accepted that. Over the next 4 years he was hospitalized repeatedly, and missed many months of school, but finally went into total remission, seeming normal and healthy and staying off all medications for about 5 years.

When he turned 10, his pediatrician recommended a booster, saying that a rise in measles cases made it dangerous for him not to be protected. Checking the PDR and other sources, I found no contraindication for kidney disease and no listing of nephrosis as a possible adverse reaction, so I agreed to it. In less than 2 weeks he relapsed, with 4+ protein in his urine, swelling, and weight gain, signs that we recognized immediately. He got worse even on Prednisone, and was admitted in hypertensive crisis, with blood in his urine, fluid in his lungs, and massive edema. On Cytoxan, high doses of Prednisone, and three other drugs, he slowly improved, but missed another 7 months of school.

It's been 2 years since that horrible episode, and he still needs Captopril daily for high blood pressure and spills 4+ protein every day. The doctor says that he sustained major kidney damage, will always need medication to control his blood pressure, and will worsen as he grows older, necessitating a transplant eventually. This time I was sure that his condition was related to the vaccine, but still the doctors didn't take me seriously, and told me it was a coincidence.

I began searching for information, and even contacted the manufacturer of the vaccine. Finally they sent me two almost identical case reports of nephrotic syndrome following the MMR vaccine. It's difficult for laypeople to get information or even ask questions, since we don't use correct medical terms and are made to feel stupid. Please tell me if my ideas are reasonable.

I don't think my son could tolerate another episode, and I think he'd have normal blood pressure and kidney function today if not for that second vaccination. I also have a great concern for other children who develop nephrotic syndrome some weeks after receiving the MMR and whose doctors never make the connection. They could all be at great risk if revaccinated. I realize that this letter has taken up a great deal of your time, and I'd appreciate any help you can give me. If we were closer, I'd make an appointment to see you in person, so please feel free to charge me. Thank you.[7]

This woman no longer doubted that her son's life had been ruined and indeed cut short by the vaccine, yet had no thought of suing the drug company that made it, the doctor who prescribed it, or the Federal Vaccine Injury Compensation Program (VICP), as she was legally entitled to do, a lack of ulterior motive that only lends further credence to her story. She wrote solely for independent validation of what she had witnessed first-hand on two separate occasions and had been forced to endure the consequences of ever since, a causal link that would be obvious to any eighth-grader of average intelligence. Yet even when the vaccine manufacturer belatedly provided two almost identical cases of their own, each of the boy's physicians independently and without hesitation continued to dismiss his misfortune as a coincidence. Today, almost twenty years later, renal failure has still not been recognized as an adverse effect of the MMR vaccine, an omission that would also have assured the boy's defeat in court, had his mother chosen that route. This glaring discrepancy between the boy's catastrophic illness and the ease with which the doctors and vaccine manufacturers escaped having to take any responsibility for it will serve to introduce the profound mystery that inspires my talk today.

According to the official guidelines, damages from a vaccine merit compensation only if they can be shown to be a necessary and predictable effect of that particular agent. With one or two exceptions, all of the listed complications are sudden, acute, and catastrophic *events* that appear full-blown within hours or at most a few days after the vaccine and result in death or permanent injury. The classic example is anaphylaxis, which oddly enough can occur after *any* vaccine, and thus has no specificity whatsoever.

Reportable Events Following Vaccination:[8]

Vaccine or Toxoid	Event	Interval (Post-Vaccine)
DTP, Pertussis,	Anaphylaxis, shock	24 hours
DPT & Polio,	Encephalopathy	7 days
DT, Tetanus Toxoid	Shock, collapse, hypotonia	7 days
	Acute complications or sequelæ	No limit
MMR	Anaphylaxis, shock	24 hours
	SSPE (encephalopathy)	15 days
Oral Polio (OPV)	Paralytic poliomyelitis	30 days
Inactivated Polio (IPV)	Anaphylaxis, shock	24 hours

As for *chronic* conditions, only two have ever occurred with sufficient frequency to be considered seriously for inclusion, namely, "DPT encephalopathy" and "autism," both of which tend to appear somewhat more gradually, with a time lag of days or weeks after the vaccine, and to follow a chronic course, like ongoing, self-sustaining *illnesses*. In both cases, physicians advocating compulsory vaccination, many with financial and other ties to the industry, have succeeded in keeping them off the list, or at least tightening the eligibility rules so drastically that almost all damage claims against them are defeated, however catastrophic the outcome.

"DPT encephalopathy" achieved considerable notoriety in the 1980's, when thousands of brain-damaged children won large court awards or settlements against the manufacturers, and this broad, nondescript entity was reluctantly accepted as a *bona fide* complication of the triple vaccine, particularly its whole-cell pertussis component. Here is a typical case, sent to me by the lawyer who represented him, involving a 3-year-old boy who reacted badly to his first DPT shot and suffered permanent brain damage after the second:

> Our firm represents a child who was born normal and healthy in every way. After his first DPT at 6 weeks, he began falling off growth charts, exhibited multiple developmental delays, and was diagnosed as "failure to thrive," but then slowly began to recover. At 5 months he received a second DPT, and his delays became much more extreme. He has never recovered. He is now 3 years old, with the mental capacity of an infant of a year and a half. I am convinced that his problems came about as a result of the DPT. In view of what happened after the first shot, he should not have had the second, or at least the pertussis component of it.[9]

While the information provided was very limited, the boy's serious and prolonged reaction to his first DPT, from which he eventually recovered, should have warned and indeed *did* warn his pediatrician against giving him the second, but it was merely postponed for a few months. This tragic pattern of a warning ignored -- a lesser version of the same illness with eventual recovery, followed by death or irreversible brain damage after a subsequent vaccination -- helped fuel a major public uproar, in response to which Congress passed the Vaccine Injury Compensation Act of 1986, which created a Federal reporting system and no-fault hearings for *all* vaccine injuries, and authorized compensation for damages at taxpayers' expense when vaccines were shown to have been at fault. In reality, however, the effect was just the opposite, a precipitous decline in the number and size of awards, a further tightening of the guidelines, and a vigorous counterattack by physicians of the vaccine establishment like this one, who rejected even the *concept* of DPT encephalopathy as essentially a coincidence:

> Dr. [Edward] Mortimer's article is the third controlled study in recent months to examine the risk of seizures and other acute neurological illnesses after the DPT. In these studies, involving 230,000 children and 713,000 vaccinations, no evidence of a causal relationship was found between the vaccine and permanent neurological illness. *It is clear from these recent studies that the major problem has been the failure to separate sequences from consequences.* Now is the last decade of the 20th Century, and it's time for the myth of "DPT encephalopathy" to end! [Italics mine: R. M.][10]

By 1996, with the scandal largely contained, the CDC and its Advisory Committee on Immunization Practices (ACIP), led by the same coterie of physician-advocates, published its official Report on DPT Encephalopathy. Rather more judicious in tone, this policy document briefly acknowledged the fact of ruined lives, but then blithely concocted three distinct levels of possible causal influence, concluded that it was impossible to tell them apart, and jumbled them all together into a tangle of obfuscations, equivocations, and government bureaucratese:

> Rare but serious neurological illnesses, including encephalitis, encephalopathy, and prolonged convulsions, have been anecdotally reported following the whole-cell DPT. *Whether the vaccine causes such illnesses or is only coincidentally related to them has been difficult to determine precisely.*

> The National Childhood Encephalopathy Study and others have provided evidence that the DPT can cause encephalopathy. This occurs rarely, but children who had a serious neurological event after DPT were significantly more likely than their controls to have chronic CNS dysfunction 10 years later and to have been given the DPT within 7 days of its onset.

> The Committee proposed three possible explanations for this association:
> 1) the illness and dysfunction could have been *caused* by DPT;
> 2) the DPT could *trigger* these events in children with brain or metabolic abnormalities who might also experience them if other stimuli such as fever or infection are present; and

3) the DPT might cause the acute event in children with underlying abnormalities that would inevitably have led to the chronic dysfunction even without it.

The data do not support any one explanation over the others. The balance of evidence was consistent with a causal relationship between the DPT and CNS diseases in children who developed acute neurological illness after the vaccine, but insufficient to determine whether it increases the overall risk of them 10 years later. SIDS is listed on death certificates as cause of death for 5000-6000 infants each year in the United States. Because the peak incidence is at 2-4 months of age, many instances of a close temporal relationship between the DPT and SIDS are to be expected by simple chance [Italics mine: R.M.].[11]

The ACIP Report gives lip service to the *possibility* of a chronic reaction, but only if the vaccine *forces* it to occur: the only type of "cause" that it allows is one powerful enough to compel the desired effect to occur in a preponderance of cases, using the same standard that Claude Bernard had proposed so long ago. According to the Report, DPT encephalopathy falls well short of it, because the authors claimed they could not distinguish between patients victimized or passively acted upon and those with pre-existing tendencies to react in the same way, either to a *precipitating* cause in those already mildly or potentially ill, or merely to one *incidental* cause among many other possibilities in those predestined to get sick.

In other words, to be recognized and compensated as such, victims must prove the absence of any pre-existing tendency to react in such ways, in spite of the fact that

1) it is famously difficult to prove a negative, and in clinical practice it is almost impossible to imagine a situation where we could know that someone is *fated* or predestined to become ill in the future;

2) *almost every illness in every patient requires both external morbid influences and individuals sensitized or at least receptive to them*; and

3) even the experts admit that they can't tell the difference.

Simply by *postulating* an ambiguity to dismiss the concept of "DPT encephalopathy," the ACIP Report also comes perilously close to disqualifying every other such claimant, both now and in the future, implying not only that *there aren't any other adverse reactions out there,* but even that *there can't be any,* by quietly relying the on same truism that their strict notion of mechanical causality had previously been invoked to rule out, that such individualizing tendencies are invariably present after all.

The Report is equally inconsistent for a second reason, that almost all of the adverse reactions that the ACIP and the courts *do* allow are acute *events,* which are extremely rare, and clearly involve a very high degree of predisposition, as we saw. On both counts, it defies ordinary experience, simple logic, and common sense to try to restrict the term "cause" to a fixed quantum of force achieving the same effect in most of the people subjected to it, when the only situations in which that standard seems usefully applicable are emergencies, like surgery, car accidents, gunshot wounds, and other traumatic injuries, or anatomic dissection of dead bodies, since they at least are no longer susceptible.

But its most important flaw is at the other end, in its *conclusion,* since even an innate or pre-existing tendency to react in a certain way by no means absolves vaccines of *some* level of causal rôle in the outcome. In any of its three hypothetical scenarios, even the one that it is virtually impossible to imagine or accept, a significant misfortune has befallen a patient as a result of being vaccinated that very probably would not have occurred if he or she had not been. By trying to disprove too much, the advocates of mandatory vaccination thus end up proving *nothing;* for whatever the extent to which a vaccine may contribute to a patient's illness, it is decidedly more than a *coincidence.*

In any case, exactly as one would expect, the same fallacy is regularly invoked to close off the debate surrounding autism, the other serious contender for inclusion in the official guidelines, an equally broad, generic, and even more prevalent form of serious brain damage in children. So named and first described by the psychiatrist Leo Kanner in 1943, curiously enough just one year after the DPT vaccine was introduced, since the 1990's it has been diagnosed with ever-increasing frequency, to the point that today, less than two decades later, it has been shown to affect tens of millions of young people at a rate that even the CDC calculates at roughly one percent. of eight-year-olds,[12] making it by far the leading cause of brain damage in American children.

Here again, the public clamor and outrage have so far been contained and to some extent dissipated by numerous studies purporting to show no causal connection with the MMR or any other specific vaccine, in the face of voluminous anecdotal evidence and well-designed experimental research to the contrary, and marshalling the very same arguments against them. As with the cases of DPT encephalopathy, these are not empirical judgments, based on actual histories of victims, but purely statistical analyses based on the policy of vaccinating *everybody*, which relegates even these millions of damaged lives to the waste-basket category of predisposed and thus already tainted individuals, whose misfortune cannot be simply imputed to any one vaccine, a conclusion that for once I actually agree with.

A specific causal link to a particular vaccine remains the "smoking gun" that both sides of the debate are looking for, whether because or in spite of the fact that the only methodology currently available all but guarantees the impossibility of ever finding it. Like the Holy Grail, the quest for specific effects of particular vaccines is a mirage, a figment of the imagination that our limited notion of cause and effect conjures up and dangles irresistibly before our eyes. Although they all occur with some frequency, even the adverse reactions that have been proposed by the anti-vaccination movement -- DPT encephalopathy, DPT and SIDS, MMR and autism, Hep B and auto-immune disease -- are all broad, generic pathological categories that are poorly defined and have been documented to follow other vaccines as well.

"Autism," for example, is largely another name for brain damage or "encephalopathy," and has also been diagnosed in DPT cases,[13] while SIDS has been reported after the Hep B,[14] and may have more to do with the special vulnerability of early infancy than the particular vaccines that happen to be administered at that time. As for Hep B and the ever-increasing roster of auto-immune diseases that have so far been linked to it, my own experience leads to the conclusion that auto-immune phenomena are an essential component of how *all* vaccines work, and tend to turn up wherever we look for them, as if indicative of chronicity itself.

This brings me to the adverse reactions that I have seen in my own practice, which are common enough to be the rule rather than the exception, involve conditions that may be latent or already manifest *before* the child is vaccinated, and are likely to be precipitated, activated, intensified, and made more chronic in the same way by *any* vaccine, often by two or more different ones in the same child. For all of these reasons, I regard them as essentially non-specific reactions to the vaccination process itself, rather than to any one particular vaccine. Without exception, they involve a definite susceptibility or pre-existing tendency of these individuals to react in a way that becomes characteristic of *them,* therefore do not qualify for compensation, and are often invisible to doctors and parents alike until the child recovers for an extended period of time, and then relapses promptly after another vaccine or combination is given.

Encompassing the full spectrum of illnesses and diseases that pediatricians and family physicians habitually deal with, and all degrees of severity, they include asthma, eczema, otitis media, sinusitis, allergies, ADD, autism, and learning and behavioral problems, as well as a variety of less common diagnoses, and even more idiosyncratic reactions that have no name at all. Like any primary immune response, they often take 14 days or more to develop, and thus fall into the category of chronic illnesses, rather than acute events, and easily fly under the radar, as we saw, but are by no means necessarily minor or trivial.

Here are a few typical cases. I'll begin with one of the simplest to recognize and easiest to understand, an 18-year-old girl whose childhood patterns of OCD and enuresis were abruptly reactivated after years of good health by an MMR booster newly required for attending college:

A patient of mine since early childhood, an 18-year-old girl was preparing to leave for college. In primary school, she had been plagued by enuresis and a variety of obsessive-compulsive symptoms, which she had overcome completely with the help of *Arsenicum album* in various potencies, remaining more or less symptom-free for over 10 years without ever having to repeat it. Within a week after the required MMR booster, her old pattern of bedwetting and OCD behavior returned in full force, and she came seeking treatment on her own for the first time. One dose of *Arsenicum album 1M* was rapidly effective, and she completed her first 2 years at a top liberal arts college with a brilliant academic record, repeating the remedy at rare intervals. She has since graduated with honors, served challenging internships in rural Latin America without major difficulty, and has not needed further treatment.[15]

Another common pattern is exemplified by this 15-month-old baby girl, who had already endured 11 ear infections and 11 rounds of antibiotics by the time I saw her:

> Otherwise in good health, a chubby girl of 15 months was brought in for repeated ear infections, which had never cleared up despite 11 rounds of antibiotics. After a good pregnancy and easy labor, her mother chose not to nurse, and the child developed her first ear infection with a fever of 103° at 2 months of age, soon after her first DPT, HiB, and polio combination. All later episodes were afebrile, most with fretting, screaming, and pulling at the ear, and were relieved by being carried about; but twice she had no symptoms whatsoever, was treated because the pediatrician found some fluid through the otoscope, and developed persistent diarrhea both times.
>
> I asked the parents to stop vaccinating her for a while, and gave her a dose of *Calcarea carb.* 200 preventively and *Pulsatilla* 30X to take as needed in the event of a flare-up. Two weeks later, she came down with a replica of her first episode, a high fever with intense screaming, which cleared up with *Pulsatilla* in a day or two. By her next visit, 3 months later, she had recovered completely and was thriving in every way. That was more than 3 years ago, an interval during which she has had no ear infections, no antibiotics, and no more shots.[16]

As often happens, the vaccine connection seemed rather tenuous at first, the only clear indication being her first episode at 2 months, after her first DPT, HiB, and polio series, after which her condition became chronic and the later shots made no further difference. What was striking about it was that the episode after homeopathic treatment was just like her first one, with fever and violent earache, and resulted in complete recovery. Hers and other such cases have taught me to regard acute illnesses with fever as a favorable sign of strong vitality and a healthy immune system that can mount a vigorous response to infection, as it seems innately programmed to do.

Another infant exhibited her own distinctive pattern of recurrent ear infections in response to two different vaccine combinations, beginning with the DPT, HiB, and polio, then even more intensely after the MMR:

> A baby girl of 10 months was brought in for otitis media, with high fever, intense earache, and loud screaming, her fifth such episode since 2 months of age, each one beginning soon after finishing the antibiotic from the previous one. Even before that, she grew fussy when her mother weaned her to go back

to work, and developed a florid rash from her milk-based formula. All of these symptoms intensified soon after her first DPT, HiB, and polio vaccinations, reaching their climax 2 weeks later in her first ear infection, with high fever and violent earache. Thereafter she got only the DT, which she didn't react to at all, but the ear infections continued unabated.

With homeopathic treatment, they stopped soon enough, but 6 months later her parents separated, and her father took her for the MMR. Three typical ear infections and three rounds of antibiotics followed in rapid succession. Again she was brought in by her mother, responded well to homeopathy, and remained in very good health overall, despite a tendency to relapse when she visited her father, who indulged her with dairy products and took her to the pediatrician for her full quota of vaccines and antibiotics. I have continued to see her at rare intervals, most recently as a college student of 18. Her ear infections are long gone, and when she does get sick, her robust immune system helps her to respond acutely and vigorously, and she recovers promptly each time.[17]

Already seriously compromised at birth, a fourth child developed persistent croup, signs of mental retardation, and other chronic complaints shortly after his first DPT and HiB, which led his mother to postpone the second round for many months, but the long wait failed to prevent a dramatic relapse as soon as he received it:

A 15-month-old boy was brought in for croup, recurrent colds, swollen glands, and developmental issues. Born to a diabetic mother, he weighed 8 lb. at birth, and spent many weeks in the Newborn ICU because of "undeveloped lungs," with cyanosis and unstable blood sugars. In the first 3 months he was also quite colicky, with a nasty diarrhea that stopped when her mother eliminated wheat from her diet. At 3 months of age, soon after his first DPT, HiB, and polio combination, he became very restless, with swollen glands and a sickly pallor that lasted for months and culminated in a prolonged episode of croup, high fever, and sunken chest, for which he was hospitalized and given IV corticosteroids. But the cough persisted for so long that the mother decided to postpone his second round of vaccinations until he recovered. At 12 months of age, she finally gave in, but the croupy cough and swollen glands reappeared within a few days, with almost exactly the same symptoms as before.

Showing a marked fear of strangers, the boy came into my office appearing subnormal, drooling profusely, with his mouth hanging open, and hiding behind his mother. After a few remedies failed to act, a single dose of *Baryta carbonica* 200 wrought such a change that the entire illness cleared up in a few days, and never returned. At follow-up a month later, his mother was ecstatic. For the first time, even in the dead of winter, there was no croup or swollen glands, he was sleeping well, and seemed much more alert, interested in his surroundings, and less fearful around strangers. That was 6 years ago, and I've not seen him since, but the experience convinced his mother not to vaccinate him again, and she recently called to tell me that he continues to thrive and develop normally, "like other children his age."[18]

My final case is that of a 4-year-old boy with severe allergic asthma since the age of two, and on meds all year round, who began a splendid recovery on remedies, even during his peak allergy season, until a DPT booster brought on an immediate and profound relapse:

Asthmatic since the age of 2, and testing positive for a broad spectrum of allergens, a 4-year-old boy was brought in for homeopathic treatment, because even a strict regimen of bronchodilators and inhaled corticosteroids had failed to prevent frequent major attacks the previous fall and winter, several of them requiring prednisone and antibiotics as well. Six weeks later, after 2 doses of *Kali iodatum* 200, he had cut his meds by half, maintained higher peak flows of 150 or more, and made it through a cold for the first time without asthma or drugs of any kind. Emotionally, too, he was calmer and less wild, even expressing remorse after a fit of rage, which he had never done before.

Early the next fall, during the peak of his allergy season, he was still doing well on half-doses of Beclovent, and had been energetic and in good health all spring and summer, with peak flows at record levels of 150-175. Almost immediately after his pre-K DPT booster, he came down with bronchitis, for which the pediatrician gave antibiotics, and his asthma and allergies returned in full force. Once again, he responded beautifully to *Kali iodatum* 200, and has continued to improve over the past 2 years, to the point that he hasn't needed to come back or take it again.[19]

In short, the adverse reactions that I witness on a routine basis are no mere *aberrations,* but predictable complications of the vaccination process itself, and thus provide valuable clues to how vaccines actually *work.* The stated purpose of all vaccines is to stimulate continuous antibody synthesis on a chronic basis, and for long periods of time, ideally for years or decades. *Chronicity* is likewise the chief feature of all my cases, and in fact the only thing they have in common, representing chronic or relapsing versions of the same broad range of diseases and illnesses seen by every pediatrician. For example, the baby girl with recurrent ear infections who responded to constitutional treatment with an *acute* episode just like her first one, followed by a complete and long-lasting cure, embodies two simple but important lessons:

1) that the immune system is "hard-wired" to mount acute and vigorous responses to infection, and

2) that the effect of vaccination is to re-program the host cells to respond *chronically,* not only to the vaccine organism, but also non-specifically to other antigens as well.

Precisely how vaccines bring this about is not entirely clear to me, even after decades of trying to figure it out. What I do know is that forcing cells of the immune system to harbor foreign antigens inside them for long periods of time will most likely result in auto-immune phenomena once their neighbors recognize them as "foreign," and eventually in various forms of chronic disease, depending on which cells, tissues, and organs are sensitized and targeted.

To appreciate what this means, compare vaccination with the process of coming down with and recovering from the corresponding acute disease, such as the measles. For measles to evolve from a scourge that kills 20% of a population exposed to it for the first time into a normal disease of childhood required centuries of adaptation, such that when I contracted it at the age of six, non-specific mechanisms were already in place that helped me and almost all of my schoolmates to recover from it with no complications or sequelæ. The natural immunity that resulted was permanent and multi-layered: partly specific, which prevented us from ever getting it again, no matter how many times we were re-exposed to it, but also *non-specific,* involving a massive, co-ordinated mobilization of every component of the immune mechanism as a whole, really a kind of graduation ceremony, certifying that our systems were primed and ready to respond acutely and vigorously to whatever other infections we might encounter in the future. On both counts, the ability to fall ill with and recover from acute diseases thus confers enormous benefits for the health of the individual, the nation, and indeed the human race as a whole.

In contrast, the cases I have presented demonstrate that the artificial immunity obtained by vaccination is *counterfeit* in both respects:

1) because the specific antibody response is only partial and temporary, and leads to no general outpouring, and

2) because to produce those precious antibodies, we must necessarily substitute chronic responses and auto-immune phenomena for the acute programming we were born with.

In other words, if children vaccinated against a particular acute disease fail to come down with it, it is because we have given them the chronic version instead, rendering them *incapable* of responding acutely, not only to it, but also non-specifically to other infections and antigenic challenges for good measure.

In much the same fashion, our unquestioning readiness to pile on as many different vaccines as we like rests on the unspoken assumption that each one acts separately on the immune system, more or less independently of the others, as the leading vaccine advocates have always contended. But the generalized, across-the-board reactions that I have been describing suggest a very different story, namely,

1) that *all* vaccines, precisely by doing what they are intended to do, promote a wide variety of auto-immune phenomena and a major escalation in the incidence and severity of the chronic diseases that correspond to them; and

2) that that effect is in some measure proportional to the total number of vaccines administered to a given individual, and the total vaccine *load* borne by the population as a whole.

The ACIP's official vaccination schedule for 2004 lists a total of 22 separate vaccination events between birth and 2 years of age, many of them with several different components:[20]

1 flu shot yearly, beginning at 6 months;
3 Hep B shots in the first 24 months, beginning at birth;
3 DPT shots at 2, 4, and 6 months, and a 4th at 24 months;
3 HiB shots at 2, 4, & 6 months, and a 4th at 12-18 months;
3 pneumo shots at 2, 4, & 6 months, and a 4th at 12-18 months;
2 IPV polio shots at 2 & 4 months, and a 3rd at 6-24 months;

1 MMR shot at 12-18 months; and
1 chickenpox shot at 12-24 months.

The same source lists 25 more separate vaccinations that are
recommended or required for children between 2 and 18 years of age:21

16 flu shots, 1 per year from 2-18 years of age;
3 or 4 Hep A shots, from 2-18 years of age (suggested);
1 DPT booster at 4-6 years;
1 DT booster at 11-12 years;
1 IPV booster at 4-6 years;
1 MMR booster at 4-6 years; and
1 chickenpox booster at 4-6 years (very likely).

That adds up to a total of 47 separate vaccinations that every child
is expected to undergo before the age of 18, with plenty more still to
come. Since 2004, several have already been added or proposed: HPV
for adolescent girls, meningococcus and rotavirus for all children of
both sexes. Many vaccines on the list have also been or soon will be
recommended and perhaps mandated for young adults and the middle-
aged and elderly, while Group A Strep, AIDS, and others are already in
the pipeline, or are planned or projected for the future, often for no more
pressing reason than our technical capacity to make them.

Finally, ever since the Clinton years, vaccines have been touted
as the most economical, efficient, and strategic use of our health-care
resources, based on what looks like a simple cost-benefit analysis, i. e.,
the ratio between the cost of the vaccination and the cost of caring for
the additional cases of the acute disease that would be expected had the
vaccine *not* been given. But once we factor in their share of the increased
incidence and severity of childhood asthma, otitis media, sinusitis, ADD,
autism, and all the rest, and calculate their share of the cost of caring for
the tens of millions so afflicted, that same cost-benefit equation will look
vastly different.

Far from being inexpensive, let alone an unmixed blessing for the
public health, vaccination represents an enormous hidden cost and risk
factor to the medical system as a whole, a hugely expensive and dangerous
experiment that has already overburdened and sickened the population,

and will undoubtedly continue to do so. Only our blind, quasi-religious faith in it, unique in all the world, will suffice to explain the scandal that the United States spends so exorbitantly on medical care, yet lags so far behind all other developed countries in every standard health measure.

3. Different Look, Same Problem: the Causal Power of Pharmaceutical Drugs.

Although vaccines highlight the limits and inconsistencies in our medical notions of causality, the same basic dilemma haunts the pharmaceutical industry as a whole, where its consequences are equally elusive, similarly hidden from view, and if anything even more pervasive and injurious.

While it played a leading rôle in the chemical revolution that gave the world qualitative and quantitative analysis, and much of organic and inorganic chemistry as we know them, the drug industry still clings religiously to the same experimental methodology that it developed in the post-Civil War era. In its first phase, crude botanical drugs such as opium, belladonna, digitalis, ergot, and coca were refined by extracting individual alkaloids with greater specificity of action -- morphine, codeine, papaverine, atropine, scopolamine, digoxin, digitoxin, ouabain, cocaine, and the like.

In the Twentieth Century, the same analytic trend yielded semisynthetic derivatives -- dilaudid, heroin, ergotrate, and many others -- and eventually wholly synthetic analogues, like meperidine, amphetamines, xylocaine, propanolol, omeprazole, alendronate, etc., each targeted to specific biochemical receptors, in order to minimize the risk of adverse or unwanted reactions -- even pleasant ones, like the wondrous euphoria of cocaine and heroin, the inexhaustible craving and demand for which upstaged and ultimately ruined their splendid contributions to medicine.

In this way, each new drug is developed for use against a particular disease, ideally a single enzyme or chemical reaction, just as diseases came to be defined more rigorously and linked to objective abnormalities of specific biochemical pathways, which it became the goal of drug treatment to inhibit or stimulate or otherwise regulate, again precisely as Claude Bernard had foreseen. As more such pathways were discovered, more and more metabolites were shown to play into them, and an ever-growing array of synthetic drugs, almost all petro-chemicals, were developed to manipulate them, Bernard's ideal of "immediate" causes that followed natural physiological pathways and could be relied upon to produce the desired effect in almost every case quickly receded from view, while even biologically active hormones were eventually replaced for the most part by a variety of synthetic analogues, derivatives, and antagonists.

Under these circumstances, the closest approximation to Bernard's *necessary* cause is in most cases merely a *sufficient* one, a drug with sufficient chemical power at a maximum dose to impose the effect by force on a statistical preponderance of cases, whatever their mechanism of action, and regardless of how an individual patient might respond to them in other ways. A well-known example from Hahnemann's time that continued throughout the Nineteenth Century, calomel and other mercurial drugs were widely used against syphilis in increasing doses until the patients salivated, then the accepted limit of tolerance. Even today, especially in the chemotherapy of cancer and other serious or life-threatening diseases, the *maximum* dose, the largest quantity that the patient can tolerate without unpalatable or toxic side-effects, remains a standard therapeutic goal, as in the case of a dear friend with ovarian cancer, who lived through her first six months of intensive, punishing chemotherapy with so few signs of toxicity that her genuinely devoted oncologist offered her a second round as a special favor.

Once the causal power of drugs could be quantified as the fraction of patients exhibiting the desired effect, it became possible and desirable to refine that measurement by comparing it to the percentage who recovered without it. Experimental tests of drug efficacy thus involved dividing subjects into two or three groups, those given the newer drug in question, and control groups, matched as closely as possible demographically and in other ways, who were treated with a more established drug or not treated at all. Just as with vaccines, to qualify as a sufficient cause of the effect in question, drugs must be shown to produce it in a majority or at least a large preponderance of patients taking it, over and above the record of their controls.

In the aftermath of World War II, this statistical exercise achieved its ultimate technical sophistication in the Random Controlled Trial, or

RCT, now generally accepted as the "Gold Standard" of drug effectiveness, in which the causal power of any drug or combination against a particular disease or abnormality is measured by randomizing the subjects into two groups, one receiving the drug, and the other only an inert imitation, with both patients and doctors kept "blinded" as to who gets which. Its potency is thus reduced to a definite, measurable quantity, the extent to which patients taking it outperform their placebo controls, while the level of effect should itself be controllable to an extent, by titrating the dose to any desired level. In this fashion, rather than an optimal *qualitative* fit with the unique features and needs of a particular patient, as homeopaths aspire to, the best drugs and the ones most diligently sought after became simply the most *potent* ones, those with the most chemical power to compel the organism to behave in whatever ways the profession determines that they should.

Almost by definition, this force will tend to be exerted in a direction that the organism shows very little natural or spontaneous inclination to go, because the "placebo effect" that they must outdo is precisely the sum of those individual tendencies and predispositions that are too subjective to define or measure, too unpredictable to control, and too idiosyncratic to merit systematic study. In other words, what we call the "placebo effect" is essentially the starved and tattered remnant of the innate self-healing capacity, the ancient *vis medicatrix naturæ,* or what little is left of it when the patient becomes an experimental subject and conditioned to expect no help at all unless graced with the tablets or capsules in question.

In the same way, modern doctors are equipped with the latest and most advanced chemical weapons to attack a vast array of diseases and abnormalities as if they were enemies on a battlefield: antibiotics to kill bacteria, anticonvulsants to control seizure activity, anti-hypertensives to force down the blood pressure, antimetabolites to seek out and destroy cancer cells, antihistamines to inhibit the allergic response, antithyroid drugs to suppress hormone secretion, bronchodilators to open constricted air passages, diuretics to compel the kidneys to excrete more urine, corticosteroids to block inflammation, insulin to substitute for a diabetic pancreas, and so forth. In advanced cases, such drugs may indeed give miraculous relief, buy valuable time, or at least do the best that can be done under adverse or extreme circumstances.

Leaving aside the ultimate question, whether most patients taking the drug will in fact *feel* better, live longer, and suffer fewer complications as a result of their treatment than without it, I will simply stipulate what is not always true in practice, that many of the drugs in common use do indeed have the power to accomplish at least some of what we ask and expect of them, to correct the abnormality in question, or at least to fight the disease process at some strategic juncture, in hopes that these more subjective, personal goals will eventually follow. But just beneath the surface of that success, as with those precious antibodies for the sake of which we vaccinate, lurks a huge built-in complication at the very heart of the system, and two other threats of equal magnitude and importance that follow directly from it.

First, when drugs really *work,* when they effectively suppress or counteract the target symptom or abnormality, the problem is likely to reappear with equal or greater intensity when the drug wears off. Using a chemical to force the issue, rather than assist whatever self-healing processes are already available, thus poses the serious risk of needing to *continue* using it for long periods of time, and always with the expectation that the original complaint or worse will reappear as soon as it is discontinued. In this fashion, what often began as an idiomatic episode in the patient's life routinely and insidiously develops into a less and less curable *chronic* illness or disease element, now *chemically* programmed, in exchange for partial and temporary relief of symptoms and the technical correction of abnormalities. Apart from acute ailments ending in death or recovery, such long-term perpetuation of the original energy disturbance also feeds into and even helps carry out the self-fulfilling prophecy that chronic diseases are by definition incurable anyway, and must therefore be controlled with drugs throughout life, removed surgically, or simply borne in silence.

One wholly predictable consequence of targeting drug treatment to specific pathological conditions is *polypharmacy,* the reliable expectation that without a unifying principle, like the "vital force" that Claude Bernard was so eager to do away with, more and more drugs will be needed to keep at bay all other identifiable diseases and abnormalities. The other is that drugs potent enough to do the things we expect them to do also have the power to act coercively on other aspects of our patients' functioning, even though these unwanted and usually undesirable "side effects" will vary quite a lot, according to the unique features and predispositions of the patient.

This is precisely where we left off with vaccines: an array of individualized responses, each indicating some degree of predisposition, which may be difficult to recognize and accept as belonging to the vaccine for that reason. In the same way, the unwanted or extra symptoms that drugs elicit or provoke are simply written off as side effects and relegated to the fine print, because each one affects a much smaller number, and may thus be regarded as an idiosyncrasy of the victim, rather than a consequence of drug action, an easy sleight-of-hand that similarly helps defeat malpractice suits against physicians and manufacturers for bad outcomes, unless specific acts of *negligence* can be traced to them.

But even though each particular side effect of a drug may seem relatively uncommon, the aggregate total of all of them combined may tell a very different story. Just as an exercise, and more or less at random, I picked out the brand-name drug Savella, or Milnacipran HCl, which was originally developed as an SNRI antidepressant, but is now marketed and used mainly for the treatment of fibromyalgia, in expensive advertisements that include the following warnings about serious side effects and possible interactions with other drugs or ailments:

1) Savella is an SNRI, similar to drugs used for depression and other psychiatric disorders. *Antidepressants increased the risk of suicidal thinking and behavior in children, adolescents, and young adults. Patients of all ages should be monitored closely for suicidality or unusual changes in behavior.*

2) *Savella is contraindicated in patients taking MAO inhibitors concomitantly. There have been reports of serious or fatal reactions* in patients started on MAOI's who were also receiving or had recently discontinued an SSRI or SNRI.

3) *Savella is contrainidicated in patients with uncontrolled narrow-angle glaucoma and should be used cautiously in patients with controlled narrow- angle glaucoma.*

4) *Development of a potentially life-threatening syndrome may occur with SRI agents, including Savella,* particularly with concomitant use of serotonergic drugs, and those that impair serotonin metabolism, such as MAOI's.

5) *SNRI's, including Savella, have been associated with cardiovascular effects, including high blood pressure, requiring immediate treatment.* Among patients who were

371

not hypertensive before, roughly twice as many receiving Savella became hypertensive as those receiving placebo. *It should be used cautiously in patients with significant hypertension or cardiac disease.*

6) *Savella should be used with caution in patients with a history of mania or seizure disorder.*

7) *Savella has been associated with mild elevations of liver enzymes (up to 3 times the upper limit of normal). Rarely, serious liver injury and fulminant hepatitis have been reported.* It should not be prescribed to alcoholics or those with chronic liver disease.

8) *Hyponatremia may occur as a result of treatment with SSRI's and SNRI's, including Savella.* Elderly patients may be at greater risk.

9) *SSRI's and SNRI's, including Savella, may increase the risk of bleeding events.* Patients should be cautioned about concomitant use with NSAID's, aspirin, warfarin, and other drugs that affect coagulation.

10) *Savella can affect urethral resistance and micturition.* Caution is advised in patients with dysuria, especially in males with obstructive uropathies, who may experience higher rates of adverse events.

11) *There are no adequate, well-controlled studies in pregnant women,* for whom it should be used only if the potential benefit outweighs the potential risk to the fetus.[22]

Needless to say, these are merely the most visible, above-ground portion of a much larger iceberg. In clinical trials, the most common adverse reactions listed were as follows:[23]

	Savella (%)	**Placebo** (%)
Nausea	37	20
Headache	18	14
Constipation	16	4
Dizziness	10	6
Insomnia	12	10
Hot flashes	12	2
Hyperhidrosis	9	2
Vomiting	7	2
Palpitations	7	2
Hypertension	7	2

URI	7	6
Tachycardia	6	1
Migraine	6	3
Dry mouth	5	2
Anxiety	5	4
Abdominal pain	3	2
Chest pain	3	2
Dyspnea	2	1
Tremor	2	1
Paresthesias	2	2
Loss of appetite	1	0
Blurred vision	1	1

Other less common reactions included the following:

Premarketing:[24]
Metabolic: weight loss, weight gain, hypercholesterolemia
Male GU: dysuria, incomplete ejaculation, erectile dysfunction, decreased libido, prostatitis, scrotal pain, testicular pain
GI: dyspepsia, GERD, diarrhea, flatulence, distention
General: fatigue, edema, irritability, fever
Infections: UTI, cystitis
Injuries: falls, contusions
Nervous system: somnolence
Psychiatric: stress, depression

Postmarketing:[25]
Blood: leukopenia, neutropenia, thrombocytopenia
Cardiac: supraventricular tachycardia
Endocrine: hyperprolactinemia
Hepatobiliary: hepatitis
Metabolic: anorexia, hyponatremia
Musculoskeletal: rhabdomyolysis
Nervous system: convulsions, Parkinsonism
Psychiatric: delirium, hallucinations
GU: acute renal failure, urinary retention

Breast: galactorrhea
Skin: *erythema multiforme,* Stevens-Johnson syndrome
Vascular: hypertensive crisis

Remember that for any side effect to make it onto this list, reluctantly compiled by the drug companies themselves, it must meet the strict standard of "cause" already alluded to, i.e., either a sudden, acute event, appearing almost immediately out of nowhere, or more chronically, in patients not obviously predisposed to it. Although individually many of them are more or less infrequent, the arithmetic sum of all of them together, and thus the risk of at least one of them occurring in any given patient, are substantial enough, when added to the various warnings, contraindications, and cross-reactions with other drugs, to make it seem like Russian roulette for *anyone* to take their chances with this still very popular drug.

Moreover, the track record of the industry virtually guarantees that when claims of actual adverse reactions mount up to the point that a drug is taken off the market, a process that consumes at least 5 years on average, the manufacturer will already have cashed out a huge profit and moved on to a whole new generation of synthetic chemicals to send up through the same process. Nor is this line-up in any way unusual: almost any brand-name drug listed in the PDR can boast of a similar profile.

In addition, instead of the usual strategy of downplaying such side-effects, several more forward-looking manufacturers have recently begun to see the advantage of *emphasizing* them, as further proof of the drug's power to do *something.* A splendid example is the recent TV ad for Cialis, a long-acting drug for impotence, impressively renamed "Erectile Dysfunction" to sound like a genuine disease, in which viewers are piously warned to beware of and seek immediate medical help for erections lasting more than four hours, a complication which to potential customers sounds a lot like hitting the jackpot.

Another way to appreciate the impact of adverse drug reactions on the general public is to highlight a particularly common or serious complication by listing the drugs known to cause it, as was done in a series of articles from the 1980's entitled "Drug Actions and Interactions," which appeared in the free tabloid *Modern Medicine.* Here are a few examples:

374

Which Drugs May Trigger Diabetes?[26]

l-Asparaginase (Elspar)	Occurs in 3-17% of recipients
Chenodeoxycholic acid (bile salt)	
Chlorpromazine (Thorazine)	Inhibits insulin secretion
Cimetidine (Tagamet)	Impaired glucose tolerance, retarded absorption
Clofibrate (Atromid)	Arginine-stimulated insulin secretion 60% lower
Contraceptives, oral	Disputed
Danazol (Danocrine)	Impaired glucose tolerance
Diazoxide (Hyperstat IV)	Hyperglycemia usual, direct effect on ß-cells
Diuretics	Hyperglycemia
Estrogens	Reduced glucose tolerance
Glucocorticosteroids	Increased gluconeogenesis, low glucose
Vitamin A	Hyperglycemia (in high doses)

Drug-Induced Thromboctyopenia:[27]

Acetaminophen	Thrombocytopenic purpura
Acetazoleamide (Diamox)	Thrombocytopenic purpura
Aspirin	Thrombocytopenia, with or without purpura
Tricyclic antidepressants	
Antineoplastic agents	Direct bone marrow toxicity, pancytopenia
Benzodiazepines	Single cases, several such drugs implicated
Cephalosporins	Allergic type, infrequent
Chloramphenicol	Associated with fatal blood dyscrasias
Chloroquine phosphate or HCl	Associated with pancytopenia
Diazoxide (Hyperstat IV)	Associated with neutropenia
Digitoxin	Specific antibodies detected
Estrogens (synthetic)	

Ethchlorvynol (Placidyl)	Recurrent episodes, ending in death (1 case)
Furosemide (Lasix)	Uncommon
Gentamicin sulfate	Rare
Gold salts	Incidence as high as 40%
Heparin	Mild decrease common, but all degrees reported
Immune sera	Toxic reactions 1 week after injection
Inandione anticoagulants	Associated with hypersensitivity reactions
Indomethacin (Indocin)	Rare form of toxicity
Insulin	Has been reported
IV Fat Emulsions	Reported in infants on long-term therapy
Iopanoic acid (Telepaque)	Allergic reactions
l-Dopa	Long-term use
Methyldopa (Aldomet)	Uncommon
NSAID's	Possibly allergic, several drugs implicated
Oxybutazone, Phenylbutazone	Associated with severe anemia
Penicillamine	Fatal TTP
Penicillin	Allergic reactions
Quinidine	Rare
Quinine	Allergic reactions
Rifampin	Allergic reaction, with severe endothelial damage
Rubella Vaccine	Thrombocytopenic purpura
Rubeola Vaccine	Thrombocytopenic purpura
Sulfonamides	Acute reactions (rare)
Sulfonylureas (oral antidiabetc)	Associated with generalized hypersensitivity
Trimethoprim/sulfamethoxazole (Bactrim, Septra)	Mild reactions common, severe ones rare

Additional side-effects from the same series include impotence (11 drugs and drug classes), infertility (15), hallucinations (38), and several others. Illustrating the perils of polypharmacy, the series also featured drug interactions, such as the following, among many others:

Oral Anticoagulants: Caution with Concurrent Drugs:[28]

Anabolic steroids	Hemorrhages dues to lowered clotting factors
Antidiabetic agents	Effects on protein binding and metabolism
Barbiturates	Decreased response to antocoagulants
Cholestyramine (Questran)	Decreased absorption of anticoagulants, Vitamin K
Clofibrate (Atromid)	Increased anticoagulation effect
Dextrothyroxine (Choloxin)	Lowered prothrombin levels
Disulfiram (Antabuse)	Inhibits anticoagulant metabolism
Glutethimide (Doriden)	Increases anticoagulant metabolism
Oxybutazone, Phenylbutazone	Inihibit anticoagulant metabolism, GI bleeding
Phenytoin (Dilantin)	Unpredictable: several interacting mechanisms
Rifampin	Stimulates liver to metabolize anticoagulants
Salicylates	Impair platelet function, lower prothrombin
Thyroid hormones	Reduce clotting factors

The point of all this is very simple. Involving so many different classes and types, the principal risk of excessive drug use is not *malpractice,* which involves fault or negligence on the part of an individual physician, but quite the opposite and immensely greater threat, an iatrogenic illness caused by medicines that are inherently dangerous, even when prescribed according to current standards, with appropriate levels of skill and genuinely informed consent. This was the shocking conclusion of a landmark study involving 815 consecutive admissions to an 80-bed medical service at a university hospital over a five-month period.[29] Of those admitted to the unit within that time, the authors found

1) that 36% suffered at least one iatrogenic complication during their stay;

2) that 9% developed complications that were seriously disabling, potentially fatal, or both; and

3) that 2% actually died as a result of such complications while still in the unit.[30]

They further stipulated that these disturbingly high figures would actually have been even higher, had they included

4) iatrogenic events suffered by the same population over the same interval, but before their admission or transfer into the unit, or after their discharge or transfer out of it, and

5) other episodes not attributable to any specific drug or procedure, such as seizures or falls in heavily medicated patients, which were written off as "incident reports," even though their medications clearly made such events more likely.[31]

In the latter part of the study, the authors tried to find out *which* drugs or procedures posed the greatest risk of serious and fatal complications, and were even more surprised to learn that it didn't make a lot of difference, that the risk depended much less on which tests were ordered, which drugs prescribed, and which surgical procedures performed, than simply on *how many,* i. e., the total number of transactions with the medical system, regardless of their specific content.[32] The obvious implication of their data is that patients are harmed much less by malpractice or how *badly* medicine is practiced, than simply by *how much* it is practiced, an admonition to which both advocates and opponents of health care reform would do well to pay heed.

4. Some Systemic Implications for Medicine as a Whole.

The ubiquity of adverse reactions to vaccines and drugs and their relative invisibility to those who manufacture and prescribe them make it easy to understand why homeopathy and other alternative approaches have become so popular with patients on the fringes of the medical system, and so easily dismissed by that establishment as ineffective, impossible, or unworthy of serious study. In pointed contrast to allopathic drugs and vaccines, which are chosen and developed for their power to *force* the organism to do what it has no natural inclination to do, homeopathy and holistic medicine in general seek to enhance the innate capacity for self-healing that is synonymous with life, perpetually at work in every patient, and encompasses those same individualizing tendencies, predispositions, and sensitivities which as physicians we were taught to ignore in our diagnoses, outperform in our research, and override in our treatment.

One important consequence of reducing patients to specimens of abstract disease categories existing in a sense apart from them has been to redefine these "entities" as simple *automatisms,* concatenated sequences of mechanisms pre-programmed to *worsen,* since the substantial and all-important capacity to *recover* remains vested in the individual patient, that least scientific of constructs, and thus quietly drops out of sight, rarely to be seen again.

Even when homeopathic remedies act curatively, the results are routinely dismissed or written off as isolated cases, possibly even miraculous at times, but nevertheless "anecdotal evidence" without scientific import, and therefore always located on the placebo side of the ledger, because medical science restricts "cause" to those interventions that force things to happen, and measures that power against the idiomatic tendency of patients to recover without them. Even in the case of well-designed RCT's that demonstrate a statistically significant benefit from homeopathic treatment, the result still "feels" unscientific and unpersuasive to most people, simply because no chemical force was exerted and no resistance overcome, just as to trained scientists its looser interpretation of causality and its reliance upon idiosyncratic elements similarly disqualify it from serious consideration as a force potent, measurable, and consistent enough to count as "hard science."

But the standard argument that homeopathic remedies are merely placebos cuts both ways. In the first place, it's simply *wrong,* since they have an equally impressive track record in the treatment of animals, newborn babies, and comatose patients, for whom the influence of suggestion is generally agreed to be negligible. Secondly, if giving placebo or natural remedies or nothing at all can achieve results equal to or better than those obtainable with suppressive drugs or crippling surgery, but without the mutilation, chronic dependence, polypharmacy, and toxicity that regularly accompany them, then it is at least an open question which method actually works better, and who of sound mind would not prefer the cheaper, gentler, and safer alternative to start with. And finally, when homeopathic remedies do act curatively, our patients rightly feel that they have healed themselves, and sometimes wonder if they might have done so without our help. But that delicious quandary is hardly cause for complaint, since I can imagine no higher compliment to be paid to a medicine than that its action cannot be distinguished from a gentle, spontaneous, long-lasting cure requiring no further treatment.

On the contrary, the irony lies wholly on the other side, that this optimal response is relegated to the placebo side of the equation, while pharmaceutical drugs are valued and considered effective only to the extent that they can overpower the physiology of as many patients for as long a time as possible. It is absurd and contemptible to boast of standards that prize brute force over elegance of fit, and subordinate healing the sick to manipulating their life functions artificially, whether for the sake of "science," ambition, or some equally abstract, hypothetical good that we are supposed to take on faith.

That is why, for the present at least, I am glad that our cures remain snugly ensconced on the placebo side of things, because until we develop a kinder, more accurate and inclusive notion of causality, that is precisely where they belong. What the nuclear physicist J. Robert Oppenheimer once told a group of psychologists seems even more apposite for the medical community as a whole:

> We inherited at the beginning of the Twentieth century a notion of the physical world as a causal one, in which every event could be accounted for if we were ingenious, a world characterized by *number,* where everything interesting could be measured, andanything that went on could be broken down and analyzed. This extremely rigid picture left out a great deal of common sense which we can now understand with a complete lack of ambiguity and phenomenal technical success. One is that the world is not completely determinate. There are predictions you can make about it, but they are purely statistical. Every event has in it the nature of a surprise, a *miracle,* or somethingyou could not

figure out. Every pair of observations taking the form "we know this and can predict that" is global and cannot be broken down. Every atomic event is individual: it is not in its essentials reproducible.[33]

This passage reminds me of a woman patient from my early years in Boston, a 34-year-old R. N. with a history of endometriosis since her teens, who consulted me to re-establish her menstrual cycle. After two courses of male hormones to suppress it, and four surgeries to remove large blood-filled cysts from her bladder and ovaries, her periods had become scanty, dark-brown, and "dead," as had any hopes of childbearing. After two or three remedies, her menses were richer and fuller, and within six months she was pregnant. When I next saw her for a different ailment eight years later, she had given birth to two healthy children after normal pregnancies and uncomplicated vaginal births, and had remained in good health ever since.[34]

While it would be absurd to attribute such an outcome to a homeopathic remedy or any other agency in precise, linear fashion, my patient has never stopped thanking me for it, which is reason enough to honor and be grateful for a process by its very nature catalytic and persuasive rather than forcible and compulsory.

For all of these reasons, instead of *competing* with the placebo effect in order to defeat it, I submit that the highest goal of medicinal treatment, whether homeopathic or otherwise, is precisely to *maximize* it, by doing everything possible to promote *healing,* rather than merely correct abnormalities, and therefore to cultivate a more intimate knowledge of our patients, rather than ignore, circumvent, or override all that they have to teach us. Much as I admire the ingenuity and dedication of my colleagues who conduct RCT's to prove the effectiveness of homeopathic treatment to the scientific world, I propose a different model for clinical research, based on *self-healing,* one that I believe is more suitable for allopathic medicine as well:

1) *Nobody is blinded:* all subjects know whether they are receiving homeopathic or allopathic treatment, having chosen it beforehand precisely because of their interest and faith in it.

2) *Nobody gets placebo:* everyone gets the treatment they selected, and the physicians who administer it are matched to them by *their* beliefs, and encouraged to use prayer, suggestion, exhortation, shamanic incantation, faith healing, laying on of hands, or whatever they or their subjects believe will most effectively assist their healing path. In other words, *each group will serve as the control of the other.*

3) *Using the totality of symptoms over time,* including subjective and objective criteria, as well as reports of family, friends, teachers, employers, etc., both *homeopathic and allopathic subjects will be followed and evaluated for a period of months or years* as to how well or badly they are measuring up in their own lives, according to their own standards and those of their community, in addition to clinical and pathological criteria, and extending beyond the acute phase to include the chronic dimension.

4) Qualified judges not doctrinally committed to either point of view will then ascertain which form of treatment comes out ahead, in which respects, and publish the results in a friendly, fair, and unbiased journal of good repute to be agreed upon in advance.[35]

A self-healing orientation in medicine will help to create the conditions under which homeopathic and allopathic points of view can collaborate and flourish in relative harmony, for both are valuable and useful, and neither by itself can accomplish everything that needs to be done. Without the scientific revolution, we would not have modern surgery, the leading edge of medical progress and quintessence of the allopathic point of view. Yet the surgical ideal also rests on a genuine paradox that cannot be ignored or set aside. As a method of assisting normal healing, whether by repairing the body when it is broken, or removing a part that is already dead, surgery unquestionably ranks among the supreme technical achievements in human history. But as the preferred method of curing *illness,* and thus the paradigm for the medical enterprise as a whole, it is a cruel travesty, a quasi-military decision to cut and burn in lieu of gentler, safer, and more authentic methods of healing the organism as a living system and the patient as a human being.

That is why for myself I prefer these aphorisms of Paracelsus, the great Renaissance physician and alchemist:

The art of healing comes from Nature, not the physician . . .
Every illness has its own remedy within itself . . .

382

A man could not be born alive and healthy were there not already a
Physician hidden in him.[36]

I interpret them roughly as follows:

Healing implies wholeness.

Derived from the same root as "whole," the English verb "to heal"
literally means to make whole [again], and suggests a basic property of
all living systems, a concerted effort of the entire organism that cannot be
accomplished by any part in isolation.

All healing is self-healing.

As an inherent function of the organism, the process of healing
goes on automatically and continuously throughout life, and tends to
complete itself spontaneously, with or without outside help. In other
words, all healing is self-healing, and the proper rôle of medicines,
surgery, physicians, and professional or designated "healers" of any kind
is simply to facilitate the natural process which is already under way, not
to alter, interfere with, or substitute for it.

Healing pertains solely to individuals.

Healing is always *possible*, but also problematic and even risky, and
can always *fail* to occur. That is because it pertains solely to individuals
in concrete, here-and-now situations, rather than to abstract diseases or
principles. In other words, it is inescapably an *art*, and can never and
should never be reduced to any technique or formula, however scientific
its foundation.[37]

As an appropriate bottom-line criterion, I conclude with a saying of
Lao-Tse:

A leader is best when people hardly know he exists,
Not so good when they obey and acclaim him,
Worst when they despise him.

Of a good leader, when his work is done and his aim fulfilled,

The people will say, "We did this ourselves."[38]

NOTES.

1. Russell, Bertrand, "The Philosophy of Logical Atomism," in *Logic and Knowledge: Essays, 1901-1950,* Allen and Unwin, London 1968, p. 193.
2. Hahnemann, S., *Organon of Medicine,* 5th Edition, trans. R. E. Dudgeon, ¶28: "As this natural law of cure [i. e., the Law of Similars] manifests itself in every pure experiment and every true observation in the world, the fact is consequently established. *It matters little what may be the scientific explanation of how it takes place, and I do not attach much importance to the attempts made to explain it .*" [Italics mine: R.M.]
3. Bernard, Claude, *An Introduction to the Study of Experimental Medicine,* trans. H. C. Greene, Dover, New York, 1957, pp. 63-65, *passim.*
4. Van Rijn, Rembrandt, *Dr. Tulp's Anatomy Lesson,* Mauritshuis Museum, the Hague, Netherlands.
5. Bernard, op. cit.
6. Bernard, *Principes de medicine expérimentale,* Paris, 1947, cited in Canguilhem, G., *The Normal and the Pathological,* trans. C. Fawcett, Zone Books, New York, 1991, p. 71.
7. Moskowitz, R., "Hidden in Plain Sight: the Rôle of Vaccines in Chronic Disease," *American Journal of Homeopathic Medicine* 98:15, Spring 2005.
8. "Reportable Events Following Vaccination," *Morbidity and Mortality Weekly Report* 37:181, April 1988.
9. Moskowitz, op. cit.
10. Cherry, J., "Pertussis Vaccine Encephalopathy: It's Time to Recognize It as the Myth That It Is," Editorial, *JAMA* 263:1679, March 1990.
11. ACIP Report on DPT Encephalopathy, *MMWR* 45:22, September 1996.
12. *JAMA* 303:602, February 2010.
13. Moskowitz, op. cit.
14. "Hepatitis B Vaccine," *The Vaccine Reaction,* Special Report, National Vaccine Information Center (NVIC), September 1988, p. 7.
15. Moskowitz, op. cit.
16. Ibid.
17. Ibid.
18. Ibid.
19. Ibid.
20. ACIP Childhood and Adolescent Immunization Schedule, *Family Practice News,* January 1, 2004, p. 9.
21. Ibid.
22. "Savella," Drug Advertisement.
23. Ibid.

24. Ibid.

25. Ibid.

26. Lipman, A., *Modern Medicine,* February 1982, p. 273.

27. Lipman, loc. cit., September 1983, p. 247.

28. Lipman, loc. cit., October 1981, p. 211.

29. Steel, K., et al., "Iatrogenic Illness on a General Medical Service at a University Hospital," *New England Journal of Medicine* 304:638, March 1981.

30. Ibid.

31. Ibid.

32. Ibid.

33. Oppenheimer, J. R., "Analogy in Science," *American Psychologist* 2:134, March 1956.

34. Moskowitz, *Resonance: the Homeopathic Point of View,* Xlibris, Philadelphia, 2001, p. 17.

35. Ibid., p. 342.

36. *Selected Writings of Paracelsus,* trans. N. Guterman, Bollingen Series, Pantheon, New York, 1958, pp. 50, 76, *passim.*

37. Moskowitz, *Resonance,* pp. 21-22.

38. Lao Tzu, *The Way of Life,* trans. W. Bynner, Putnam, New York, 1944, pp. 34-35.

Bibliography

Books.
1. *Homeopathic Medicines for Pregnancy and Childbirth,* 288 pp., Index, North Atlantic, Berkeley, 1992; German version, *Homöopathie für Schwangerschaft und Geburtshilfe,* Haug, Heidelberg, 1998.
2. *Resonance: The Homeopathic Point of View,* 372 pp., with Epilogue & Appendix, Xlibris, Philadelphia, 2001; German version, *Das Resonanzgesetz der Heilung,* Kai Kröger Verlag, Groß Wittensee, 2012.
3. *Plain Doctoring: Selected Writings, 1983-2013,* 397 pp., with Bibliography, CreateSpace, Charleston, SC, 2013.

Articles.
1. "Drug Reactions and Biological Individuality," *Homeotherapy* 3:1, August 1977.
2. "When *Not* to Give a Remedy," *Journal of the AIH* 73:11, March 1980.
3. "Homeopathic Remedies vs. the Placebo Effect," *Homeotherapy* 6:99, July-August 1980.
4. "Homeopathic Reasoning," Lecture to Symposium, "Homeopathy: the Renaissance of Cure, San Francisco, April 1980; published in *Homeotherapy* 6:135, September 1980.
5. "Two Obstetrical Remedies," *Homeopathy Today,* July 1981.
6. "Homeopathic Remedies in Pregnancy and Childbirth," *Homeopathy Today,* January 1983.
7. "*Magnesia Phosphorica,*" *Homeopathy Today,* February 1983.
8. "The Case Against Immunizations," *Journal of the AIH* 76:7, March 1983; reprinted as NCH and UK Society of Homœopaths pamphlets; included in Robert Mendelsohn, ed., *Dissent in Medicine,* Contemporary Books, Chicago, 1985.
9. Vague, Long-Term Diagnosis: the *Nocebo* Effect," *Journal of the AIH* 76:26, March 1983.

10. "Peculiar and Characteristic Symptoms," *Homeopathy Today,* April 1983.

11. "Postscript on Immunizations," *Journal of the AIH* 76:101, September 1983.

12. "Unvaccinated Kids: What's Next for Them (and Us)?" *Mothering* Magazine, January 1987.

13. "AIDS: Chronic Immune Failure," *Resonance* (Journal of the American Foundation for Homeopathy), January 1988.

14. "Some Thoughts on the Malpractice Crisis," *British Homœopathic Journal* 77:17, January 1988; reprinted in *Journal of the AIH* 81:22, March 1988, and *The Homœopath* (Journal of the UK Society of Homeopaths), September 1992.

15. "What Is Homeopathy?" in Robin Larsen, ed., *Emanuel Swedenborg: a Continuing Vision,* Swedenborg Foundation, New York, 1988, p. 475.

16. "Is There More than One Correct Remedy?" *Resonance*, January 1989.

17. "More on *Similia Similibus Curentur,*" *Journal of the AIH* 82:22, March 1989.

18. "Hospital Ethics Committees: the Healing Function," *HEC Forum* 1:309, January 1990; reprinted in Stuart Spicker, ed., *The Hospital Ethics Committee Experience,* Kluwer, 1998.

19. "Options in Homeopathic Self-Care," *East-West Journal,* January 1990.

20. "Two Childbirth Remedies," *Journal of the AIH* 83:72, September 1990; reprinted in *British Homœopathic Journal* 79:206, October 1990; German version, *Zeitschrift für Klassische Homöopathie,* 1991.

21. "Whose Life Is It, Anyway? Some Thoughts about the Doctor-Patient Relationship," *Chrysalis* (Journal of the Swedenborg Foundation) 6:103, Summer 1991.

22. "Vaccination: a Sacrament of Modern Medicine," lecture to the Society of Homeopaths Annual Conference, 1991; published in *Journal of the AIH* 84:96, December 1991; reprinted in *The Homœopath* 12:137, March 1992.

23. "Ethics in Homeopathic Practice," lecture to the AIH Conference, 1993; published in *Journal of the AIH* 86:238, December 1993.

24. "Vaccinations," in Barbara Katz Rothman, ed., *Encyclopedia of Childbearing,* Oryx Press, Phoenix, 1993.

25. "Childhood Ear Infections," lecture to the AIH Conference, 1994; published in *Journal of the AIH* 87:137, Autumn 1994; reprinted in *The Homœopath,* 1994.

26. "Homeopathy," with Jennifer Jacobs, M. D., in *Fundamentals of Complementary and Alternative Medicine,* Marc Micozzi, ed., Churchill Livingstone, London, 1995.

27. "Plain Doctoring," *Resonance* 19:30, March-April 1997.

28. "Hahnemann's Achievement and Legacy," *American Homeopath* 6:65, Summer 2000.

29. "To Have and Have Not: Homeopathy in Cuba," *Journal of the AIH* 93:59, Summer 2000; reprinted in *Homeopathy Today,* July-August 2000, and *New England Journal of Homeopathy* 9:115, Spring-Summer 2000.

30. "Illness as Metaphor (with Apologies to Susan Sontag)," *Journal of the AIH* 94:176, Autumn 2001.

31. "Innovation and Fundamentalism in Homeopathy," *American Journal of Homeopathic Medicine* (reborn AIH Journal) 95:91, Summer 2002; reprinted in *Simillimum* (Journal of Homeopathic Academy of Naturopathic Physicians) 15:17, Fall 2002.

32. "Epiphany: the Quantum Mechanics of the Spiritual Life," published as "Housecalls," *Chrysalis Reader,* Swedenborg Foundation, New York, December 2002.

33. "The Fundamentalist Controversy: an Issue That Won't Go Away," lecture to Society of Homeopaths Annual Conference, May 2003; published in *American Journal of Homeopathic Medicine* 97:28, Spring 2004, reprinted in *The Homeopath,* Winter 2004.

34. "Hidden in Plain Sight: the Rôle of Vaccines in Chronic Disease," lecture to the 60th LIGA Congress, Berlin, 2005; published in *American Journal of Homeopathic Medicine* 98:15, Spring 2005.

35. "Advisory on Bird Flu," *American Journal of Homeopathic Medicine* 99:16, Spring 2006.

36. "Diagnosis," *American Journal of Homeopathic Medicine* 102:7, Spring 2009, and 102:56, Summer 2009; reprinted in *Medical Studies* (Netherlands) 2:121, 2010.

37. "Vaccines, Drugs, and Other Causes: a Homeopath Looks at the Medical System," lecture to 65th LIGA Congress, Los Angeles, May 2010; published in *American Journal of Homeopathic Medicine* 103:214, Winter 2010, and 104:13, Spring 2011.
38. "Hidden in Plain Sight: Vaccines as a Major Risk Factor for Chronic Disease," abridged version of op. cit., *AJHM,* 2005, *American Journal of Homeopathic Medicine* 106:107, Fall 2013.
39. "Some Thoughts on the Beginnings of Life," *Spectrum,* Spring 2013; reprinted in *American Journal of Homeopathic Medicine* 106:147, Winter 2013.

Case Reports.

1. "Plague and Pregnancy: a Case Report," with Jonathan Mann, M. D., *Journal of the AMA* 237:1854, 25 April 1977.
2. "A Sampling of Animal Cases," *Homœopathic Links* 16:15, Spring 2003.
3. "A Wound Heals - after 25 Years," *Homeopathy Today,* February 2007.
4. "A 42-Year-Old Man with Bronchiectasis," *American Journal of Homeopathic Medicine* 102:78, Summer 2009.
5. "An Autistic Boy," *American Journal of Homeopathic Medicine* 102:117, Autumn 2009.
6. "A Woman with Lupus, and a Whole Lot More," *American Journal of Homeopathic Medicine* 103:22, Spring 2010.

Reviews.

1. Book Review: Dana Ullman and Stephen Cummings, *Everybody's Guide to Homeopathic Medicines, Homeopathy Today,* March 1985.
2. Book Review: Adelaide Suits, *Brass Tacks: an Oral Biography, Homeopathy Today,* December 1985.
3. Book Review: Alain Horvilleur, *The Family Guide to Homeopathy, Homeopathy Today,* May 1987.
4. Conference Review: "The Scientific Sessions," 42nd LIGA Congress, Washington, May 1987, *Homeopathy Today,* July-August 1987.

5. Book Review: Larry Dossey, *Beyond Illness, Chrysalis* (Journal of the Swedenborg Foundation) 4:117, Spring 1989.

6. Book Review: Catherine Coulter, *Portraits of Homeopathic Medicines,* Volume 2, **Homeopathy Today,** April 1989.

7. Book Review: George Vithoulkas, *A New Model of Health and Disease,* **Homeopathy Today,** January 1993.

8. Book Review: George Vithoulkas, *Materia Medica Viva,* Volume 1, **Journal of the AIH** 86:257, December 1993.

9. Book Review: Harris Coulter, *The Controlled Clinical Trial,* **Journal of the AIH** 86:254, December 1993.

10. Book Review: Roger Morrison, *Desktop Guide to Keynotes and Confirmatory Symptoms,* **Homeopathy Today,** January 1994.

11. Video Review: Julian Winston, *The Faces of Homeopathy,* **Journal of the AIH** 88:158, Spring 1995.

12. Book Review: Nancy Herrick, *Animal Mind, Human Voices: Provings of Eight New Animal Remedies,* **Homeopathy Today,** January 1999.

13. Book Review: Roger Morrison, *Desktop Guide to Physical Pathology,* **Homeopathy Today,** April 1999.

14. Book Review: Julian Winston, *The Faces of Homeopathy,* **Homeopathy Today,** October 1999.

15. Book Review: Judyth Reichenberg-Ullman and Robert Ullman, *Rage-Free Kids,* **Homeopathy Today,** July-August 2000.

16. Book Review: A. U. Ramakrishnan and Catherine Coulter, *A Homeopathic Approach to Cancer,* **Homeopathy Today,** November 2001; reprinted in **Homœopathic Links** (Netherlands) 15:60, Spring 2002.

17. Book Review: Julian Winston, *The Heritage of Homeopathic Literature,* **Homeopathy Today,** April-May 2002.

18. Book Review: Isaac Golden, *Homeoprophylaxis,* **American Journal of Homeopathic Medicine** 99:149, Summer 2006.

19. Seminar Review: Russell Malcolm, "Introduction to Homeopathy" and "The Bowel Nosodes," **American Journal of Homeopathic Medicine** 102:27, Spring 2009.

20. Book Review: Dana Ullman, *The Homeopathic Revolution,* **Journal of Alternative and Complementary Therapies** 16:517, April 2010.

21. Book Review: Massimo Mangialavori, *Praxis, Spectrum of Homeopathy* (Germany), 2010, p. 134; reprinted in *American Journal of Homeopathic Medicine* 104: 218, Winter 2011.
22. Book Review: Catherine Coulter, "The Power of Vision: a Life of Samuel Hahnemann," *Spectrum*, Spring 2012, reprinted in *Homeopathy Today,* Spring 2012.
23. Book Review: Rajan Sankaran, *The Synergy in Homeopathy,* *American Journal of Homeopathic Medicine* 105:138, Autumn 2012.
24. Seminar Review: Karl Robinson, et al., "Prafull Vijayakar's Predictive Homeopathy," *American Journal of Homeopathic Medicine* 106:56, Summer 2013.

Obituaries

1. "Henry Waters, 1899-1986," *Homeopathy Today,* July-August 1986.
2. "Elinore Peebles, 1897-1992," *Homeopathy Today,* October 1992.
3. "Maesimund Panos, M. D., 1912-1999: Stateswoman, Friend, Mother of Us All," *Homeopathy Today,* October 1999.
4. "Julian Winston, 1941-2005, In Loving Memory," *Homeopathy Today,* July-August 2005.
5. "In Memoriam: Christine Luthra, M. D. (1951-2006)," *Homeopathy Today,* November-December 2006.
6. "Harris Coulter (1932-2009): Devoted Scholar, Keen Intellect, Soldier for the Cause," *American Journal of Homeopathic Medicine* 103:7, Spring 2010.
7. "David Warkentin (1951-2010): An Appreciation," *American Journal of Homeopathic Medicine* 103: 179, Winter 2010.

Political Statements.

1. "On Lay Prescribing," *Homeopathy Today,* April 1982.
2. President's Message, *Homeopathy Today,* June 1985.
3. President's Message, "Lay Practice," *Homeopathy Today,* October 1985.
4. President's Message, *Homeopathy Today,* January 1986.
5. "Homeopathy on the Line," *Homeopathy Today,* April 1986.

6. President's Report, *Homeopathy Today,* September 1986.
7. Open Letter to President Clinton, *Homeopathy Today,* February 1993.

Letters and Rebuttals.

1. "The Great Malpractice Scandal," *Santa Fe Reporter,* 16 April 1981.
2. Open Letter to Prof. Harold Morowitz, in reply to his article, "Much Ado about Nothing," in *Hospital Practice,* July 1982, *Homeopathy Today,* October 1982.
3. Reply to letter from John Coker, *Homeopathy Today,* September 1984.
4. Letter to the Editor, "Sample Living Will Addendum," *Journal of the AIH* 85:10, March 1992.
5. Open Letter to Gerald Weissman, M. D., in reply to his article, "Dancing with Fairies, Sucking with Vampires," in *MD Magazine,* November 1992, *Homeopathy Today,* March 1993.
6. "Animal Testing in Homeopathy," Open Letter to Jennifer Jacobs, M. D., and the Homeopathic Research Network, *Journal of the AIH* 88:8, Spring 1995.
7. "More on Vaccinations," Letter to the Editor, *Mothering* Magazine, Spring 1997.
8. Reply to letter from Domenick Masiello, D. O., *Homeopathy Today,* December 2000.
9. "For Homeopathy: a Practicing Physician's Perspective," in rebuttal to Kevin Smith's article, "Against Homeopathy: a Utilitarian Perspective," in *Bioethics* (UK), February 2011, *American Journal of Homeopathic Medicine* 104:125, Autumn 2011; German version, *Homöopathie Zeitschrift,* 2012, p. 99.

Lectures.

1. "Homeopathic Reasoning," lecture to Symposium, "Homeopathy: the Renaissance of Cure, San Francisco, April 1980; published in *Homeotherapy* 6:135, September 1980.
2. "Whose Birth Is It, Anyway?" lecture to Cæsarean Prevention Movement Conference, Newark, 1984; CPM videotape.

3. "What Homeopathy Can Teach, and What It Has to Learn," lecture to NCH Annual Conference, 1986, summarized in *Homeopathy Today,* September 1986.

4. "Poverty in the Midst of Plenty: American Homeopathy in 1987," Lecture to NCH Annual Conference, 1987, summarized in *Homeopathy Today,* October 1987; NCH audiotape.

5. "How Can It All Be Done?" lecture to NCH Annual Conference, 1987, summarized in *Homeopathy Today,* September 1987; NCH audiotape.

6. "Beyond Curing," Julia Green Memorial Lecture, NCH Summer School, July 1988, NCH audiotape.

7. "Vaccination: a Sacrament of Modern Medicine," lecture to Society of Homeopaths Annual Conference (UK), 1991; published in *Journal of the AIH* 84:96, December 1991; reprinted in *The Homœopath* (UK)12:137, March 1992.

8. Homeopathic Philosophy Lecture Series, NCH Summer School, 1991, 1992; NCH audiotapes.

9. "Childhood Ear Infections," lecture to AIH Conference, 1994; published in *Journal of the AIH* 87:137, Autumn 1994; reprinted in *The Homœopath* (UK), 1994.

10. "Illness as Conflict, Health as Resolution," lecture to Boston Graduate School of Psychoanalysis Annual Conference, Santa Fe, 1997, unpublished.

11. "Samuel Hahnemann: the Man and His Impact," lecture at Centenary of the Hahnemann Monument, Washington, May 2000, AIH audiotape.

12. "Hidden in Plain Sight: the Rôle of Vaccines in Chronic Disease," lecture to 60th LIGA Congress, Berlin, 2005; published in *American Journal of Homeopathic Medicine* 98:15, Spring 2005.

13. "Vaccines, Drugs, and Other Causes: a Homeopath Looks at the Medical System," lecture to 65th LIGA Congress, Los Angeles, May 2010; published in *American Journal of Homeopathic Medicine* 103:214, Winter 2010, and 104:13, Spring 2011.

Panels and Symposia.

1. "Malpractice," *Firing Line,* William F. Buckley, moderator, WNET, New York, October 1982, WNET videotape.
2. Symposium, "Vaccination: The Issue of Our Time," *Mothering* Magazine, Spring 1996.
3. "The Vaccination Debate," with Andrew Weil, M. D., *Natural Health,* November-December 1997.
4. "Report on Bioterrorism," AIH Bioterrorism Committee, *American Journal of Homeopathic Medicine* 96:94, Summer 2003.

Miscellaneous.

1. Memoir, "Why I Became a Homeopath," *Homeopathy Today,* December 1982.
2. Interview with Peggy O'Mara, *Mothering,* April 1988.
3. Memoir, "Why I Became a Homeopath," *Journal of the AIH* 89:74, Winter 1996; reprinted in *The Homœopath* (UK),1997, p. 712.
4. "What Is Homeopathy?" unpublished patient handout, 1996.
5. Interview with Jane Ryan, *New England Journal of Homeopathy* 9:83, Spring-Summer 2000.
6. "Advisory on Anthrax," unpublished patient handout, 2002.
7. "Advisory on Smallpox," unpublished patient handout, 2002.
8. Foreword, Nancy Herrick, *Sacred Plants, Human Voices: Provings of Seven New Plant Remedies,* Hahnemann Clinic Publishing, San Francisco, 2003.
9. "Hidden in Plain Sight," expanded version of op. cit., *AJHM,* 2005, unpublished.
10. "Advisory on Swine Flu," unpublished patient handout, 2009.

About the Author:

Richard Moskowitz earned his B. A. from Harvard in 1959, Phi Beta Kappa, and his M. D. from New York University in 1963. After a graduate fellowship in Philosophy at the University of Colorado, he interned at St. Anthony's Hospital in Denver, and has been in private practice since 1967.

Attending over 600 home births in the 1970's, he studied Japanese acupuncture with Sensei Masahilo Nakazono in Santa Fe, and classical homeopathy with many teachers, notably Prof. George Vithoulkas in Greece and Dr. Rajan Sankaran in India. He has practiced homeopathic medicine more or less exclusively since 1974.

Author of two books and numerous articles on homeopathy, midwifery, and natural medicine, Dr. Moskowitz has served as President of the National Center for Homeopathy (1985-86), as Secretary of the American Institute of Homeopathy (2007-present), and has taught and lectured widely. He lives and practices in the Boston area.

* 9 7 8 1 4 8 2 3 3 8 0 1 0 *